Acute Care Neuroconsultation and Neurorehabilitation Management

Amy K. Wagner • Justin Weppner
Editors

Acute Care Neuroconsultation and Neurorehabilitation Management

Springer

Editors
Amy K. Wagner
Department of Physical Medicine and Rehabilitation
University of Pittsburgh School of Medicine
Pittsburgh, PA, USA

Justin Weppner
Virginia Tech Carilion School of Medicine
Edward Via College of Osteopathic Medicine
Roanoke, VA, USA

ISBN 978-3-031-42829-6   ISBN 978-3-031-42830-2 (eBook)
https://doi.org/10.1007/978-3-031-42830-2

This Springer imprint is published by the registered company Springer Nature Switzerland AG
The registered company address is: Gewerbestrasse 11, 6330 Cham, Switzerland

Paper in this product is recyclable.

Contents

Contributors

Christian Aponte-Lopez, MD Baylor Scott and White Institute for Rehabilitation, Dallas, TX, USA

Heather Asthagiri, MD Department of Physical Medicine and Rehabilitation, University of Virginia, Charlottesville, VA, USA

Amy O. Bowles, MD Department of Rehabilitation Medicine, Brooke Army Medical Center (BAMC), Joint Base San Antonio, San Antonio, TX, USA

Department of Physical Medicine and Rehabilitation, Uniformed Services University of the Health Sciences, Bethesda, MD, USA

Rong Tina Chen, MD Carle Foundation Hospital, Urbana, IL, USA

Kerry DeLuca, MD Department of Physical Medicine and Rehabilitation, University of Pittsburgh School of Medicine, Pittsburgh, PA, USA

Michelle Didesch, MD Confluence Health, Central Washington Hospital and Clinics Campus, Wenatchee, WA, USA

Selina Doncevic, MSN, RN, CRRN United States Department of Veterans Affairs, Washington, DC, USA

Walter Reed National Military Medical Center, Bethesda, MD, USA

Blessen C. Eapen, MD Department of Physical Medicine and Rehabilitation, VA Greater Los Angeles Health Care System, Los Angeles, CA, USA

Division of Physical Medicine and Rehabilitation, Department of Medicine, David Geffen School of Medicine at UCLA, Los Angeles, CA, USA

Gary Galang, MD Department of Physical Medicine and Rehabilitation, University of Pittsburgh School of Medicine, Pittsburgh, PA, USA

Aileen Giordano, MD Parham Doctors Hospital, Richmond, VA, USA

William Ide, MD Department of Physical Medicine and Rehabilitation, University of Virginia, Charlottesville, VA, USA

Kennedy Krieger Institute, Baltimore, MD, USA

Department of Physical Medicine and Rehabilitation, Johns Hopkins University School of Medicine, University of Virginia, Baltimore, MD, USA

Shannon B. Juengst, PhD The Institute for Rehabilitation Research (TIRR), Memorial Hermann Hospital Brain Injury Research Center (BIRC), Houston, TX, USA

Michael Kryger, MD Department of Physical Medicine and Rehabilitation, Penn State University College of Medicine, Hershey, PA, USA

Julie Lanphere, DO Intermountain Medical Center, Murray, UT, USA

Mark Linsenmeyer, MD Department of Physical Medicine and Rehabilitation, Sunnyview Rehabilitation Hospital, Schenectady, NY, USA

Gerald J. Nora, MD Medrina, Chicago, II, USA

Department of Physical Medicine and Rehabilitation, Medical College of Wisconsin, Milwaukee, WI, USA

Komal Patel, DO James A. Haley Veterans' Hospital and Clinics, U.S. Department of Veterans Affairs, Tampa, FL, USA

Mary Miller Phillips, MD Baylor Scott and White Institute for Rehabilitation, Dallas, TX, USA

Shanti M. Pinto, MD Department of Physical Medicine and Rehabilitation, University of Texas - Southwestern, Dallas, TX, USA

Geoffrey Smith, MD St. Mary's Hospital Rehabilitation Unit, Mayo Clinic, Rochester, MN, USA

Neurological Rehabilitation Division, Department of Physical Medicine and Rehabilitation, Mayo Clinic, Rochester, MN, USA

Melissa Sutcliffe, PhD Division of Pediatric Rehabilitation Medicine Center, Department of Physical Medicine and Rehabilitation, Children's Hospital of Pittsburgh of UPMC, Pittsburgh, PA, USA

Anne Tita, MD Allina Health, Minneapolis, MN, USA

Amy K. Wagner, MD Department of Physical Medicine and Rehabilitation, University of Pittsburgh School of Medicine, Pittsburgh, PA, USA

Justin Weppner, DO Virginia Tech Carilion School of Medicine, Edward Via College of Osteopathic Medicine, Roanoke, VA, USA

Chapter 1
Introduction and Rationale

Justin Weppner and Amy K. Wagner

Introduction

The American Academy of Physical Medicine and Rehabilitation's "PM&R Bold" initiative outlines the vision for the future of physiatry. The vision is clear that "in the future … The physiatrist will be a recognized leader across the Rehabilitation Care Continuum with expertise in managing utilization of resources to achieve maximal patient outcome" [1]. In the acute setting, physiatric involvement focusing on impairments prepares the patient for rehabilitation and enhances post-acute management. Consultations are common, essential components of medical care, but several studies have found that the quality and effectiveness of consultations are variable [2–6]. In any setting, ineffective consultations diminish the quality of patient care and education and frustrate clinicians, patients, and their families. Forty years ago, the "ten commandments" of high-quality consults were outlined by Goldman and colleagues [7]. While these recommendations focused on the role of the consultant, Goldman noted that effective consultation is a bidirectional process requiring effective communication and framing of the consult request from the referring provider. Consulting physicians should respect care plans established jointly with referring physicians but, when necessary, must always exercise their independent clinical judgment in patients' best interest. The consulting physician

J. Weppner (✉)
Virginia Tech Carilion School of Medicine, Edward Via College of Osteopathic Medicine, Roanoke, VA, USA
e-mail: jlweppner@carilionclinic.org

A. K. Wagner
Department of Physical Medicine and Rehabilitation, University of Pittsburgh School of Medicine, Pittsburgh, PA, USA
e-mail: wagnerak@upmc.edu

A. K. Wagner, J. Weppner (eds.), *Acute Care Neuroconsultation and Neurorehabilitation Management*, https://doi.org/10.1007/978-3-031-42830-2_1

should always carefully and respectfully explain recommendations to the referring physician and obtain concurrence for significant procedures such as botulinum toxin injections or when requesting additional consultants. For persons with acquired brain injury, effective consultation that supports safe transitions of care leads to decreased acute care length of stay [8]. This handbook aims to provide the tools needed to support the consulting physiatrist to maximize function and outcome for persons with neurologic injury.

Improving Compliance with Consult Recommendations

Depending on the setting, compliance with consultant recommendations is achieved 54% to 95% of the time [9–13]. To improve compliance with recommendations, the consultant must understand the central reason for the consultation, and the consultation request needs to be clearly stated, understood, and fully addressed [3, 11, 13]. Consults must be completed promptly to ensure that recommendations are followed. In general, all consultations should be completed within 24 h, preferably on the same day the consult was placed. If delays are anticipated, they should be communicated to the referring provider in a timely fashion [2]. The organization of recommendations is also vital, and they should be definitive, precise, and prioritized in order of importance [2, 3, 9, 14]. The number of recommendations should be limited to five or fewer, and highlighting essential or critical recommendations also improves compliance by the referring provider [10–12, 15]. When monitoring consult compliance, therapeutic recommendations are more likely to be followed than diagnostic recommendations [2, 11]. The consultant should closely monitor diagnostic recommendations, and careful communication should be performed to ensure that needed diagnostic testing is completed. Consultation recommenations to start therapy are less likely to be followed than those to continue or discontinue treatment [2, 11]. Frequent follow-up visits documented with progress notes are vital in improving compliance with the consultant's recommendations [2, 15]. When the consultant no longer needs to follow the patient, they should provide written communication indicating that they are signing off the case and make arrangements to ensure continuity of care with a follow-up plan to meet the patient's rehabilitation needs at discharge from the acute hospital.

Coordination of Care

PM&R physicians play a critical role in caring for patients with functional impairments and must work closely with discharge planners and rehabilitation liaisons to ensure optimal outcomes for these patients. Discharge planners are responsible for coordinating the transition of patients from the hospital to post-acute care, while rehabilitation liaisons are responsible for coordinating rehabilitation services for patients. Effective communication and collaboration between PM&R consultants and these professionals are essential for ensuring that patients receive appropriate care and support. According to Vargas et al. [16], the involvement of PM&R physicians in discharge planning is associated with reduced readmission rates and improved patient outcomes. Poor communication and collaboration between PM&R physicians, discharge planners, and rehabilitation liaisons can have several negative consequences for patients. For instance, inadequate communication between healthcare providers during transitions of care can result in medication errors, delays in treatment, and adverse events [17]. Poor communication can also lead to misunderstandings about patient needs and preferences, resulting in suboptimal care and outcomes [18]. Furthermore, poor collaboration and coordination among healthcare providers can lead to fragmented care, unnecessary readmissions, and increased healthcare costs [19]. Therefore, physiatrists should actively engage with discharge planners and rehabilitation liaisons to ensure patients receive the best possible care and outcomes.

The "Treatment Teams: Roles and Goals" chapter of this handbook defines the roles and responsibilities of the acute care rehabilitation team. This chapter outlines the key team members, including the physiatrist, physical therapists, occupational therapists, speech therapists, and other healthcare professionals, and their specific roles and goals in the patient's rehabilitation process. Importantly, the chapter emphasizes the crucial role of the physiatrist in leading the team and ensuring that each team member works together collaboratively to provide the highest quality care to the patient. By defining the team's roles and goals, this chapter sets the foundation for effective communication, collaboration, and coordination among team members. The consulting physiatrist must partner with acute care therapists to establish rehabilitation goals and treatment plans for optimal care. Effective collaboration between physiatry consultants and therapy services, including occupational therapy, physical therapy, and speech therapy, is essential for establishing acute care rehabilitation goals and maximizing patient outcomes. Physiatry consultants should work closely with therapy services to determine the patient's functional abilities, goals, and needs in order to develop a comprehensive rehabilitation plan tailored to the patient's specific condition and circumstances. Studies have shown that collaborative care models that involve physiatry consultants can lead to improved patient outcomes, including shorter lengths of stay, reduced healthcare costs, and improved functional status [8, 20]. Effective communication and coordination between PM&R consultants and therapy services can help ensure that patients receive appropriate care, minimize the risk of complications, and optimize the transition from acute care.

The physiatry consultant should also collaborate with patients and families and assume an essential role in educating patients and their families about rehabilitation goals and strategies. One key aspect of this education is teaching families how to be effective advocates for their loved ones' care and rehabilitation. The "Resources and Advocacy" chapter provides detailed and essential advocacy information that can support patients with neurologic injuries and their families during the rehabilitation process. Families can play a vital role in supporting the patient's rehabilitation goals by providing emotional support, encouraging adherence to treatment plans, and communicating with healthcare providers about the patient's progress and needs. Physiatrists should engage families in the rehabilitation process and provide them with information about the patient's condition, treatment plan, and goals for recovery. This education should be tailored to the family's needs and level of understanding and should involve clear communication about the patient's prognosis, potential complications, and expected outcomes. Family involvement in rehabilitation can improve patient outcomes, including shorter hospital stays, reduced readmissions, and improved functional status [21]. Physiatrists need to recognize the vital role of families in the rehabilitation process and provide them with the knowledge and resources they need to support their loved one's recovery.

Physiatry consultants play a crucial role in helping patients recover from injuries or illnesses and regain their independence. Coordinating care with liaisons, discharge planners, acute care therapists, and families ensure that the patient receives comprehensive and holistic care, addressing all aspects of their physical, emotional, and social well-being. By setting rehabilitation goals with acute care therapists and educating and partnering with families, PM&R consultants empower patients to achieve their maximum potential and regain function as quickly as possible. Overall, the interdisciplinary approach of PM&R consultations is essential for improving patient outcomes and enhancing their quality of life.

Ten Factors for Effective Consultation [6, 7]

Gain a Thorough Understanding of Your Referral Team

Ask the requesting physician how you can best help them if a specific question is not apparent. It is of paramount importance for the consultant to determine precisely why the consultation was requested. Consider both the question that the primary service asked and the question they should have asked to prepare the patient for rehabilitation. A physiatry consultant may be asked to make post-acute care recommendations to facilitate a safe transfer to the next level of care. When assessing the patient, the requesting physician's question should be answered, but other questions that should have been asked should also be considered. For example, a patient with a traumatic brain injury (TBI) may have spasticity and bracing needs that also should be addressed by the consulting physiatrist. While it is essential to identify and answer the clinical question requested by the requesting physician, it is just as vital to address other clinical questions that better prepare the patient with neurologic injury for post-acute care.

Without effective communication, the consultant's response may not adequately answer the question and convey other significant findings identified by the consultant that need to be addressed. The need for direct communication to minimize the potential for misunderstanding has been highlighted in studies exploring the disagreement between the requesting physician and consultant about the primary reason for the consultation in 14% of cases [3], and a second study revealing that no specific questions were asked in 24% of consults and that the consultant ignored detailed questions in 12% of cases [14]. Direct consultant-to-referring provider communication via phone or electronic messaging ensures that the referring provider can answer any questions about a consultant's proposed plan of care.

Establish Urgency

The consultant must determine whether the consultation is emergent, urgent, or elective, and a timely response is important to improve compliance with recommendations [2]. Urgent or emergent consultations need to be seen promptly, and elective in-patient consultations should usually be answered the same day as requested, but in all cases, within 24 h.

Look for Yourself

Consultants are most effective when they are willing to gather data independently. While a significant amount of data is available in the electronic medical record, the consulting physiatrist should not expect definitive conclusions and meaningful interventions based solely on the assessment of data already in the medical chart. Pertinent historical and physical examination data should be obtained independently by the consultant. Due to the physiatrist's orientation to function, the consultant may obtain overlooked information such as previous and current level of functioning, home setup and layout, and caregivers available for training. Specialized examinations such as the JFK Coma Recovery Scale-Revised and International Standards for Neurological Classification of Spinal Cord Injury may be performed to inform post-acute care decision-making and prognosis. Typically, completing a consult in person results in better, more individualized care to maximize function, reduce complications, inform prognosis, and make specific and tailored post-acute care recommendations.

Be as Brief as Appropriate

The consultant's report should be informative yet concise [6, 7]. Encapsulate the case from your point of view. Documentation should be as succinct as possible; however, it should contain adequate accounting of your medical and rehabilitation decision-making, particularly if your discussion could be surprising or unfamiliar to other clinicians.

Be Specific, Thorough, and Descend from Thy Ivory Tower to Help When Requested

Leave as many specific recommendations as needed to answer the consultation and ask the requesting physician if they need help with order writing. Leaving a long list of suggestions decreases the likelihood that any of them will be followed, including the crucial recommendations [15]. Explicit language should be used, and recommendations should be prioritized, precise, and preferably limited to five [11, 12, 15]. When recommending medications, consultations are more likely to be effective if recommendations are specific regarding drug dose, frequency, route, and indication [2, 5]. Recommendations felt to be "critical" are more likely to be followed, as are therapeutic recommendations, when compared to diagnostic recommendations [2, 10–12, 15].

Provide Contingency Plans and Discuss Their Execution

Consultants should anticipate potential problems, document contingency plans, and provide an after-hours point of contact to help execute the consult recommendations if requested [6, 7]. The physiatrist must remember that, regardless of the quality of the initial assessment and proposed plan, neurologic injuries are dynamic and initial recommendations may be irrelevant over the course of the acute hospitalization depending on patient progress [7]. Consultants should anticipate potential patient complications that might be expected after neurologic injury, and a brief description of therapeutic options to reduce these complications may reduce the hospital length of stay and prepare the patient for transfer to the next level of care [8].

Thou May Negotiate Joint Title to Thy Neighbor's Turf

Physiatrists can and should comanage any facet of patient care that the requesting physician desires within their scope of physiatric practice, and frank institutional discussions defining which specialty is responsible for what aspects of patient care are needed to promote an effective and efficient health system. For example, at some institutions, psychiatrists manage agitation following acquired brain injury. In contrast, at other institutions, this role is performed by physiatrists, and institutional discussions defining these roles help reduce conflict among providers serving patients with neurologic injuries.

The physiatry consultant should be careful to address the problem they were called for and refrain from conflicting with other specialists if a clinical question lies outside their domain. The consultant must consider that more than one diagnostic or therapeutic approach is appropriate for many patients with neurologic injuries. Suppose the strategy chosen by the requesting physician seems as reasonable as the one the physiatry consultant would typically pursue. In that case, it is more appropriate for the consultant to indicate agreement with this course than to go to great lengths to describe a different but equivalent plan [7].

Teach with Tact and Pragmatism

Judgments on leaving references should be tailored to the requesting physician's specialty, training level, and the consult's urgency [6, 7]. Consultants should share their expertise and insight into the case clearly without condescension. References cited or discussed with the referring physician should be brief, pertinent, current, and have a direct clinical bearing on the patient's problems.

Talk Is Essential

There is no substitute for direct personal contact with the primary physician after a consultation, especially if the consultant thinks the recommendations are crucial or controversial. For example, if the consultant finds a patient hypoxic and tachycardic with clinical concern for a pulmonary embolus, this critical information should be directly communicated with the referring physician. While the implementation of the electronic medical record has facilitated communication, surveys have reported that 67% of medical providers consider verbal communication as the best or second-best method of communication [22], with many studies documenting the importance of verbal communication between the consultant and the requestor [4, 6, 7, 22, 23]. The evidence suggests that the advantage of verbal communication between consultant and requester is that it increases the likelihood that provider-to-provider contact will be accurate, comprehensive, and completely understood [22].

Provide Appropriate Follow-Up

Consultants should recognize the appropriate time to fade into a background role, but that time is seldom the same day the consultation note is signed. The consultant's responsibilities rarely end with the initial physiatry consultation. Appropriate follow-up visits with documentation in the chart improve compliance with recommendations and may improve care [2, 15]. The patient's severity of the injury, level of arousal, functional status, medical stability, and readiness for discharge will dictate the frequency and duration of follow-up management by the consultant. Frequent written follow-up is desirable; when the patient's problems are not active, the consultant should discuss signing off with the requesting physician beforehand. The consultant should sign off in writing when they no longer need to follow the patient, and arrangements for post-acute rehabilitation and long-term PM&R follow-up after discharge should be documented.

Conclusion

The physiatrist providing consultation to persons with neurologic injury should identify the pertinent medical problems and potential complications, maximize patient function, inform prognosis, make specific and tailored post-acute care recommendations, and communicate effectively with the referring provider. Effective communication is essential to the consultation process, and the role of the consultant should be defined through direct contact with the referring clinician. The requesting provider should clearly state the questions to be answered by the consultant. Given the high frequency of misunderstanding between consultants and referring clinicians, direct communication is important and likely will prevent misinterpretation. Compliance with consultant recommendations improves when the consultant makes fewer recommendations. The number of recommendations should be limited, preferably to five or fewer. The consultant should respond to the consultation within 24 h and create precise, relevant recommendations. When the consultant no longer needs to follow the patient, a note should be written indicating they are signing off the case. Arrangements should be made to ensure comprehensive rehabilitation care and physiatry follow-up for the patient after discharge. This handbook provides the knowledge needed to support timely and efficient transitions of care for persons with neurologic injury to decrease lengths of stay and hospital readmissions and to prepare patients for post-acute rehabilitation. By providing real-life cases and practical guidance, this handbook will equip consultants with the tools and knowledge they need to make informed decisions and provide effective care to patients with neurologic injuries. Whether dealing with complex diagnoses, challenging comorbidities, or difficult rehabilitation goals, this handbook offers practical strategies for consultants to overcome these obstacles and achieve the best possible outcomes for their patients. Ultimately, this handbook will serve as a valuable resource for physiatry consultants who are dedicated to providing the highest quality care to patients with neurologic injuries.

References

1. American Academy of Physical Medicine and Rehabilitation. Rehabilitation care continuum practice area. https://www.aapmr.org/about-aapm-r/visioning-pm-r-bold/acute-post-acute-care-practice-area. Accessed 18 Jan 2023.
2. Horwitz RI, Henes CG, Horwitz SM. Developing strategies for improving the diagnostic and management efficacy of medical consultations. J Chronic Dis. 1983;36(2):213–8. https://doi.org/10.1016/0021-9681(83)90096-6.
3. Lee T, Pappius EM, Goldman L. Impact of inter-physician communication on the effectiveness of medical consultations. Am J Med. 1983;74(1):106–12. https://doi.org/10.1016/0002-9343(83)91126-9.
4. Lo E, Rezai K, Evans AT, et al. Why don't they listen? Adherence to recommendations of infectious disease consultations. Clin Infect Dis. 2004;38(9):1212–8. https://doi.org/10.1086/383315.
5. Popkin MK, Mackenzie TB, Hall RC, Garrard J. Physicians' concordance with consultants' recommendations for psychotropic medication. Arch Gen Psychiatry. 1979;36(4):386–9. https://doi.org/10.1001/archpsyc.1979.01780040028002.
6. Salerno SM, Hurst FP, Halvorson S, Mercado DL. Principles of effective consultation: an update for the 21st-century consultant. Arch Intern Med. 2007;167(3):271–5. https://doi.org/10.1001/archinte.167.3.271.
7. Goldman L, Lee T, Rudd P. Ten commandments for effective consultations. Arch Intern Med. 1983;143(9):1753–5.
8. Weppner JL, Linsenmeyer MA, Wagner AK. Effects of an acute care brain injury medicine continuity consultation service on health care utilization and rehabilitation outcomes. PM R. 2021;13(11):1227–36. https://doi.org/10.1002/pmrj.12563.
9. Klein LE, Levine DM, Moore RD, Kirby SM. The preoperative consultation. Response to internists' recommendations. Arch Intern Med. 1983;143(4):743–4.
10. Ballard WP, Gold JP, Charlson ME. Compliance with the recommendations of medical consultants. J Gen Intern Med. 1986;1(4):220–4. https://doi.org/10.1007/BF02596186.
11. Sears CL, Charlson ME. The effectiveness of a consultation. Compliance with initial recommendations. Am J Med. 1983;74(5):870–6. https://doi.org/10.1016/0002-9343(83)91079-3.
12. Pupa LE, Coventry JA, Hanley JF, Carpenter JL. Factors affecting compliance for general medicine consultations to non-internists. Am J Med. 1986;81(3):508–14. https://doi.org/10.1016/0002-9343(86)90307-4.
13. Ferguson RP, Rubinstien E. Preoperative medical consultations in a community hospital. J Gen Intern Med. 1987;2(2):89–92. https://doi.org/10.1007/BF02596302.
14. Rudd P, Siegler M, Byyny RL. Perioperative diabetic consultation: a plead for improved training. J Med Educ. 1978;53(7):590–6.
15. Mackenzie TB, Popkin MK, Callies AL, Jorgensen CR, Cohn JN. The effectiveness of cardiology consultation. Concordance with diagnostic and drug recommendations. Chest. 1981;79(1):16–22. https://doi.org/10.1378/chest.79.1.16.
16. Vargas C, Deane J, Granger C, Ottenbacher K. The role of physical medicine and rehabilitation physicians in acute care: a report from the Society of Academic Physiatrists, the American Academy of Physical Medicine and Rehabilitation, and the Association of Academic Physiatrists. Am J Phys Med Rehabil. 2017;96(9):664–9.
17. Kripalani S, LeFevre F, Phillips CO, Williams MV, Basaviah P, Baker DW. Deficits in communication and information transfer between hospital-based and primary care physicians: implications for patient safety and continuity of care. JAMA. 2007;297(8):831–41. https://doi.org/10.1001/jama.297.8.831.
18. O'Leary KJ, Wayne DB, Haviley C, Slade ME, Lee J, Williams MV. Improving teamwork: impact of structured interdisciplinary rounds on a medical teaching unit. J Gen Intern Med. 2010;25(8):826–32. https://doi.org/10.1007/s11606-010-1345-6.

19. Coleman EA, Parry C, Chalmers S, Min SJ. The care transitions intervention: results of a randomized controlled trial. Arch Intern Med. 2006;166(17):1822–8. https://doi.org/10.1001/archinte.166.17.1822.
20. Langton-Frost N, Orient S, Adeyemo J, et al. Development and implementation of a new model of care for patients with stroke, acute hospital rehabilitation intensive services: leveraging a multidisciplinary rehabilitation team. Am J Phys Med Rehabil. 2023;102(2S Suppl 1):S13–8. https://doi.org/10.1097/PHM.0000000000002132.
21. Gonçalves-Bradley DC, Lannin NA, Clemson LM, Cameron ID, Shepperd S. Discharge planning from hospital. Cochrane Database Syst Rev. 2016;2016(1):CD000313. https://doi.org/10.1002/14651858.CD000313.pub5.
22. Boulware DR, Dekarske AS, Filice GA. Physician preferences for elements of effective consultations. J Gen Intern Med. 2010;25(1):25–30. https://doi.org/10.1007/s11606-009-1142-2.
23. Haldis TA, Blankenship JC. Telephone reporting in the consultant-generalist relationship. J Eval Clin Pract. 2002;8(1):31–5. https://doi.org/10.1046/j.1365-2753.2002.00313.x.

Chapter 2
Treatment Teams: Roles and Goals

Kerry DeLuca

Chapter Objectives
1. Understand the physiatrist's role as the acute care rehabilitation team leader.
2. Describe the impact of the consulting physiatrist on systems of care to improve functional outcomes for persons with acquired brain injury and spinal cord injury.

Introduction

Physical Medicine and Rehabilitation (PM&R) physicians provide acute care consultations with the primary goal of improving patient and systems of care outcomes. PM&R consultation provides leadership and coordination of the acute care rehabilitation process by providing expertise in managing relevant neurological and medical issues impacting patient function and participation in therapy and determining an appropriate level of post-acute rehabilitation care. There is some evidence that PM&R acute care consultation in the population with traumatic brain injury (TBI) has been associated with improved patient outcomes and shorter acute care lengths of stay [1–3]. This chapter will explore the role of the acute care interdisciplinary treatment team and its impact on systems of care for the rehabilitation of persons with neurologic disabilities.

K. DeLuca (✉)
Department of Physical Medicine and Rehabilitation, University of Pittsburgh School of Medicine, Pittsburgh, PA, USA
e-mail: delucakg3@upmc.edu

A. K. Wagner, J. Weppner (eds.), *Acute Care Neuroconsultation and Neurorehabilitation Management*, https://doi.org/10.1007/978-3-031-42830-2_2

Acute Care Team

Care for the patient with severe ABI and spinal cord injury often begins in the intensive care unit (ICU). The team caring for the patient may initially include neuro critical care medicine (CCM) specialists, neurosurgeons, trauma surgeons, neurologists, ICU nursing, dieticians, respiratory therapists, care managers, and social workers. Patients with less severe acquired brain or spinal cord injuries may be cared for the on the neurosurgical or neurologic step-down units or wards where the team may include neurosurgeons, neurologists, trauma surgeons, other medical or surgical specialists, nurses who specialize in the care of patients with neurologic conditions, nutrition and respiratory therapists, care managers, and social workers.

Acute Care Rehabilitation Team

The rehabilitation team in the acute care hospital may include occupational therapy (OT), physical therapy (PT), speech-language pathology (SLP), and a PM&R consultant (physiatrist).

Physiatrists are physicians who have completed residency training in PM&R. The physiatrist evaluates the patient's functional impairments and recommends appropriate rehabilitation interventions. To do this, the physiatrist must understand multiple issues, including the patient's clinical condition, hospital course, and current function. In addition, the physiatrist identifies conditions that may be limiting the patient's function and recommends appropriate treatment.

The physical therapist (PT) specializes in treating patients with conditions that limit their ability to move and perform functional activities [4]. PTs focus on functional mobility retraining and therapeutic exercise [5]. Mobility often begins in conjunction with nursing staff, starting with bed mobility, with progression to sitting at edge of bed, standing, and transfers to a chair when appropriate. Progression to ambulation is introduced when medically appropriate, with close attention to patient tolerance, weight-bearing and range of motion restrictions, and vital sign stability.

The occupational therapist (OT) may initially be focused on splinting and positioning of patients with impaired consciousness and limited mobility. As appropriate, the OT evaluates the patient's ability to participate in activities of daily living (ADLs), also assessing cognition and functional mobility. Treatment includes ADL retraining and therapeutic exercise. They also evaluate impairments of upper limb mobility/function and evaluate potential need for adaptive equipment [6]. OTs often treat spasticity using static hand, wrist and elbow splinting. Special attention is paid to weight-bearing status and range of motion restrictions of the upper limb.

Speech and language pathologists (SLPs) assess multiple functional domains, including speech/language, swallowing, and cognition/communication. Evaluation may include assessment of voice, language disorders (including aphasias), or motor speech disorders (including dysarthria or apraxia). For patients with severe communication impairments, SLP recommendations may include compensatory communication strategies including assistive technology. SLPs also evaluate patients for prosthetic or adaptive devices for communication, such as tracheostomy speaking valves or artificial larynges. Swallowing evaluation may include non-instrumental (clinical) assessment as well as instrumental (e.g., videofluoroscopic) assessment. Swallowing interventions may include muscle retraining exercises and modification of handling and swallowing of solids, liquids, and saliva [7].

All rehabilitation team members work with each other and with nursing staff to maximize the patient's function. This collaborative approach to care, often initiated in the neurotrauma ICU, has been shown to improve patient's mobilization and decrease length of stay [8]. Physiatrists leading the acute care rehabilitation team for persons with ABI reduce acute hospital lengths of stay, prepare the patient for rehabilitation with fewer unplanned acute care transfers, and increase the likelihood of emerging from a minimally conscious state during inpatient rehabilitation [3]. Current guidelines from the American Heart Association/American Stroke Association recommend that evaluation of a stroke survivor's rehabilitation needs is best performed by an interprofessional team that can include a physician with expertise in rehabilitation as well as nurses, PTs, OTs, and SLPs [9].

Physiatry and the Acute Care Consultation

Interfacing Systems of Care

The physiatrist may be consulted to evaluate a patient's rehabilitation needs early in the acute care stay. This evaluation often starts in the ICU, where care by acute care therapists (i.e., PTs, OTs, SLPs) may have already been initiated. The physiatrist assesses the patient and recommends additional therapy services when needed. Communication with the acute care medical and surgical teams is important, with special focus on medical issues that may be limiting the patient's ability to participate in therapies.

The physiatrist works closely with the acute care therapists, discussing issues including the patient's tolerance of the therapy program and potential barriers to activity progression. The fundamental purpose of the acute care rehabilitation team is the same as the inpatient rehabilitation team, with each discipline contributing unique perspectives to serve and advocate for individuals recovering from ABI or spinal cord injury (SCI) [10].

The physiatrist also communicates frequently with the care manager and/or social worker in the acute care setting. The care manager usually has a nursing background and facilitates the transition between acute care and post-acute settings. Communication between the physiatrist and care manager/social worker in the acute care setting often includes discussion of social supports, home setting, prior function, and anticipated rehab course, taking into considerations any mobility restrictions (for example, weight-bearing restrictions) and other considerations that might affect discharge to the community. The physiatrist, with knowledge of the entire continuum of rehabilitation care, integrates all this information in determining which level of post-acute care is most appropriate for the patient.

A rehabilitation liaison performs activities and duties related to preadmission assessment screening and works as an intermediary between the physiatry consult team and the care managers to evaluate patients for possible inpatient rehabilitation care. This collaboration facilitates a smooth transition from the acute care hospital to the inpatient rehabilitation facility. The rehabilitation liaison functions in several roles, including practitioner, educator, advocate, and consultant. As a practitioner, the rehabilitation liaison conducts on-site, or record review screening for patients and completes all required preadmission screening documentation to support that inpatient rehabilitation services are appropriate, reasonable, and necessary. As a consultant, the liaison is an expert at assessing discharge plan feasibility, rehabilitation regulations, and external payor requirements, which help the physiatrist guide rehabilitation services across the continuum of care. Liaisons serve as an essential resource to educate patients, family members, and caregivers on external payers and rehabilitation program benefits and services available to maximize patient access to appropriate rehabilitation facilities.

Integrating Clinical Care Teams

The physiatry consultant evaluating patients for neurologic injury, whether traumatic or nontraumatic, must understand the expected functional impairments associated with the patient's medical or surgical condition(s) and anticipate possible complications that may adversely affect the patient's function. They should communicate with the primary team, other consultants, nursing staff, therapy staff, and care managers to minimize adverse effects of medical conditions on the patient's function, prevent complications, and optimize recovery.

Structured weekly interdisciplinary neurotrauma rounds provide a forum for providers from different disciplines to add their perspective to the care of individual patients; they also enhance communication among providers outside that setting. In a survey of PM&R departments in Level I trauma centers, 76% of respondents participated in multidisciplinary rounds with the trauma service [11].

Physiatrists integrate information about the patient's function with input from the medical and surgical teams to anticipate the patient's short-term and long-term rehabilitation needs. The physiatrist must understand all the post-acute rehabilitation options and determine which would be the most appropriate for the patient. Communication with patients (when able), family, and other caregivers is vital so that the physiatrist understands the patient's wishes and goals to arrange appropriate rehabilitation resources to work toward these goals.

Clinical Evaluation and Management

The physiatrist can assist the acute care primary team in evaluating and managing multiple issues including agitation [12], spasticity, pain, neurostimulation [1], and neurogenic bowel/bladder [3]. Clear and prompt communication with the primary team is important, as are regular follow-up visits with adjustment of the regimens as indicated. Recommendations for splinting/positioning, therapy timing, and involvement of additional therapy disciplines may be made, as appropriate.

Patient Safety and Quality Care Goals

Patient safety is a key principle. For patients who are deemed to be appropriate inpatient rehabilitation candidates, physiatrists anticipate issues that may preclude the patient from participating in inpatient rehabilitation and seek to have these addressed prior to rehabilitation transfer. Communication with primary teams regarding medical issues often occurs. Physiatrists also communicate with acute care therapists regarding patient's tolerance for exercise, with attention to vital signs during therapy sessions. Per Centers for Medicare and Medicaid Services (CMS) guidelines, a candidate for inpatient rehabilitation should be able to tolerate at least 3 h of therapies 5 days per week and show potential for meaningful functional progress in a prescribed period of time [13].

A key goal for the acute care physiatry consultant is to minimize early transfers from the inpatient rehabilitation facility back to the acute care hospital. Physiatrists and rehabilitation liaisons work to identify issues during the acute care stay that may cause early transfer from the inpatient rehab facility (Hammond, Pinto) [3, 14, 15]. When appropriate, the PM&R consult team communicates those concerns directly to the primary team, asking for additional medical evaluation and management. The goal is to minimize early transfers from inpatient rehabilitation back to acute care, in order to position the patient to be successful in the rehabilitation setting and beyond. Patients with TBI who were readmitted to acute care during their inpatient rehabilitation stay have been shown to have increased rehabilitation length of stay and decreased likelihood of discharge home [14].

Transitions of Care and Integrative Care Planning

The work of the acute care PM&R consultant and acute care rehab team often focuses on the transition from the acute care hospital to the post-acute setting. The consultant must understand all post-acute rehabilitation options—outpatient therapies, home therapies, skilled nursing facilities, long-term acute care hospitals, and inpatient rehabilitation facilities.

When determining the most appropriate level of post-acute rehabilitation care for a patient, communication between the physiatry consultant, patient (if able), family or decision-maker, primary team, therapists, and care manager/social worker is key, as all members of the team contribute information and insight to the decision-making process. The acute care physiatrist integrates information about the patient's current function, participation in therapies, ongoing medical issues, anticipated medical interventions/treatments, functional trajectory, and anticipated rehabilitation goals with their own assessment of the patient to make the most appropriate post-acute rehabilitation recommendation for each individual patient.

If the patient's clinical picture is complicated by ongoing medical care (i.e., cancer treatment), the physiatrist should obtain details about future medical plans to make the most appropriate recommendations that address the patient's rehabilitation needs in the context of their ongoing medical care and personal goals.

If the patient has need for ongoing therapies in at least two disciplines (PT, OT, SLP), is able to tolerate/participate in three or more hours of therapies per day, has medical complexity warranting ongoing rehabilitation nursing and physician care, and is expected to make measurable functional improvement in a prescribed period of time, the patient would be an appropriate candidate for inpatient rehabilitation [13]. Once the appropriate level of post-acute rehabilitation is determined, the physiatrist discusses the recommendation with the patient, family, and appropriate team members.

Depending on the patient's situation, s/he may not be an appropriate candidate for inpatient rehabilitation and may need therapies in a less-intensive level of care. If the patient is deemed safe to return home with family or other support for supervision and physical assistance, discharge with home therapies may be appropriate. For the patient to be deemed safe and ready for discharge to home, a provider must consider several factors beyond the medical determinants. These factors include (1) patient cognitive status, (2) patient activity level and functional status, (3) the nature of the patient's current home and suitability for the patient's conditions, (4) availability of family or caregiver support, (5) ability to obtain medications and services, (6) availability of transportation from hospital to home and for follow-up visits, (7) availability of services in the community to assist the patient with ongoing care [16–18]. Approximately three-quarters of hospitalized patients can return to their home environment following discharge [19]. For discharge home, patients, with help from family or other caregivers if available, should be able to (1) obtain and administer medications, (2) demonstrate safe mobility and transfers, (3) perform activities of daily living, and (4) manage nutritional needs [18, 20, 21]. If the patient has reliable transportation, outpatient therapies may be an option. If the patient needs continued nursing care and supervision in a less-intense setting, continued therapies can be done in the skilled nursing facility setting. If the patient has ongoing medical acuity requiring daily medical management but is cleared for discharge from the acute care hospital, continued therapies in the Long-Term Acute Care Hospital (LTACH) may be appropriate. Patients in the LTACH setting often have multiple and complex medical issues, which may include mechanical ventilation and/or frequent tracheostomy management.

For patients who are not candidates for inpatient rehabilitation, recommendations should be made for appropriate PM&R outpatient clinic visits when needed. The physiatry consultant should assure that recommendations for follow-up appointments or services are placed in the patient's discharge paperwork.

Outcomes

Patients with TBI who were treated with a formalized early rehabilitation program during the acute care stay have been reported to have improved cognition and decreased length of stay. Also, these programs involve families in the treatment and discharge planning process, helping to ease the transition from trauma center to rehabilitation facility [22]. Literature supports improved outcomes with PM&R consultation during the acute hospitalization. In the TBI population, PM&R consultation resulted in significantly better Functional Independence Measures (FIM) scores with transfers and locomotion and significantly shorter length of stay [2]. In another study of TBI patients, patients treated at a trauma center with a physiatrist as part of the acute care team had greater improvement than those coming from a trauma center without physiatrist care [1]. A recent review concluded that the limited studies regarding early physiatry consultation during acute care have all demonstrated improvements in outcome measures within each study's select population [23].

Case Illustration

A 28-year-old male with no significant medical history presented with muscle weakness to the trauma bay following a motor vehicle collision (MVC). The patient was a seat-belted driver who experienced a brief loss of consciousness after being rear-ended by a car traveling 70 miles per hour. In the trauma bay, the patient was alert and oriented with a Glasgow Coma Scale Score of 15 and no movement or sensation below the C6 level. The trauma service performed a digital rectal exam and noted decreased anal tone and no anal sensation. Cervical spine imaging showed bilateral facet dislocations at the C6–7 level with evidence of cervical spinal cord damage. No other significant injuries were identified on initial trauma imaging. Neurosurgery was consulted, and the patient was taken to the operating room emergently with open reduction of the facet dislocation with combined anterior and posterior approach cervical fusion. The patient's hospital course was uncomplicated, and he was extubated on hospital day 2. He passed a speech therapy bedside swallow and was started on a regular diet. PM&R was consulted on hospital day 3 for general rehabilitation management of the SCI and post-acute care recommendations.

On assessment, the patient had no motor or sensation below the C6 level and was an American Spinal Injury Association (ASIA) Impairment Scale Score of C6 ASIA A. The patient did not report any symptoms of a TBI, and bedside cognitive testing was in the normal range. Social history revealed that the patient lived in a one-story home with one step to enter with his spouse and 2-year-old child. His spouse did not work and was available for supervision, physical assistance, and family training. A foley catheter remained in place, and the physiatrist recommended removing the foley catheter and initiating an every-4-h intermittent catheterization program, once intravenous fluid resuscitation with injury and post-operative management were completed. Examination revealed absent rectal tone and leaking of feces on the bed under the patient, and a bowel program with a daily bisacodyl suppository after dinner was recommended. Lungs were clear, and respiratory therapy followed the patient with chest therapy. Review of systems revealed new onset of headaches since MVC, with light sensitivity and intermittent nausea, as well as poor sleep initiation and bouts of anxiety. At the bedside, nursing reported no skin breakdown and stated that they were performing turns every 2 h. The PM&R consult service placed an order for Pressure Relief Ankle Foot Orthoses (PRAFOs) to protect the integrity of the ankles and heels. Physical therapy and occupational therapy had not evaluated the patient, and the consulting physiatrist coordinated with the primary service to place therapy referrals. In addition to oxycodone and acetaminophen already prescribed by the primary service, recommendations for ondansetron PRN for headache and nausea were made as well as melatonin for sleep. Patient education was provided regarding concurrent post-concussive symptoms and care, as well as the need for ongoing symptom monitoring and management as the patient transitions to acute inpatient rehabilitation care.

On hospital day 5, the PM&R consult service was contacted by the physical therapist managing the patient. She reported that the patient had significant orthostatic hypotension that impacted the patient's ability to mobilize out of bed and participate in acute care therapies. The PM&R team re-evaluated the patient at bedside and ordered compression ace wraps to bilateral lower extremities and an abdominal binder when up and out of bed. The patient was doing well with intermittent catheterizations, with volumes of 300–400 mL. However, it was noted that the bisacodyl suppositories were not administered with nursing documenting "not indicated." The nurse caring for the patient was identified and reported that the suppository was not being administered because the patient had several small incontinent bowel movements. Collegial education was provided on the importance of the bowel regimen and that the incontinent bowel movements likely reflected overflow incontinence. Instruction was provided on the importance of the bowel program to promote continence. The patient was a good candidate for acute interdisciplinary inpatient rehabilitation, which was documented in the medical record.

The social worker was notified and coordinated with the rehabilitation liaison for insurance authorization for inpatient rehabilitation. The patient was admitted to acute inpatient rehabilitation on hospital day 7 and discharged home with his family following a 4-week inpatient rehabilitation stay.

Conclusion

The culture of PM&R is oriented to an interdisciplinary team-based approach to patient management, and physiatrists are proficient in both communication and collaboration with other medical specialists, interdisciplinary teams, patients, and families. Inpatient physiatrists are skilled at running patient and family meetings and discussing complex medical and rehabilitation issues, including challenging discharge planning. Physiatrist impact patient care in the acute setting by decreasing lengths of stay, reducing inpatient rehabilitation acute care transfers, increasing the likelihood of emerging from disordered consciousness in inpatient rehabilitation, and improving patient preparation to participate in an intensive interdisciplinary rehabilitation program. The consulting physiatrist serves as a leader of the acute care rehabilitation team, assisting medical and surgical teams in guiding the patient and family through the rehabilitation continuum of care and orchestrating discharge plans to support comprehensive patient rehabilitation to maximize the patient's function and ability to return to the community.

References[1]

1. Greiss C, Yonclas P, Jasey N, et al. Presence of a dedicated trauma center physiatrist improves functional outcomes following traumatic brain injury. J Trauma Acute Care Surg. 2016;80:70–5.
2. Wagner AK, Fabio T, Zafonte RD, et al. Physical medicine and rehabilitation consultation: relationships with acute functional outcome, length of stay, and discharge planning after traumatic brain injury. Am J Phys Med Rehabil. 2003;82(7):526–36.
3. Weppner JL, Linsenmeyer MA, Wagner AK. Effects of an acute care brain injury medicine continuity consultation service on health care utilization and rehabilitation outcomes. PM R. 2021;13(11):1227–36. https://doi.org/10.1002/pmrj.12563.
4. Smith B, Fields C, Fernandez N. Physical therapists make accurate and appropriate discharge recommendations for patients who are acutely ill. Phys Ther. 2010;90(5):693–703.
5. Malone D, Ridgeway K, Nordon-Craft A, et al. Physical therapist practice in the intensive care unit: results of a national survey. Phys Ther. 2015;95(10):1335–44.
6. Bondoc S, Lashgari D, Hermann V. American Occupational Therapy Association fact sheet: occupational therapy's role in acute care. https://www.aota.org/About-Occupational-Therapy/Professionals/RDP/AcuteCare.aspx. Accessed 26 Jan 2022.
7. American Speech-Lanuage-Hearing Association. Preferred practice patterns for the profession of speech-languge pathology. https://www.asha.org/policy/pp2004-00191/. Accessed 26 Jan 2022.
8. Kajs-Wyllie M, Holnar V, Tragger R Jr. Enhancing recovery via NeuroRehab rounds. J Neurosci Nurs. 1993;25(3):153–7.
9. Winstein CJ, Stein J, Arena R, et al. Guidelines for adult stroke rehabilitation and recovery: a guideline for healthcare professional for the American heart Association/American stroke association. Stroke. 2016;47:e98–e169.

[1] Key References [1–3, 9].

10. Joint Committee on Interprofessional Relations Between the American Speech-Language-Hearing Association and Division 40 (Clinical Neuropsychology) of the American Psychological Association. Structure and function of an interdisciplinary team for persons with acquired brain injury. https://www.asha.org/policy/gl2007-00288/. Accessed 26 Jan 2022.
11. Melchiorre PJ. Status of physiatry and physical medicine and rehabilitation departments in adult level 1 trauma centers. Arch Phys Med Rehabil. 1998;79:62.
12. Rosati DL. Polypharmacologic intervention in brain injury agitation. Am J Phys Med Rehabil. 2002;81(2):90–3.
13. Centers for Medicare & Medicaid Services. Inpatient hospital services covered under part A. Section 110: inpatient rehabilitation facility (IRF) services. 100–02 medicare benefit policy manual. 2021. https://www.cms.gov/Regulations-and-Guidance/Guidance/Manuals/Downloads/bp102c01.pdf
14. Hammond FM, Horn SD, Smout RJ, et al. Readmission to an acute care hospital during inpatient rehabilitation for traumatic brain injury. Arch Phys Med Rehabil. 2015;96(8 Suppl 3):S293–303.
15. Pinto SM, Galang G. Venous thromboembolism as predictor of acute care hospital transfer and inpatient rehabilitation length of stay. Am J Phys Med Rehabil. 2017;96(6):376–3.
16. Kane RL. Finding the right level of posthospital care: "we didn't realize there was any other option for him". JAMA. 2011;305(3):284–93. https://doi.org/10.1001/jama.2010.2015.
17. Tsai P, Bao GC. The safe discharge. J Palliat Med. 2018;21(10):1533–4. https://doi.org/10.1089/jpm.2018.0058.
18. Soong C, Daub S, Lee J, et al. Development of a checklist of safe discharge practices for hospital patients. J Hosp Med. 2013;8(8):444–9. https://doi.org/10.1002/jhm.2032.
19. Agency for Healthcare Research and Quality. Facts and figures 2006. Healthcare Cost and Utilization Project (HCUP). Agency for Healthcare Research and Quality. https://www.hcup-us.ahrq.gov/reports/factsandfigures/2007/exhibit1_4.jsp. Accessed 9 Jan 2023.
20. Wong SP, Sharda N, Zietlow KE, Heflin MT. Planning for a safe discharge: more than a capacity evaluation. J Am Geriatr Soc. 2020;68(4):859–66. https://doi.org/10.1111/jgs.16315.
21. Wright JR, Koch-Hanes T, Cortney C, et al. Planning for safe hospital discharge by identifying patients likely to fall after discharge. Phys Ther. 2022;102(2):pzab264. https://doi.org/10.1093/ptj/pzab264.
22. Mackay L. Benefits of a formalized traumatic brain injury program within a trauma center. J Head Trauma Rehabil. 1994;9(1):11–9.
23. Tam AKH, Berbrayer D, Robinson LR. What should be the role of physiatrist in early acute care rehabilitation? Current literature, models of care, and thoughts for the future. Am J Phys Med Rehabil. 2016;95:225–9.

Chapter 3
Conducting the History and Physical Exam: A Neurorehabilitation Consultant Guide

Michael Kryger, Rong Tina Chen, and Justin Weppner

Chapter Objectives

1. This chapter will provide an overview of the important elements of the history and physical (H&P) exam to solicit and perform when consulting on a patient with neurologic impairments in the acute care setting. The primary goal is to provide a comprehensive review of these elements, including a discussion of their purpose, their validity, and implications to neurorehabilitation.

Introduction

Patient history and physical (H&P) exam are extremely important components of a neurorehabilitation consultant's assessment, allowing for the formulation of a plan of care. The history gives clues regarding a patient's presentation, comorbidities, and social support system, all of which may impact rehabilitation goals. The physical exam allows the consultant to identify specific physical, cognitive, and functional impairments that can be barriers to independence and should be a focus of

M. Kryger (✉)
Department of Physical Medicine and Rehabilitation, Penn State University College of Medicine, Hershey, PA, USA
e-mail: mkryger@pennstatehealth.psu.edu

R. T. Chen
Carle Foundation Hospital, Urbana, IL, USA
e-mail: Tina.Chen@Carle.com

J. Weppner
Virginia Tech Carilion School of Medicine, Edward Via College of Osteopathic Medicine, Roanoke, VA, USA
e-mail: jlweppner@carilionclinic.org

A. K. Wagner, J. Weppner (eds.), *Acute Care Neuroconsultation and Neurorehabilitation Management*, https://doi.org/10.1007/978-3-031-42830-2_3

rehabilitation. Also key to the history and physical exam is the identification of medical and neurorehabilitation conditions and complications that can be treated and/or managed with neurorehabilitation consultant input. By identifying key elements of the H&P exam, the consultant will be able to contribute to medical management as well as determine the most appropriate setting for rehabilitation.

Principles of History Taking

History of Present Illness

The History of Present Illness (HPI) narrative describes the patient's onset of symptoms, change in health over time, and what brought them to the hospital. This history forms the basis for the differential diagnosis (DDx) and allows the examiner to narrow their line of questioning over the course of the clinical encounter. Traditionally, using open-ended interview questions regarding presentation often builds rapport [1]. However, patients with neurological injury are often unable to participate fully in the H&P exam due to their compromised neurological and injury status.

As with the entire H&P, a systematic approach is recommended to gather information effectively. Options include the OPQRST (Onset, Pain, Quality, Referral, Severity, Time frame) [2] or OLDCART (Onset, Location Duration, Characteristics, Aggravating factors, Relieving factors, Treatments) [3] mnemonics. These systems document timing of symptom presentation, characteristics and location of the symptoms, and what has worsened or improved symptoms. An HPI may also include a hospital course up to the point of consultation, to describe testing or surgeries that have been performed, as well as any diagnoses that have been established.

The HPI can help narrow a DDx and help formulate a rehabilitation plan. Symptom timing can inform the DDx. For example, an abrupt onset change in strength may suggest a cardioembolic stroke, whereas a more gradual onset may suggest an ischemic stroke [4]. Duration of illness and use of paralytics may help discern whether a patient is at risk for deconditioning or critical illness myopathy. Location of pain may identify an injured segment along the neural axis.

Past Medical, Surgical, and Family Histories

Obtaining a comprehensive list of other medical conditions and surgeries the patient has undergone is crucial in forming a DDx. Many medical conditions put patients at risk for secondary conditions or complications commonly encountered by the neurorehabilitation consultant. For example, a history of diabetes, atrial fibrillation, or dyslipidemia increases stroke risk [5]. If a patient had a previous spinal fusion and presents with new back pain, then hardware failure or adjacent level disease may be considered. The timing of these histories can also be significant. Long-standing diabetes carries a higher risk of peripheral neuropathy [6]. A patient 1-month status post-spinal cord injury (SCI) with worsening spasticity is expected; a patient 10-years status post-SCI with worsening spasticity could be the consequence of late effect complications such as a tethered cord or syringomyelia [7]. Knowing the past medical and surgical history is also essential in justifying the medical complexity warranting inpatient rehabilitation and what type of medical care to expect. Family history is an important consideration, as it may help refine the DDx if a condition exists in other family members. Even when the diagnosis has already been established, or family history is not relevant to their presentation (such as in traumatic cases), family history should be determined to anticipate other risk factors.

Medications

A medication review and update are helpful in building a picture of a patient's chronic illnesses and should match the past medical history in addition to the current presentation. Medication errors and adverse reactions are very common, so it is important to ensure that the current regimen is appropriate. In addition, the abrupt stoppage of some medications during acute hospitalization could have serious consequences or adverse effects. For example, ~14–31% of geriatric patients receive potentially inappropriate medications based on Beer's Criteria that may have contributed to their injury or condition [[8, 9]. When a patient presents after a fall, a medication review is essential to assist in an etiologically driven assessment identifying root causes for the fall and guiding workup to evaluate for conditions like orthostasis, syncope, ataxia, dizziness, etc. [10] Medication reviews are important in patients with altered mental status for similar reasons.

Social History

The neurorehabilitation consultant's documentation often has an emphasis on social history compared to a traditional H&P, as patient recovery potential and discharge plans are often influenced by social determinants of health, socioeconomic resources, and social supports [11].

Home Environment

The home environment is often described as the type of dwelling, number of steps inside and outside the house, availability of elevators and handrails, availability of first floor set up (either temporary or permanent), and presence of accessibility/safety measures such as bathroom grab bars and seated shower. This information can help the neuro-consultant formulate rehabilitation goals and consider the likelihood of returning home.

Support System

Patients with neurologically induced functional loss often require cognitive, physical, and behavioral assistance. It is important to identify available caregivers and what care they can provide in a community setting. Religion and spirituality can also be associated with better health outcomes [12] and may help some patients adjust to new disabilities.

Vocational Activities

A patient's educational background, work history, and leisure activities are important parts of their identity. Knowing this information can help determine the patient's ability to return to work and recreation, and may be used to direct goal-oriented and personalized therapy programs. Premorbid physical activity can predict disability progression in patients with neurological diseases [13].

Substance Use

Obtaining a substance use history is important, and should include tobacco, alcohol, and illicit drugs, detailing frequency, quantity, and last use. These pieces of the history are often contributing factors in traumatic and anoxic brain injuries [14]. A history of substance abuse portends a higher risk of recurrent use, especially when new disability can lead to increased pain and emotional instability [15]. Confirming histories via toxicology reports or family corroboration may be necessary, as some patients may be misleading about the extent of substance use or unable to provide this history due to neurological compromise.

Other Social Factors

The burden of medical cost can be overwhelming regardless of background. While these factors should not impact medical management of the patient, knowing a patient's health insurance, financial resources, and potential litigations or incarceration is important as these issues can affect family supports and discharge planning, and therefore, should be considered when discussing rehabilitation.

Functional History

Delineating premorbid functional status is essential to rehabilitation management and goal setting. Standardized instrumentation such as functional independence measure (FIM) can be useful if available. Recent updates to Center for Medicare Services guidelines advise the use of new quality indicators to describe functional abilities and goals [16, 17]. These scores are meant to be used across healthcare settings for consistency. The most recent physical, occupational, and speech therapy assessments during acute hospitalization should be documented to help determine goals and appropriate setting for rehabilitation.

Mobility

Mobility assessments should reflect the ability to move about in one's environment, which includes bed mobility, transfers, household and community ambulation, and driving. The consultant should ask about the use of assistive devices such as transfer board, cane, walker, wheelchair, orthoses, etc., and whether these devices are functional and with appropriate dimensions to optimize utility for each patient. Ambulation can be characterized by distance/time walked and if uneven surfaces (i.e., stairs, curbs, slopes) can be managed. Weight bearing and range of motion precautions should be considered as should fall history (e.g., the number and frequency of falls and near falls), if any injuries or hospitalizations resulted, and whether an etiology was determined. The consultant should also ask about driving, which can be crucial for community independence. Depressive symptoms rise in elderly people who have stopped driving [18]. Also, driving status may indicate a baseline impairment that requires further investigation.

Activities of Daily Living

Activities of daily living (ADLs) are essential to the history and should include information on self-care activities of eating, grooming, bathing/showering, dressing, toileting, and hygiene. Instrumental ADLs include care of others, meal preparation, financial management, medication management, shopping, driving, and household activities such as cleaning, laundry, and yard work. If a certain activity cannot be completed, the clinician should document how and why this area of function is limited.

Cognition/Communication

Deficits in baseline cognition and communication skills can interfere with the rehabilitation plan and potential. It is important to gather information from family and friends as patients with cognitive deficits are often unaware of their impairments and can downplay these deficits. Other premorbid function, such as native language and hearing function should be explored, and may require translators or augmentative communication devices during the H&P exam.

Review of Systems (ROS)

The ROS is the process of asking brief yes/no questions regarding any other significant symptoms from every organ system to ensure that nothing else has been missed. It can be tailored to symptoms expected based on the DDx, however, a systematic approach is recommended to avoid missing any other diagnoses. The 14 systems recognized by the Centers for Medicare and Medicaid Services (CMS) include:

1. Constitutional symptoms
2. Eyes
3. Ears, nose, mouth, throat
4. Cardiovascular
5. Respiratory
6. Gastrointestinal
7. Genitourinary
8. Musculoskeletal
9. Integumentary
10. Neurological
11. Psychiatric
12. Endocrine
13. Hematologic/Lymphatic
14. Allergic/Immunologic.

Principles of the Physical Exam

The physical exam allows the neurorehabilitation consultant to paint a picture of how the patient functions, and the information garnered aids in diagnosis. Physical exam findings can assist in determining what types of impairments the patient presents with, what to focus on in rehabilitation, and what to expect regarding recovery. It is also very important in determining the most appropriate rehabilitation care setting.

Inspection and Palpation

The process of examination begins with observation upon entering the patient's room—evaluating general appearance, body habitus, disposition, level of arousal, spontaneous activity, or malaise. History taking can be useful in assessing the patient's speech, cognition, memory, and judgment. Inspection can involve multiple different items, depending on the diagnosis. For example, examine the skin for rashes or joint swelling if there is concern of a rheumatologic condition. The examiner may assess muscle mass, twitches, tremors, or fasciculations if there is concern for a neuromuscular, movement, or motor neuron disorder. The examiner may also identify asymmetry, swelling, bruising, or unexpected deformities to evaluate any further injury in a multi-trauma patient. Palpation, the use of touch to assess a patient, can confirm deformity seen on inspection, evaluate for any underlying masses or edema, determine if there is a "step-off" injury of the spinal column, and identify a musculoskeletal source of pain.

Strength Testing

Manual muscle testing (MMT) is performed on 5-point scale (Table 3.1). One should test the primary plane of motion for each major myotome, including shoulder abduction, elbow flexion/extension, wrist flexion/extension, grip, hip flexion, knee flexion/extension, and ankle dorsiflexion/plantarflexion. Other MMT may be warranted based on symptoms and diagnosis. The spinal cord strength exam require very specific motion testing to assess each spinal nerve (see "The ISNCSCI Exam" below). With each higher level of strength, there is a greater likelihood of regaining function in the context of SCI [19, 20].

Table 3.1 Grading scales for manual muscle testing and muscle stretch reflex

Name of test	Grading scale	
Manual muscle test	0	No movement muscle contraction
	1	Visible or palpable muscle contraction without movement
	2	Active movement through full available range of motion (ROM) with gravity eliminated
	3	Active movement through full available ROM against gravity
	4	Active movement through full available ROM against gravity and with moderate resistance
	5	Active movement through full ROM against gravity and with maximal resistance
Muscle stretch reflex	0	No response, often a sign of lower motor neuron process
	1	Diminished by present
	2	Normal
	3	More brisk than usual
	4	Hyperactive with clonus

Subtle weakness may require forceful resistance by the examiner, or functional tasks such as squatting and heel-raise while standing. Less resistance may be indicated for patients who are frail, or with other conditions such as pain, vascular injuries, or weight-bearing restrictions. In contrast, volitional strength testing may be limited by a variety of conditions that require advanced clinical acumen to differentiate etiology of the apparent weakness. For example, spasticity, as well as heterotopic ossification, can physically limit strength testing over joints through their full range of motion (ROM). Critical illness neuromyopathy (CINM) may limit MMT participation in someone with cognitive abilities to participate. Language deficits due to receptive aphasia or motor planning deficits due to apraxia can also limit patient ability to participate in MMT. Furthermore, primary sensory deficits (e.g., visual cortex injury or sensory nerve damage from hypoxic ischemic brain injury (HIBI) may limit ability to follow commands required for MMT, as well as other parts of the physical exam.

Range of Motion Testing

Patients with neurologic disorders are at risk for reductions in joint function and ROM. Causes include rotator cuff disease, severe spasticity, contractures, or heterotopic ossification. Each joint should be extended, flexed, and compared side-to-side to determine any functional restriction. The neurorehabilitation consultant should describe ROM using angles and specify the direction of loss to ensure clear documentation (for example, "Lacking 30° of knee extension"). It is also important to be aware of any ROM restrictions due to surgeries or concurrent wound/injuries.

Cranial Nerve Exam

Cranial Nerve (CN) exam tests the function of CN I-XII. CN I is often omitted due to practicality. See Table 3.2 for specific evaluations.

Table 3.2 Cranial nerve examination

Nerve	Evaluations	Comments
I: Olfactory	Common hospital room items such as alcohol swabs, coffee, and other food items can be used. Avoid irritating items	The olfactory nerve is often injured in head traumas, and can be associated with fracture of the cribriform plate. Hyposmia and anosmia can be an early sign of Parkinson's disease [21].
II: Optic	Both visual acuity and visual fields should be tested. For visual fields, all four quadrants should be tested with one eye covered at a time	Optic neuropathy can be a result of trauma, tumors, CNS pathology, or metabolic and toxic insults. Its function is closely associated with that of CN II, IV, and VI

Table 3.2 (continued)

Nerve	Evaluations	Comments
III: Oculomotor	CN II-VI are best tested together. Assess eye position at rest. Then assess movements in the six cardinal directions. The target (usually a finger at arm's length) is moved in an "H" shape. CN II and III are involved in the pupillary light reflex; a normal reflex results in constriction of both pupils when light is shone in either eye.	Innervates superior/inferior/medial rectus, inferior oblique, and levator palpebrae superioris muscles.
IV: Trochlear		Innervates Lateral Rectus Muscle
VI: Abducens		Innervates Lateral rectus muscle
V: Trigeminal	Sensory	Trigeminal neuralgia is characterized by severe pain along the distribution of trigeminal nerves
	– Test light touch, pinprick, or temperature sensation in each of the three sensory branches bilaterally: Ophthalmic (forehead), maxillary (cheeks), and mandibular (jaw)	
	Motor	
	– Innervates muscles of mastication	
	– Clench jaw to palpate masseter and temporalis	
	– Open mouth to test pterygoids. Mouth will deviate toward the weak side	
	Corneal reflex tests the ophthalmic branch (afferent) and the facial nerve (efferent)	
VII: Facial	Motor	A central lesion typically only affects the lower face. A peripheral lesion, such as Bell's palsy, will affect both the upper and the lower face
	– Smile/show both upper and lower teeth (orbicularis oris)	Usually, only motor functions are tested clinically
	– Raise eye brows (frontalis)	
	– Close eyes tightly against examiner's attempt to open them (orbicularis oculi)	
	– Puff out cheeks (buccinators)	
	Sensory	
	– Provides sensation to the anterior 2/3 of the tongue	
	– Innervates the stapedius	

(continued)

Table 3.2 (continued)

Nerve	Evaluations	Comments
VIII: Vestibulocochlear	Hearing	Vestibular dysfunction can present in patients with trauma, stroke, or medication toxicity; vestibular therapy should be considered
	– Tested by rubbing fingers next to each ear	
	– Tuning forks can be utilized for more detailed sensorineural hearing loss evaluation (Weber and Rinne tests)	
	Vestibular	
	– Test for nystagmus, which can be vertical, horizontal, or rotary	
IX: Glossopharyngeal	Inspect the soft palate for elevation symmetry	Prolonged intubation can cause laryngeal injuries and vocal fold dysmotility, which may cause dysphonia [23]
X: Vagus	Inspect if the uvula is midline	The presence of a gag reflex does not eliminate risk of aspiration [24]
	– In UMN lesion, uvula deviates to the ipsilateral side of the lesion	
	– In LMN lesion, uvula deviates toward the contralateral side of the lesion	
	Hoarseness is often associated with injury to the recurrent laryngeal nerve	
	Gag reflex assesses sensation provided by the glossopharyngeal nerve and palatal contraction initiated by the vagus nerve	
XI: Accessory	Trapezius—have the patient shrug shoulders and assess for strength and symmetry	
	Sternocleidomastoid—Ask the patient to turn their head against resistance. The ipsilateral muscle turns the head to the contralateral side	
XII: Hypoglossal	Protrude tongue	Tongue fasciculation is common in patients with amyotrophic lateral sclerosis
	– In central process such as stroke, tongue deviates to the contralateral side of the lesion	
	– In peripheral hypoglossal nerve lesion, tongue deviates to the ipsilateral side of the lesion	
	Assess for tongue fasciculation	

Sensory Exam

Superficial sensation encompasses light touch, pain, and temperature sensation. The consultant may assess light touch using a wisp of cotton, pain sensation using a safety pin, and temperature sensation using ice cubes or water.

Deep sensation includes proprioception and vibration. Proprioception is tested with the examiner moving a distal joint vertically—usually the distal phalange of the finger or the toe—and asking the patient to identify the direction of movement. When completing this portion of the examination, the clinician should grasp the phalange on the sides instead of the nailbed to avoid the confounding sensation associated with vertical pressure. Vibratory sensation is a sensitive and specific measure in detecting diabetic peripheral neuropathy [25]. A 128-Hz tuning fork is placed on a bony prominence (e.g., malleoli). The duration of vibration is measured. If normal, the examiner and the patient should feel vibrations cease at the same time. It is important to compare sensation side-to-side or affected dermatomes versus unaffected dermatomes.

Cognition/Mental Status

Level of Consciousness

Disorders of consciousness, including coma, unresponsive wakefulness syndrome (UWS), and minimally conscious state (MCS), are states where consciousness has been affected by damage to the brain. A person in a coma appears asleep and shows no signs of being awake or aware. The patient will lie with closed eyes, have no sleep-wake cycles, and not respond to their environment, voices, or pain. In contrast, UWS is when a person is awake but shows no signs of awareness. A person in a UWS may open their eyes, have evidence of sleep-wake cycles, and have basic reflexes such as blinking when startled by a loud noise. MCS is a condition of severely altered consciousness in which minimal but definite behavioral evidence of self or environmental awareness is demonstrated. To diagnose MCS, limited but discernible evidence of self or environmental awareness must be demonstrated on a reproducible or sustained basis by one or more of the following behaviors: following simple commands, inconsistent gestural or verbal yes/no responses, and intelligible verbalization. Arousal with intense stimuli such as sternal rub and minimal voluntary movement describes stupor. A lethargic patient may fall asleep easily but also arouse [26]. A conscious patient is awake, eyes open, and responds appropriately to various stimuli. Emergence from MCS is characterized by the reliable and consistent demonstration of one or both of the following: (1) accurate functional interactive communication or (2) functional object use, such as bringing a comb to the head or a pencil to a sheet of paper. The JFK Coma Recovery Scale is a tool that assesses six domains of cognitive function, and can assist in prognostication, documenting incremental changes in neurological exam associated with neurostimulant trials and/or the development of complicating conditions, and functional goal setting [27].

Orientation

The four components of orientation are person, place, time, and situation. Acute illness, hospitalization, and stress can account for temporary and minimal loss of orientation. Typically, time awareness is first to be lost and orientation to self is last [26].

Attention

Month Backwards Test (MBT) is a simple yet sensitive tool for evaluating attention [28]. It correlates highly with other attention tests such as trail making test and serial sevens but eliminates some confounding issues such as lower educational background. Often, practitioners will start by asking the patient to recite the months of the year in forward order. Once that response is established, performance with backward order can be compared. Alternatively, days of week forward/backward may be appropriate for individuals who cannot perform the MBT or are easily frustrated by the difficulty of this test.

Memory

Both immediate and delayed recall should be tested. The clinician should ask the patient to immediately repeat three words to evaluate immediate recall. The Centers for Medicare & Medicaid Services advises using "sock," "blue," and "bed." Five minutes later, patient should be asked to recall the same three words to assess delayed memory recall. If a patient is unable to remember, categorical cues (e.g., "a color" for the word "blue") or multiple choices can be used to stimulate recall [29].

Abstraction

Abstraction can be tested by interpreting common proverbs such as "you can't judge a book by its cover," and describing similarities such as "How are a train and a plane similar?" Concrete responses, or lack of response, may indicate neurological pathology, though cultural and educational backgrounds should be taken into consideration when interpreting patient answers [26].

General Assessment Tools

The Montreal Cognitive Assessment (MoCA) is an extensively validated 30-point general cognition screening tool; a score of 26 or above is normal [30]. A similar tool is the Folstein Mini-Mental State Examination, where a score of 24/30 or above is normal [31]. Both tests have 30 items, and are meant to take about 5–10 min, however, in someone with cognitive impairments, they can be time-consuming and taxing. The clock drawing test is a quicker alternative that tests executive functioning, sequencing, visual-spatial functioning, and memory [32].

Speech

Fluency, comprehension, repetition, phonation, and motor planning are all parts of speech evaluation.

Aphasia

Aphasia is the impairment of language utilization due to an injury to the brain. It is characterized in terms of fluency, comprehension, repetition, and prosody (Fig. 3.1). Testing should start with simple words and progress to more complex sentences and commands. Reading and writing should also be assessed if patients are physically and cognitively able. Aphasia testing documentation should descriptively review these component areas of language. Other common speech errors should be noted and include paraphasias (incorrect word substitution), anomia (word finding difficulties), neologisms (creating new words), and echolalia (repetition of the same word).

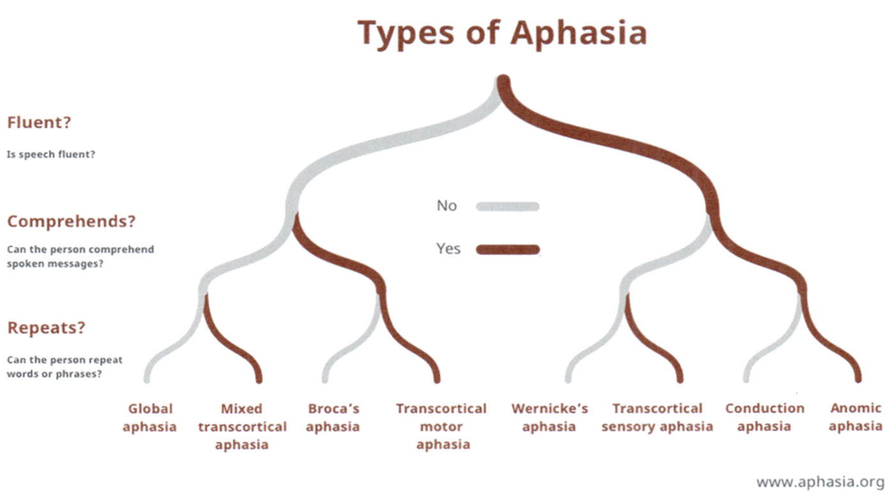

Fig. 3.1 Determining aphasia type based on fluency, comprehension and repetition

Dysarthria

Dysarthria is impaired articulation. Types of dysarthria include ataxic, hypokinetic, hyperkinetic, spastic, and flaccid (Table 3.3). Dysarthrias can be evaluated by listening to spontaneous speech production and by asking the patient to produce specific sounds such as "ga" (laryngeal consonants), "mm" (labial consonants), and "ta" (lingual consonant) [26].

Other Disorders

Dysphonia is impaired sound production, often caused by vocal cord dysfunction because of neurological insult or laryngeal trauma including intubation. Verbal or oromotor apraxia is characterized by motor planning deficits leading to disorganized speech, dysphagia, and oral/facial manipulation difficulty [26].

Table 3.3 Types of dysarthria

	Flaccid	Spastic	Ataxic	Hypokinetic	Hyperkinetic
Pathophysiology	– Hypotonia	– Hypertonia	– Hypotonia	– Hypokinesia	– Hyperkinesia
			– Dysmetria		
Articulation	– Distorted pressure consonants and vowels	– Imprecise consonants	– Distorted vowels	– Imprecise consonants	– Distorted vowels
	– Slow rate	– Slow movement	– Slow articulatory breakdowns	– Dysfluencies	– Irregular articulatory breakdowns
		– Slow rate	– Telescoping	– Increased or variable rate	– Variable rate
			– Slow speech		
Phonation	– Hoarse and breathy	– Harsh and strained	– Breathy, harsh, and strained	– Breathy and harsh	– Breathy and strained
		– Pitch breaks	– Voice tremor	– Reduced loudness	– Intermittent voice arrests
			– Pitch breaks		
Prosody	– Monopitch	– Monopitch	– Prolonged phonemes	– Monopitch	– Prolonged silences
	– Monoloudness	– Monoloudness		– Monoloudness	
	– Prolonged phonemes	– Short phrases		– Short rushes of speech	
Resonance	– Hypernasality	– Hypernasality	– Intermittent hypo-hyper nasality	– Mild hypernasality	– Irregular velopharyngeal incompetence
	– Nasal emissions				
Respiration	– Inhalatory stridor	– Paradoxical breathing	– Excessive loudness variations	– Reduced vital capacity	– Sudden involuntary inspirations or expirations
	– Reduced max phonation time				

Apraxia is the inability to perform sequenced, coordinated motor programs. Apraxia of speech is an important type of apraxia that can be present in those with neurological compromise. Apraxia of speech may not specifically involve word finding or comprehension difficulties, but fluency can be significantly impacted, with sound distortions and slow speech rate. It can present separately, or in addition to other speech disorders, making it sometimes difficult to parse out which speech disorder is most prominent [33]. When compared with dysarthria, error variability may facilitate distinguishing between apraxia and dysarthria. It is argued that individuals with apraxia demonstrate more significant variability in sound-level errors, meaning errors are less predictable when compared with dysarthria [34]. Moreover, the oral mechanism evaluation for an individual with apraxia is generally unremarkable, but dysarthrias may be associated with facial, labial, or lingual weakness and reduced range of motion, especially if there is cranial nerve involvement. Additionally, a speech therapist may administer the apraxia of speech rating scale (ASRS) and provide an additional tool for quantifying the presence and severity of apraxia of speech [35].

Coordination, Balance, and Gait

If data from allied health professionals suggest that the patient can safely stand up (based on therapy notes on cognition and strength), then evaluating balance and gait can be very helpful. Romberg's test, in which a patient stands with his or her feet close together and closes their eyes, tests the body's proprioception and vestibular systems [36]. If the patient cannot stand, cerebellar dysfunction may be assessed with rapid alternating movements and extremity coordination evaluation. When appropriate, gait analysis can identify weakness and bracing needs.

Much like apraxia of speech, apraxia of the limb is often a difficult diagnosis, as those with apraxia may have other more prominent deficits, such as sensory loss, motor weakness, ataxia, upper motor neuron lesions, neglect, etc. There are several different apraxia types, including ideomotor, limb-kinetic, conceptual, and ideational. Each have different features related to sequencing and movement errors. There are multiple tests focused particularly on testing limb apraxia, such as coin rotation and imitation tasks [37].

Upper Motor Neuron Lesion Evaluation

Upper motor neuron (UMN) lesions occur proximal to the alpha motor neuron, resulting in decreased descending inhibition. Causes include stroke, brain injury, spinal cord injury, demyelinating disease, motor neuron disease, and cerebral palsy. UMN syndrome can result in spasticity, dystonia, and hyperactive reflexes.

Spasticity

Spasticity is velocity dependent change in muscle tone. It can manifest from days to months after onset of injury. Changes in a person's baseline spasticity may indicate other systemic issues such as infection or wound. Spasticity can be qualitatively measured by the Modified Ashworth Scale (see Chap. 8).

Dystonia

Dystonia is sustained muscle contraction and posturing. For example, torticollis is caused by dystonic neck muscles pulling the head and neck. Diagnosis relies on visual inspection and history. Dystonias can lead to pain and impaired motor function.

Muscle Stretch Reflex

Muscle Stretch Reflex (MSRs) can be tested by tapping over the muscle tendon with a reflex hammer. Commonly tested locations include biceps, brachioradialis, triceps, pronator teres, patella, medial hamstring, and achilles. The reflexes are influenced by various factors, including age, sex, and examiner's techniques [38, 39]. Aging affects muscle stretch reflexes at different levels of the proprioceptive reflex arc, including degenerative changes in muscle spindle receptors, functional deficiency within the muscle spindle primary afferent pathway, changes in corticospinal excitability, loss of motor neurons and loss of muscle mass and strength [40]. In general, the limb should be in a relaxed position, midway between extension and flexion. If a response is difficult to illicit, one can try to change limb position to put in into slight tension. If a patient cannot relax, distraction methods can be used. MSR grading is described in Table 3.1 [41].

Abnormal Reflexes

Babinski's sign is tested by applying a stimulus to the sole of the foot. A normal response (plantar reflex) would be toe flexion or lack of extension. Up-going Babinski (extension of the big toe and fanning of other toes) suggest an upper motor neuron injury and corticospinal tract dysfunction [42]. Hoffmann's sign (tapping or flicking the distal phalanx of the middle finger with resulting flexion of the thumb) may indicate corticospinal tract dysfunction at the level of the cervical spine. Unlike Babinski's sign, a positive Hoffman's reflex can be observed in normal individuals, and thus, this finding must be considered in the context of other neurological exam findings to determine its relevance to the clinical presentation [43]. These reflexes may assist in determining the level of an injury.

The ISNCSCI Exam

The International Standards for the Neurological Classification of Spinal Cord Injury (ISNCSCI) Exam (previously known as the "ASIA" Exam for the American Spinal Injury Association) is an extensively validated method to examine and classify patients who have experienced SCI [44]. The exam documents sensation and strength at every accessible dermatome and myotome of the spinal cord to determine the dysfunctional spinal pathways. After the examination, a worksheet is used to determine the ASIA Impairment Scale, a Grade of A through E, and the most caudal intact level of the spinal cord (Table 3.4). The exam can be a very important tool to determine possible medical complications, provide expectations to family, and formulate a rehabilitation and medical plan. A grade of A, in which there is no sacral sparing, is considered a complete injury and has the worst prognosis for recovery. The incomplete injuries, B through E, indicate progressively better prognoses and chance of ambulation [44]. The level of the injury can also play an important role in formulating rehabilitation goals; the more rostral the level, the more assistance the patient will need with mobility and activities of daily living.

The main components of the ISNCSCI Exam are light touch testing, pinprick testing, and manual muscle testing. Light touch testing is performed by comparing sensation from a wisp of cotton over the face to the various dermatomes and can be graded as 0 (no sensation), 1 (altered), and 2 (normal). Pinprick testing examines the patient's discrimination between sharp and dull. It is graded as 0 (no sensation/no discrimination between sharp and dull), 1 (altered sensation, but can differentiate between sharp and dull), and 2 (normal). MMT uses the traditional 0 through 5 scale, with a few differences. Deep anal pressure, voluntary anal contraction, and dermatomes around the anus are also tested; their total absence indicates a complete injury. The Exam Form (Fig. 3.2) details every dermatome testing location and manual muscle testing, as well as test grading [45].

Table 3.4 ASIA Impairment Scale (AIS) Grade (Adapted from ISNCSCI Form)

AIS grade	Injury type	Description
A	Complete	No sensory or motor function at sacral levels S4–S5
B	Sensory incomplete	Sensory but no motor function is preserved below the neurological level, and includes sensation at S4–S5
C	Motor incomplete	Motor function preserved below the neurologic level, but more than half of the key muscles below the neurologic level are less than grade 3
D	Motor incomplete	Moto function preserved below the neurologic level, and at least half of the key muscles below the neurologic level are grade 3 or greater
E	Normal	Patient with SCI that now has normal sensation and motor function at all levels tested

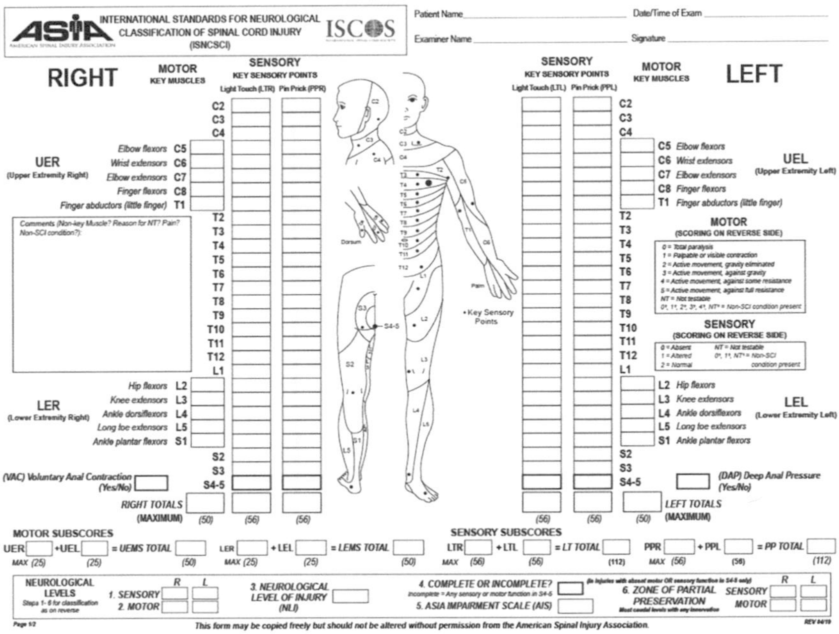

Fig. 3.2 International Standard for Neurological Classification of Spinal Cord Injury Worksheet

Other Important Reflexes After SCI

While not formal parts of the ISNCSCI exam, the bulbocavernosus reflex can be clinically important in differentiating between UMN and LMN lesions. In men, the bulbocavernosus reflex is elicited by squeezing the glans of the penis [46]. In women, it is elicited by tapping or squeezing the clitoris [47]. A somewhat less intrusive option is to gently tug on a foley catheter, if inserted. The anal wink reflex is elicited by testing pinprick sensation at the mucocutaneous junction of the anus (which is already done as part of the ISNCSCI exam, however, not explicitly to test the reflex). As a result of any of these tests, there should be contraction of the anal sphincter. The absence of this reflex suggests a LMN injury [48]. The cremaster reflex is elicited in males by stroking the inner thigh, resulting in the retraction of the ipsilateral testicale [49]. It is one of the early reflexes to return following spinal shock, along with the bulbocavernosus reflex [50].

Summary and Key Points

- The neurorehabilitation consult H&P goes beyond the normal medical H&P with a special focus on elements relevant to functional impairment and disability. It is critical to formulating the appropriate individualized rehabilitation plan and discharge.
- Home environment and functional histories in mobility, ADLs, I-ADLs, and cognition/communication are unique elements of the neurorehabilitation consultant's H&P.
- Obtaining history and performing a physical exam can be challenging due to cognitive and communication impairments inherent to the patient population.
- A thorough neurologic and musculoskeletal exam is essential in eliciting impairments, developing a differential diagnosis, and determining a rehabilitation plan.
- The ISNCSCI exam is a validated and specialized diagnostic and prognostic tool for SCI patients.
- For persons with disorders of consciousness, the JFK Coma Recovery Scale assists with determining the level of consciousness, which helps guide prognosis and treatment planning for this patient population.
- The Montreal Cognitive Assessment Score (MoCA) is a brief screening tool designed to assess various cognitive domains, which is a sensitive test for cognitive impairment in the TBI population.

References[1]

1. Makoul G. Essential elements of communications in medical encournters: the Kalamazoo consensus statement. Acad Med. 2001;76(4):390–3.
2. Thomas SA. Spinal stenosis: history and physical examination. Phys Med Rehabil Clin N Am. 2003;14:29–39.
3. Summers S. Evidence-based practice part 2: reliability and validity of selected acute pain instruments. J Perianesth Nurs. 2001;16(1):35–40.
4. American Medical Association. CPT 2015 professional edition. Chicago: AMA; 2015.
5. Arboix A, Garcia-Eroles L, Massons J, Oliveres M, Pujades R, Targa C. Atrial fibrillation and stroke: clinical presentation of cardioembolic versus atherothrombotic infarction. Int J Cardiol. 2000;73(1):33–42.
6. Goldstein L, Adams R, Alberts M, et al. Primary prevention of ischemic stroke: a guideline from the American Heart Association/American Stroke Association Stroke Council: cosponsored by the Atherosclerotic Peripheral Vascular Disease Interdisciplinary Working Group; Cardiovascular Nursing Council; Clinical Cardiology Council; Nutrition, Physical Activity, and Metabolism Council; and the Quality of Care and Outcomes Research Interdisciplinary Working Group. Circulation. 2006;113(24):e873–923.
7. Adler A, Boyko E, Ahroni J, Stensel V, Forsberg R, Smith D. Risk factors for diabetic peripheral sensory neuropathy. Results of the Seattle Prospective Diabetic Foot Study. Diabetes Care. 1997;20(7):1162–7.

[1] Key References [1, 8, 12, 25].

8. Campagnolo D, Kirshblum S, Nash M, Heary R, Gorman P, editors. Spinal cord medicine. 2nd ed. Philadelphia: Lippincott Williams & Wilkins; 2011.
9. Gallagher PF, Barry PJ, Ryan C, Hartigan I, O'Mahony D. Inappropriate prescribing in an acutely ill population of elderly patients as determined by Beers' Criteria. Age Ageing. 2008;37(1):96–101.
10. Barnett K, McCowan C, Evans JM, Gillespie ND, Davey PG, Fahey T. Prevalence and outcomes of use of potentially inappropriate medicines in older people: cohort study stratified by residence in nursing home or in the community. BMJ Qual Saf. 2011;20(3):275–81.
11. Masud T, Morris R. Epidemiology of falls. Age Ageing. 2001;30(S4):3–7.
12. Nguyen V, PrvuBettger J, Guerrier T, et al. Factors associated with discharge to home versus discharge to institutional care after inpatient stroke rehabilitation. Arch Phys Med Rehabil. 2015;96(7):1297–303.
13. Mueller P, Plevak D, Rummans T. Religious involvement, spirituality, and medicine: implications for clinical practice. Mayo Clin Proc. 2001;76(12):1225–35.
14. Motl R, Dlugonski D, Pilutti L, Sandroff B, McAuley E. Premorbid physical activity predicts disability progression in relapsing-remitting multiple sclerosis. J Neurol Sci. 2012;323(1–2):123–7.
15. Corrigan J. Substance abuse as a mediating factor in outcome from traumatic brain injury. Arch Phys Med Rehabil. 1995;76:302–9.
16. Smedema S, Ebener D. Substance abuse and psychosocial adaptation to physical disability: analysis of the literature and future directions. Disabil Rehabil. 2009;32(16):1311–9.
17. Centers for Medicare & Medicaid Services. Federal Register: Medicare and Medicaid Programs; CY 2018 Home Health Prospective Payment System Rate Update and CY 2019 Case-Mix Adjustment Methodology Refinements; Home Health Value-Based Purchasing Model; and Home Health Quality Reporting Requirements. In: US Department of Health and Human Services, editor. Vol 822017:51676.
18. Center for Medicare & Medicaid Services. Inpatient rehabilitation facility—patient assessment instrument. In: US Department of Health and Human Services, ed. Version 4.0 ed2020.
19. Marottoli R, Mendes de Leon C, Glass T, et al. Driving cessation and increased depressive symptoms: prospective evidence from the New Haven EPESE. Established Populations for Epidemiologic Studies of the Elderly. J Am Geriatr Soc. 1997;45(2):202–6.
20. Feys H, De Weerdt W, Nuyens G, van de Winckel A, Selz B, Kiekens C. Predicting motor recovery of the upper limb after stroke rehabilitation: value of a clinical examination. Physiother Res Int. 2000;5(1):1–18.
21. Doty RL. Olfaction in Parkinson's disease. Parkinsonism Relat Disord 2007;13:S225–8
22. Marino R, Graves D. Metric properties of the ASIA motor score: subscales improve correlation with functional activities. Arch Phys Med Rehabil. 2004;85(11):1804–10.
23. Colton House J, Noordzij JP, Murgia B, Langmore S. Laryngeal injury from prolonged intubation: a prospective analysis of contributing factors. Laryngoscope. 2011;121(3):596–600.
24. Palmer JB, Drennan JC, Baba M. Evaluation and treatment of swallowing impairments. Am Fam Physician. 2000;61(8):2453–62.
25. Martin CL, Waberski BH, Pop-Busui R, et al. Vibration perception threshold as a measure of distal symmetrical peripheral neuropathy in type 1 diabetes: results from the DCCT/EDIC study. Diabetes Care. 2010;33(12):2635–41.
26. Braddom R, Chan L, Harrast M, editors. Physical medicine & rehabilitation. 4th ed. Philadelphia: Saunders/Elsevier; 2011.
27. Giacino J, Kalmar K, Whyte J. The JFK Coma Recovery Scale-Revised: measurement characteristics and diagnostic utility. Arch Phys Med Rehabil. 2004;85(12):2020–9.
28. Meagher J, Leonard M, Donoghue L, et al. Months backward test: a review of its use in clinical studies. World J Psychiatry. 2015;5(3):305–14.
29. Centers for Medicare & Medicaid Services. Inpatient rehabilitation facility quality reporting program: technical specifications for reporting assessment-based measures for IRF-PAI 1.4 and 1.5. 2017. https://www.cms.gov/Medicare/Quality-Initiatives-Patient-Assessment-

Instruments/IRF-Quality-Reporting/Downloads/IRF-QRP-Technical-Specifications-for-Reporting-Assessment-Based-Measures.pdf. Accessed 7 Feb 2022.
30. Nasreddine Z, Phillips N, Bedirian V, et al. The Montreal Cognitive Assessment, MoCA: a brief screening tool for mild cognitive impairment. J Am Geriatr Soc. 2005;53(4):695–9.
31. Burton L, Tyson S. Screening for cognitive impairment after stroke: a systematic review of psychometric properties and clinical utility. J Rehabil Med. 2015;47(3):193–203.
32. Scanlan J, Borson S. The Mini-Cog: receiver operating characteristics with expert and naive raters. Int J Geriatr Psychiatry. 2001;16(2):216–22.
33. Botha H, Josephs KA. Primary progressive aphasias and Praxia of speech. Continuum. 2019;25(1):101–27.
34. Miller N. Variability in speech dyspraxia. Clin Linguist Phon. 1992;6(1–2):77–85.
35. Strand EA, Duffy JR, Clark HM, Josephs K. The Apraxia of Speech Rating Scale: a tool for diagnosis and description of apraxia of speech. J Commun Disord. 2014;51:43–50.
36. Khasnis A, Gokula R. Romberg's test. J Postgrad Med. 2003;49(2):169–72.
37. Heilman KM. Upper limb apraxia. Continuum. 2021;27(6):1602–23.
38. Lim K-S, Bong Y, Chaw Y, Ho K, Kwok K. Wide range of normality in deep tendon reflexes in the normal population. Neurol Asia. 2009;14:21–5.
39. Chandrasekhar A, Abu Osman NA, Tham LK, Lim KS, Wan Abas WA. Influence of age on patellar tendon reflex response. PLoS One. 2013;8(11):e80799.
40. Romanovsky D, Mrak RE, Dobretsov M. Age-dependent decline in density of human nerve and spinal ganglia neurons expressing the α3 isoform of Na/K-ATPase. Neuroscience. 2015;310:342–53.
41. Walker HK. Deep tendon reflexes. In: Walker HK, Hall WD, Hurst JW, editors. Clinical methods: the history, physical, and laboratory examinations. Boston: Butterworths; 1990.
42. Isaza Jaramillo SP, Uribe Uribe CS, Garcia Jimenez FA, Cornejo-Ochoa W, Alvarez Restrepo JF, Roman GC. Accuracy of the Babinski sign in the identification of pyramidal tract dysfunction. J Neurol Sci. 2014;343(1–2):66–8.
43. Tejus M, Singh V, Ramesh A, Kumar V, Maurya V, Madhugiri V. An evaluation of the finger flexion, Hoffman's and platar reflexes as markers of cervical spinal cord compression—a comparative clinical study. Clin Neurol Neurosurg. 2015;134:12–6.
44. Kirshblum S, Waring W III. Updates for the international standards for neurological classification of spinal cord injury. Phys Med Rehabil Clin N Am. 2014;25(3):505–17.
45. American Spinal Injury Association. International Standards for Neurological Classification of Spinal Cord Injury (ISNCSCI). Richmond, VA: The American Spinal Injury Association; 2019.
46. Bors E, Blinn KA. Bulbocavernosus reflex. J Urol. 1959;82(1):128–30.
47. Wester C, FitzGerald MP, Brubaker L, Welgoss J, Benson JT. Validation of the clinical bulbocavernosus reflex. Neurourol Urodyn. 2003;22(6):589–91; discussion 591–582.
48. Kirshblum S, Eren F. Anal reflex versus bulbocavernosus reflex in evaluation of patients with spinal cord injury. Spinal Cord Ser Cases. 2020;6:2.
49. Mellick LB, Mowery ML, Al-Dhahir MA. Cremasteric reflex. In: StatPearls. Treasure Island, FL: StatPearls Publishing; 2021.
50. Ko HY, Ditunno JF Jr, Graziani V, Little JW. The pattern of reflex recovery during spinal shock. Spinal Cord. 1999;37(6):402–9.

Chapter 4
Neurorehabilitation Testing, Metrics, and Procedures in Acquired Brain Injury

Gerald J. Nora

Introduction

After a brain injury, there are various testing methods and clinical scales used to assess neurological and traumatic pathology. In addition to physical exam skills, radiologic studies are a critical tool in managing and predicting outcomes for acquired brain injury (ABI), while neurophysiological and biomarker testing complement these studies. Medical and surgical specialists use various clinical grading instruments to evaluate injury severity and recovery level. However, some tools simplify the details and sacrifice specificity. It is important for physiatrists to understand these limitations in clinical grading instruments when discussing outcomes and goals with patients' families and other disciplines. Although serum biomarkers are being researched, most are still in the early stages of development. As an acute care physiatry consultant, it is crucial to be familiar with these modalities and how they can work together to provide a comprehensive understanding. This information can help guide expectations for patients and the primary medical or surgical team while following the hospital course.

G. J. Nora (✉)
Medrina, Chicago, IL, USA

Department of Physical Medicine and Rehabilitation, Medical College of Wisconsin, Milwaukee, WI, USA
e-mail: jerry.nora@medrina.com

A. K. Wagner, J. Weppner (eds.), *Acute Care Neuroconsultation and Neurorehabilitation Management*, https://doi.org/10.1007/978-3-031-42830-2_4

Radiologic Testing and Prognostication

Computed Tomography in Stroke

The speed and availability of computed tomography (CT) imaging means that it is often the first radiological test used in evaluating a neurological patient. Neuroimaging is crucial to many ABI protocols. For example, the head CT is the sine qua non for stroke patients, allowing physicians to distinguish between ischemic and hemorrhagic strokes, as well as their extent of insult. For an ischemic infarction with no sign of hemorrhagic conversion, the patient may be evaluated for thrombolysis therapy. CT perfusion studies are newer methods to assess any ischemic penumbra, which may be salvaged by intraarterial therapy (Fig. 4.1) [2]. If a CT scan of the head detects blood, it can be the result of a bleed into an ischemic stroke (hemorrhagic conversion) or a primary bleed. A CT angiogram (CTA) may be used at that time to help gauge the likelihood of hematoma expansion or the presence of an aneurysm [3]. In the case of a subarachnoid hemorrhage, bleeding in the corpus callosum is associated with a 50-fold relative risk of poor outcome [4].

CT in Anoxic Brain Injury

In anoxic brain injury, a CT scan can quantify lack of differentiation between gray and white matter, which reflects cytotoxic edema (Fig. 4.2). For example, the cutoff for the gray-white-matter ratio (GWR) can vary from 1.2 to 1.5, below which suggests a "poor outcome" where the patient requires assistance for activities of daily living (ADLs) and mobility, in studies measuring outcomes at either discharge from the ICU [6, 7] or 6 months post-injury [7]. Caution should be applied regarding CT

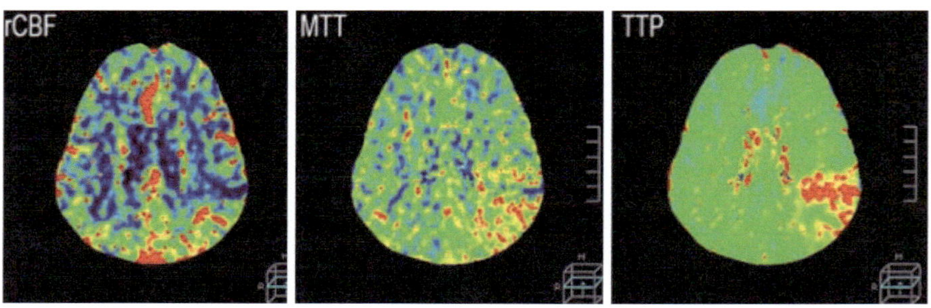

Fig. 4.1 CT Perfusion study showing regional cerebral blood flow (rCBF), mean transit time (MTT), and time to peak (TTP). The reduced CBF, and increased MTT and TTP indicated ischemia in the left middle carotid artery (MCA) territory [1]

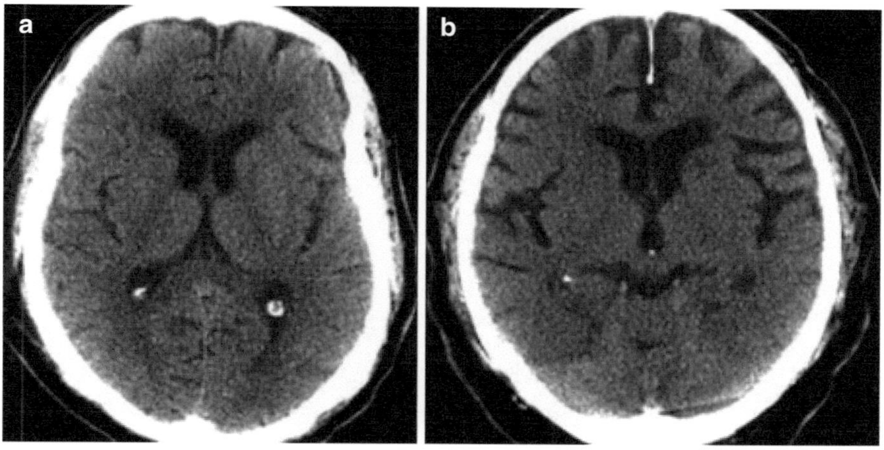

Fig. 4.2 CT scans of a normal (**a**) and post-arrest (**b**) brain. The gray-white differentiation appreciated in the normal brain has been largely eliminated by post-hypoxic edema in (**b**) [5]

scans obtained within 24 h of injury, especially among patients placed under a hypothermia protocol [7], due to potential alterations in blood flow and perfusion caused by the hypothermia protocol. The dynamic nature of brain injuries during this critical timeframe can lead to evolving physiological changes that may impact the accuracy of CT scan findings. Additionally, the cumulative radiation exposure from multiple scans must be carefully considered, balancing the benefits of imaging against the potential risks to the patient.

CT in Traumatic Brain Injury (TBI)

While imaging may guide surgical decisions, long-term prognostication on the broad spectrum of traumatic findings is difficult. Subsequent scans can be used to track evolution of hematomas, hygromas, pneumocephalus, and hydrocephalus—so the consulting physician should have a low threshold to request a new scan if a patient has an unexpected decline. There is active ongoing research to create systematic classifications for radiologic findings of TBI, using the presence of bleeding, volume of blood, and other characteristics (e.g., hydrocephalus or midline shift) and correlate these with outcome [8]. There is some indication that this grading correlates both with Glasgow Coma Score (GCS) on arrival and also with significantly lower Extended Glasgow Outcome Scale (GOSE) score with more severe radiological grades, albeit in a single trauma center, so further validation is necessary [9].

Magnetic Resonance Imaging

Magnetic resonance imaging (MRI) uses magnetic fields and electromagnetic pulses to map soft tissues in the body, typically water and fat. In newer devices with stronger magnets this provides a much finer-grained image of the anatomy and physiology of a patient's brain, albeit at the cost of increased time to obtain the imaging and requires the patient to hold still.

MRI in Stroke

An MRI may be useful when a patient has no clear stroke on a CT scan of the head, one reason being that it can better differentiate whether there is evidence of older subacute or chronic strokes. MRI is also more sensitive with the detection of hemorrhagic conversion of an ischemic stroke [10], which may guide the initiation of deep venous thrombus (DVT) chemical prophylaxis and/or anticoagulation. For non-aneurysmal hemorrhagic strokes, patients may require a follow-up MRI—with and without contrast—once the blood has reabsorbed to rule out the presence of a neoplasm.

MRI in ABI

In anoxic injuries, MRI can detect cytotoxic edema in more specific regions of the brain and can reveal heterogeneities in structures affected by the injury. Using the apparent diffusion coefficient (ADC) and diffusion weighted imaging (DWI), perfusion abnormalities can be tracked with the former and cellular injury with the latter [11]. Depressed ADC levels are associated with reduced probability of eye opening at 1 week after return of spontaneous circulation (ROSC) and long-term severe disability, with "severe" meaning requiring help for self-cares and mobility [12]. Though it can improve outcomes, hypothermia can confound the use of MRI, as ADC may be lowered by hypothermia, making the injury look artificially worse—at least 36 h should elapse after rewarming to avoid this hypothermia artifact [13].

Additionally, MRI has demonstrated value in detecting small bleeds that are not visible in CT. MRI is of particular interest for detecting diffuse axonal injury (DAI)—damage to the axonal tracts in white matter—that is likely due to rotational shearing associated with TBI. Grading with respect to DAI corresponds with location of shearing: grade I is cortical, grade II extends into the corpus callosum, and grade III in the brain stem [14]. While higher grades of DAI are associated with increased risk of poor outcome [15, 16], a "good" outcome was still found in 37% of grade III cases in one systematic review [15].

Transcranial Doppler Ultrasound

While originally used to monitor post-procedural cerebral blood flow in aneurysm patients, clinicians are beginning to apply transcranial doppler (TCD) ultrasound elsewhere. Ultrasound (US) is a bedside procedure that does not use radiation and quantifies perfusion in the anterior circulatory system of the brain—e.g., the internal carotid and anterior cerebral arteries (ACA) and middle cerebral arteries (MCA) [17]. A recent study found an association of increased "pulsatility" of the MCA, which is associated with arterial stenosis and cerebral blood flow autoregulation, as a predictor of poorer outcomes in ischemic stroke patients [18]. TCD may better direct blood pressure management in stroke patients; TCD-managed patients were found to have a higher percentage of good outcome at 90 days post-stroke than patients with traditional blood pressure management [19]. New applications, which are still in varying degrees of validation, include bedside monitoring of intracranial pressure (ICP) in brain injury [20], as well as detection and monitoring of intracranial hemorrhage and midline shift [17]. Given the complexities of obtaining TCD data, it is important to monitor trends over time rather than relying on one snapshot of the patient's circulation [17].

Bedside Evaluation of Stroke Patients

In stroke care, there are standard bedside evaluations to judge the severity of illness and function of the patient in the earliest phases of medical care.

National Institutes of Health Stroke Scale

The best-known grading system for ischemic stroke is the NIHSS (Table 4.1), which is graded from 0 (asymptomatic) to 42 (severe stroke), measuring the patient's level of consciousness, verbal responses, command following, and language, motor, and sensory symptoms [22]. A score >10 is a common criterion for intraarterial thrombectomy [23]; score <8 is associated with favorable functional outcomes with no or minimal deficits [24, 25]; and a score of ≥14 is associated with an increased likelihood of institutionalization [26].

The NIHSS is not without its drawbacks; acknowledged pitfalls include the relative weighting of cortical stroke symptoms versus the brainstem, and divergent outcomes have been observed among stroke patients with identical scores. For instance, right hemiparesis, dysarthria, and facial droop can produce an identical NIHSS value as a patient with all the same features except aphasia instead of facial droop. The latter, however, was found to have a higher mortality in a subgroup analysis [27]. Looks can also be deceiving with "mild" strokes. Sixty-five percent of patients

Table 4.1 NIH stroke scale (Public domain [21])

NIH STROKE SCALE

Patient Identification. ___ ___-___ ___ ___-___ ___ ___

Pt. Date of Birth ___ ___/___ ___/___ ___

Hospital ____________________(___ ___-___ ___)

Date of Exam ___ ___/___ ___/___ ___

Interval: [ ] Baseline [ ] 2 hours post treatment [ ] 24 hours post onset of symptoms ±20 minutes [ ] 7-10 days [ ] 3 months [ ] Other ____________________(___ ___)

Time: ___ ___:___ ___ [ ]am [ ]pm

Person Administering Scale ____________________

Administer stroke scale items in the order listed. Record performance in each category after each subscale exam. Do not go back and change scores. Follow directions provided for each exam technique. Scores should reflect what the patient does, not what the clinician thinks the patient can do. The clinician should record answers while administering the exam and work quickly. Except where indicated, the patient should not be coached (i.e., repeated requests to patient to make a special effort).

Instructions	Scale Definition	Score
1a. Level of Consciousness: The investigator must choose a response if a full evaluation is prevented by such obstacles as an endotracheal tube, language barrier, orotracheal trauma/bandages. A 3 is scored only if the patient makes no movement (other than reflexive posturing) in response to noxious stimulation.	0 = **Alert;** keenly responsive. 1 = **Not alert**; but arousable by minor stimulation to obey, answer, or respond. 2 = **Not alert**; requires repeated stimulation to attend, or is obtunded and requires strong or painful stimulation to make movements (not stereotyped). 3 = Responds only with reflex motor or autonomic effects or totally unresponsive, flaccid, and areflexic.	____
1b. LOC Questions: The patient is asked the month and his/her age. The answer must be correct - there is no partial credit for being close. Aphasic and stuporous patients who do not comprehend the questions will score 2. Patients unable to speak because of endotracheal intubation, orotracheal trauma, severe dysarthria from any cause, language barrier, or any other problem not secondary to aphasia are given a 1. It is important that only the initial answer be graded and that the examiner not "help" the patient with verbal or non-verbal cues.	0 = **Answers** both questions correctly. 1 = **Answers** one question correctly. 2 = **Answers** neither question correctly.	____
1c. LOC Commands: The patient is asked to open and close the eyes and then to grip and release the non-paretic hand. Substitute another one step command if the hands cannot be used. Credit is given if an unequivocal attempt is made but not completed due to weakness. If the patient does not respond to command, the task should be demonstrated to him or her (pantomime), and the result scored (i.e., follows none, one or two commands). Patients with trauma, amputation, or other physical impediments should be given suitable one-step commands. Only the first attempt is scored.	0 = **Performs** both tasks correctly. 1 = **Performs** one task correctly. 2 = **Performs** neither task correctly.	____
2. Best Gaze: Only horizontal eye movements will be tested. Voluntary or reflexive (oculocephalic) eye movements will be scored, but caloric testing is not done. If the patient has a conjugate deviation of the eyes that can be overcome by voluntary or reflexive activity, the score will be 1. If a patient has an isolated peripheral nerve paresis (CN III, IV or VI), score a 1. Gaze is testable in all aphasic patients. Patients with ocular trauma, bandages, pre-existing blindness, or other disorder of visual acuity or fields should be tested with reflexive movements, and a choice made by the investigator. Establishing eye contact and then moving about the patient from side to side will occasionally clarify the presence of a partial gaze palsy.	0 = **Normal.** 1 = **Partial gaze palsy;** gaze is abnormal in one or both eyes, but forced deviation or total gaze paresis is not present. 2 = **Forced deviation,** or total gaze paresis not overcome by the oculocephalic maneuver.	____

Rev 10/1/2003

Table 4.1 (continued)

NIH STROKE SCALE

Patient Identification. __ __-__ __ __-__ __ __

Pt. Date of Birth __ __/__ __/__ __

Hospital ____________________(__ __-__ __)

Date of Exam __ __/__ __/__ __

Interval: [ ] Baseline [ ] 2 hours post treatment [ ] 24 hours post onset of symptoms ±20 minutes [ ] 7-10 days
[ ] 3 months [ ] Other ____________________(__ __)

3. Visual: Visual fields (upper and lower quadrants) are tested by confrontation, using finger counting or visual threat, as appropriate. Patients may be encouraged, but if they look at the side of the moving fingers appropriately, this can be scored as normal. If there is unilateral blindness or enucleation, visual fields in the remaining eye are scored. Score 1 only if a clear-cut asymmetry, including quadrantanopia, is found. If patient is blind from any cause, score 3. Double simultaneous stimulation is performed at this point. If there is extinction, patient receives a 1, and the results are used to respond to item 11.	0 = **No visual loss.** 1 = **Partial hemianopia.** 2 = **Complete hemianopia.** 3 = **Bilateral hemianopia** (blind including cortical blindness).	____
4. Facial Palsy: Ask – or use pantomime to encourage – the patient to show teeth or raise eyebrows and close eyes. Score symmetry of grimace in response to noxious stimuli in the poorly responsive or non-comprehending patient. If facial trauma/bandages, orotracheal tube, tape or other physical barriers obscure the face, these should be removed to the extent possible.	0 = **Normal** symmetrical movements. 1 = **Minor paralysis** (flattened nasolabial fold, asymmetry on smiling). 2 = **Partial paralysis** (total or near-total paralysis of lower face). 3 = **Complete paralysis** of one or both sides (absence of facial movement in the upper and lower face).	____
5. Motor Arm: The limb is placed in the appropriate position: extend the arms (palms down) 90 degrees (if sitting) or 45 degrees (if supine). Drift is scored if the arm falls before 10 seconds. The aphasic patient is encouraged using urgency in the voice and pantomime, but not noxious stimulation. Each limb is tested in turn, beginning with the non-paretic arm. Only in the case of amputation or joint fusion at the shoulder, the examiner should record the score as untestable (UN), and clearly write the explanation for this choice.	0 = **No drift;** limb holds 90 (or 45) degrees for full 10 seconds. 1 = **Drift;** limb holds 90 (or 45) degrees, but drifts down before full 10 seconds; does not hit bed or other support. 2 = **Some effort against gravity;** limb cannot get to or maintain (if cued) 90 (or 45) degrees, drifts down to bed, but has some effort against gravity. 3 = **No effort against gravity;** limb falls. 4 = **No movement.** UN = **Amputation** or joint fusion, explain: ____________ **5a. Left Arm** **5b. Right Arm**	 ____ ____
6. Motor Leg: The limb is placed in the appropriate position: hold the leg at 30 degrees (always tested supine). Drift is scored if the leg falls before 5 seconds. The aphasic patient is encouraged using urgency in the voice and pantomime, but not noxious stimulation. Each limb is tested in turn, beginning with the non-paretic leg. Only in the case of amputation or joint fusion at the hip, the examiner should record the score as untestable (UN), and clearly write the explanation for this choice.	0 = **No drift;** leg holds 30-degree position for full 5 seconds. 1 = **Drift;** leg falls by the end of the 5-second period but does not hit bed. 2 = **Some effort against gravity;** leg falls to bed by 5 seconds, but has some effort against gravity. 3 = **No effort against gravity;** leg falls to bed immediately. 4 = **No movement.** UN = **Amputation** or joint fusion, explain: ____________ **6a. Left Leg** **6b. Right Leg**	 ____

Rev 10/1/2003

Table 4.1 (continued)

NIH STROKE SCALE

Patient Identification. ___ ___-___ ___ ___-___ ___ ___

Pt. Date of Birth ___ ___/___ ___/___ ___

Hospital ____________________(___ ___-___ ___)

Date of Exam ___ ___/___ ___/___ ___

Interval: [ ] Baseline [ ] 2 hours post treatment [ ] 24 hours post onset of symptoms ±20 minutes [ ] 7-10 days
[ ] 3 months [ ] Other ____________________(___ ___)

7. Limb Ataxia: This item is aimed at finding evidence of a unilateral cerebellar lesion. Test with eyes open. In case of visual defect, ensure testing is done in intact visual field. The finger-nose-finger and heel-shin tests are performed on both sides, and ataxia is scored only if present out of proportion to weakness. Ataxia is absent in the patient who cannot understand or is paralyzed. Only in the case of amputation or joint fusion, the examiner should record the score as untestable (UN), and clearly write the explanation for this choice. In case of blindness, test by having the patient touch nose from extended arm position.	0 = **Absent.** 1 = **Present in one limb.** 2 = **Present in two limbs.** UN = **Amputation** or joint fusion, explain: ________	____
8. Sensory: Sensation or grimace to pinprick when tested, or withdrawal from noxious stimulus in the obtunded or aphasic patient. Only sensory loss attributed to stroke is scored as abnormal and the examiner should test as many body areas (arms [not hands], legs, trunk, face) as needed to accurately check for hemisensory loss. A score of 2, "severe or total sensory loss," should only be given when a severe or total loss of sensation can be clearly demonstrated. Stuporous and aphasic patients will, therefore, probably score 1 or 0. The patient with brainstem stroke who has bilateral loss of sensation is scored 2. If the patient does not respond and is quadriplegic, score 2. Patients in a coma (item 1a=3) are automatically given a 2 on this item.	0 = **Normal;** no sensory loss. 1 = **Mild-to-moderate sensory loss;** patient feels pinprick is less sharp or is dull on the affected side; or there is a loss of superficial pain with pinprick, but patient is aware of being touched. 2 = **Severe to total sensory loss;** patient is not aware of being touched in the face, arm, and leg.	____
9. Best Language: A great deal of information about comprehension will be obtained during the preceding sections of the examination. For this scale item, the patient is asked to describe what is happening in the attached picture, to name the items on the attached naming sheet and to read from the attached list of sentences. Comprehension is judged from responses here, as well as to all of the commands in the preceding general neurological exam. If visual loss interferes with the tests, ask the patient to identify objects placed in the hand, repeat, and produce speech. The intubated patient should be asked to write. The patient in a coma (item 1a=3) will automatically score 3 on this item. The examiner must choose a score for the patient with stupor or limited cooperation, but a score of 3 should be used only if the patient is mute and follows no one-step commands.	0 = **No aphasia;** normal. 1 = **Mild-to-moderate aphasia;** some obvious loss of fluency or facility of comprehension, without significant limitation on ideas expressed or form of expression. Reduction of speech and/or comprehension, however, makes conversation about provided materials difficult or impossible. For example, in conversation about provided materials, examiner can identify picture or naming card content from patient's response. 2 = **Severe aphasia;** all communication is through fragmentary expression; great need for inference, questioning, and guessing by the listener. Range of information that can be exchanged is limited; listener carries burden of communication. Examiner cannot identify materials provided from patient response. 3 = **Mute, global aphasia;** no usable speech or auditory comprehension.	____
10. Dysarthria: If patient is thought to be normal, an adequate sample of speech must be obtained by asking patient to read or repeat words from the attached list. If the patient has severe aphasia, the clarity of articulation of spontaneous speech can be rated. Only if the patient is intubated or has other physical barriers to producing speech, the examiner should record the score as untestable (UN), and clearly write an explanation for this choice. Do not tell the patient why he or she is being tested.	0 = **Normal.** 1 = **Mild-to-moderate dysarthria;** patient slurs at least some words and, at worst, can be understood with some difficulty. 2 = **Severe dysarthria;** patient's speech is so slurred as to be unintelligible in the absence of or out of proportion to any dysphasia, or is mute/anarthric. UN = **Intubated** or other physical barrier, explain:____________	____

Rev 10/1/2003

Table 4.1 (continued)

N I H
STROKE
SCALE

Patient Identification. ___ ___-___ ___ ___-___ ___ ___

Pt. Date of Birth ___ ___/___ ___/___ ___

Hospital ____________________(___ ___-___ ___)

Date of Exam ___ ___/___ ___/___ ___

Interval: [ ] Baseline [ ] 2 hours post treatment [ ] 24 hours post onset of symptoms ±20 minutes [ ] 7-10 days
[ ] 3 months [ ] Other ______________________________(___ ___)

11. Extinction and Inattention (formerly Neglect): Sufficient information to identify neglect may be obtained during the prior testing. If the patient has a severe visual loss preventing visual double simultaneous stimulation, and the cutaneous stimuli are normal, the score is normal. If the patient has aphasia but does appear to attend to both sides, the score is normal. The presence of visual spatial neglect or anosagnosia may also be taken as evidence of abnormality. Since the abnormality is scored only if present, the item is never untestable.	0 = **No abnormality.** 1 = **Visual, tactile, auditory, spatial, or personal inattention** or extinction to bilateral simultaneous stimulation in one of the sensory modalities. 2 = **Profound hemi-inattention or extinction to more than one modality;** does not recognize own hand or orients to only one side of space.	____

____

____

Rev 10/1/2003

Table 4.1 (continued)

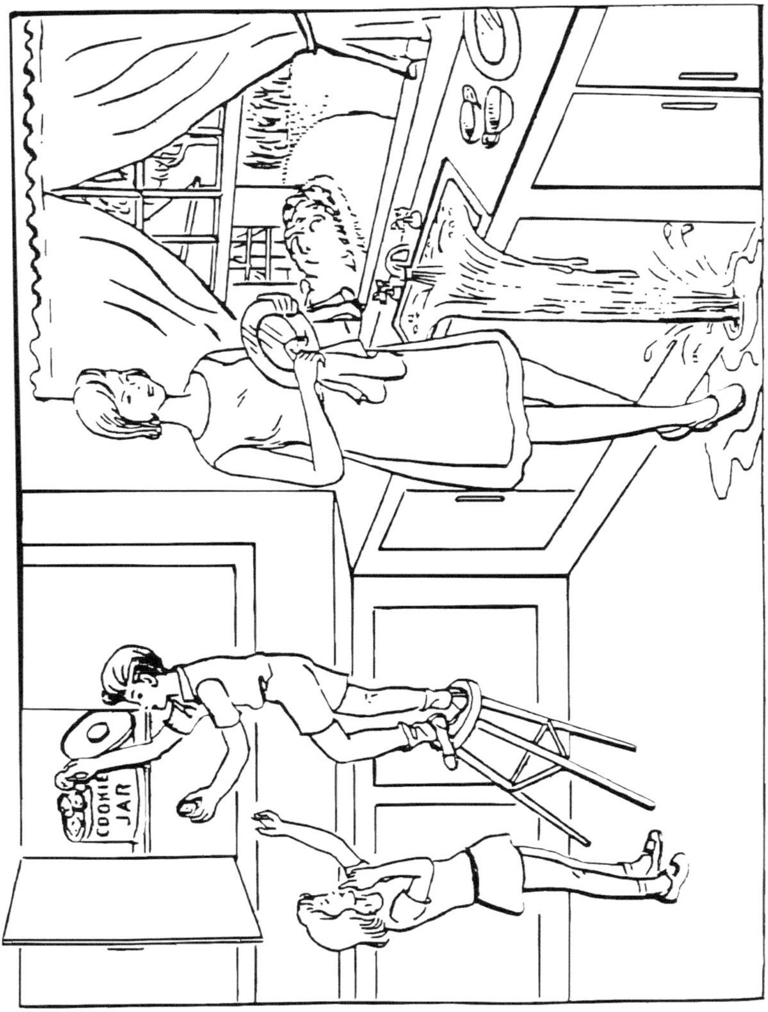

Table 4.1 (continued)

You know how.

Down to earth.

I got home from work.

Near the table in the dining room.

They heard him speak on the radio last night.

Table 4.1 (continued)

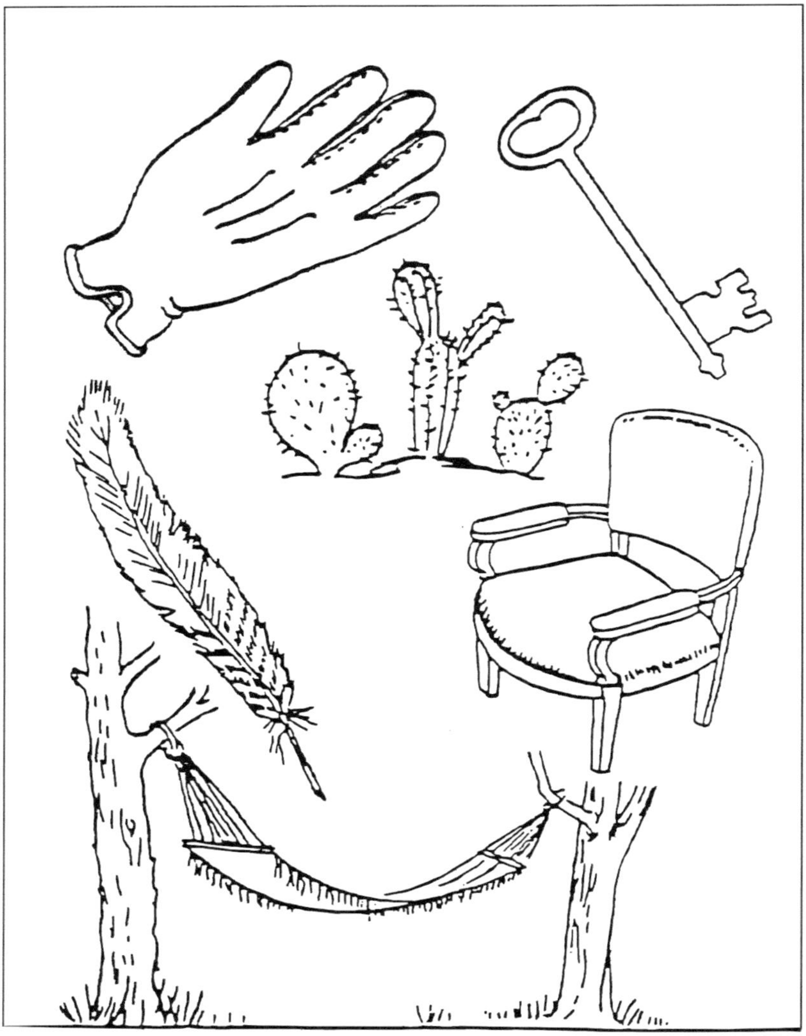

Table 4.1 (continued)

MAMA
TIP – TOP
FIFTY – FIFTY
THANKS
HUCKLEBERRY
BASEBALL PLAYER

with an NIHSS of <5 were discharged home without care, while those who failed to go home had deficits primarily in ambulation and swallowing [28]. A physiatrist can be an important advocate for patients with these deceptively minor symptoms: even if the patient does not proceed to inpatient rehabilitation, closer outpatient follow-up can be arranged in addition to other appropriate therapies.

Hunt and Hess Scale

The Hunt and Hess Scale (H-H) (Table 4.2), is used to stratify aneurysmal bleed on an ordinal scale from I (asymptomatic, mild headache, or nuchal rigidity) to V (coma, decerebrate posturing) [30]. If the patient has evidence of vasospasm or severe systemic comorbidity, the score is increased by one, though this scoring feature is not consistently applied [29]. A recent metanalysis found significant variability in the definition of a good outcome with H-H grading [31], and another meta-analysis of "poor grade" (H-H IV or V) showed a favorable outcome in 37% of pooled patients [32].

Table 4.2 Hunt and Hess scale [29] for grading subarachnoid hemorrhage

Grade
I. Asymptomatic and minimal headache or nuchal rigidity
II. Moderate–severe headache or nuchal rigidity and CN palsy
III. Drowsy, confused, or mild focal deficit
IV. Stupor, moderate–severe hemiparesis, possible decerebrate rigidity
V. Deep coma, decerebrate rigidity, "moribund appearance"

CN cranial nerve

Functional Grading in Neurological Patients

The following evaluations are used to track outcomes in neurological patients, traumatic or nontraumatic. Their scales are presented in parallel in Table 4.3 to help the reader compare their similarities and limitations.

Modified Rankin Score

The neurocritical care literature often measures post-acute outcomes with the modified Rankin Score (mRS) (Table 4.3), which quantifies function from 0 (asymptomatic) to 6 (dead). A moderately disabled person at a level of 3 is described as being able to walk but requiring some assistance, whereas a severely disabled person at an mRS of 5 is bedridden and incontinent, requiring constant care [34]. A person who is ambulatory but episodically incontinent does not readily fall into one category, which may be why the interrater reliability in the mRS is modest, particularly in larger studies [35]. In a study of geriatric stroke patients, higher pre-stroke mRS scores (i.e., higher baseline degree of disability) was predictive of post-stroke inpatient rehabilitation, while lower mRS (<2) was associated with discharge home [36].

The mRS has no clear predictive value for mortality prediction or even necessarily for post-hospital disposition, perhaps reflecting socioeconomic variability in obtaining assistive technology and services [37]. The mRS less sensitive is also functional gains in hemorrhagic stroke survivors in the year post-discharge, suggesting that it may present a more pessimistic picture than reality [38]. This limitation could reflect the relatively coarse-grained nature of the mRS scoring, the problems with inter-observer reliability, and the necessity of using a proxy (as opposed to the patient) for answering questions in the case of more severe disability [39].

Table 4.3 Glasgow outcome scale-extended and modified Rankin scale

Glasgow outcome scale extended [41]	Modified Rankin scale [46]
1. Dead	6. Dead
2. Vegetative state	5. Severe disability
No command following or simple speech.	*Bedridden, requiring constant nursing care*
3. Severe disability (lower)	4. Moderate severe disability
May not be left unattended in home.	*Needs help for walking and self-cares*
4. Severe disability (upper)	3. Moderate disability
May be alone at home up to 8 h	*Walks unaided; needs help with some care*
Require assistance in community	2. Slight disability
5. Moderate disability (lower)	*Not at baseline but able to care for self*
Sheltered employment; rare participation in previous community activities	1. No significant disability
	Has some symptoms but fully at baseline
6. Moderate disability (upper)	0. Asymptomatic
Limited employment	
7. Good recovery (lower)	
Full employment and independence with some symptoms	
8. Good recovery (upper)	
Asymptomatic	

Extended Glasgow Outcome Scale

The most common long-term functional grading scale in neurotrauma is the Extended Glasgow Outcome Scale (GOSE) (Table 4.4). The GOSE divides outcome as dead, vegetative, severe disability, moderate disability, and good recovery, with the latter three categories subdivided into upper and lower levels. The original GOS did not subdivide these categories [40]. The coarse nature of the instrument was meant to create an easy-to-use instrument for outcomes in research, though standardizing the interview used to gather the data for the GOSE grading help the inter-user reliability [41]. Research suggests that the correlation between post-traumatic amnesia (PTA) and GOSE was stronger than that of PTA and GCS—with more than two-thirds of patients with PTA over 7 days (i.e., a severe TBI) having severe disability at 5 to 10 months post-injury [42]. The GOSE score can be converted to the original GOS, which in turn is comparable to the mRS. [43]

Table 4.3 Glasgow coma scale [33]

Eye opening
1. None
2. To pressure
3. To speech
4. Spontaneous
Verbal response
1. None
2. Sounds
3. Words
4. Confused
5. Oriented
Best motor response
1. None
2. Extension
3. Abnormal flexion
4. Withdrawal to pain
5. Localizing
6. Command following

Cerebral Performance Category

The Cerebral Performance Category (CPC) (Table 4.4) is a grading tool for cardiac arrest survivors, ranked on a scale from 1 (normal) to 5 (brain death). As can be seen in the table, it is the most coarse-grained of the three scales, and has been criticized for its relative inability to distinguish between mild and moderate disability [44] and poor correlation with subjective or objective measures of disability and quality of life [45]. The consulting physiatrist should also keep in mind that even well-characterized scales like the mRS are hardly infallible predictors of the future for patients. Attention could be called to the implicit "ableism" of calling the outcome where a patient needs help at home "poor," even though many such patients have rich and rewarding lives.

Grading Consciousness and Cognition

Grading consciousness began with the venerable Glasgow Coma Scale in neurotrauma and has expanded with other common instruments, including the Pittsburgh Cardiac Arrest Categories and the Coma Recovery Scale-Revised, the latter of which is used in both traumatic and anoxic brain injury. Grading consciousness and cognition in acute care is at least partially driven by the desire to prognosticate functional outcomes.

Glasgow Coma Scale

The most commonly used instrument for grading consciousness in TBI is the Glasgow Coma Scale (GCS), which grades verbal, motor, and ocular function on a numeric scale with higher score classified as mild and lower classified as severe (Table 4.3) [33]. While the GCS is readily administered, the same score can describe any number of brain injury patterns observed on imaging [47], and GCS score is poorly correlated with long-term outcomes [48]. Consideration should be given to confounding issues such as vision and hearing deficits, sedation, illicit drug or alcohol use at the time of injury, or end-organ dysfunction, each of which can affect neurologic scoring. Intubation status, and the use of paralytics with intubation can also confound neurologic scoring.

Coma Recovery Scale-Revised

In patients with disorders of consciousness (DoC), the Coma Recovery Scale Revised (CRS-R) (Table 4.5) is the standard measure for distinguishing between coma, unresponsive wakefulness (UWS, now the preferred term for "vegetative state"), and minimally conscious (MCS) [49]. Coma is a state of profound unconsciousness characterized by the absence of wakefulness, awareness, and purposeful responses to the environment. Patients in a coma do not exhibit voluntary movements, demonstrate signs of consciousness, or respond to external stimuli. It remains unclear if individuals in a coma can appreciate pain as suffering. The primary goals of care in a coma focus on stabilizing the patient, managing their medical condition, and identifying the underlying cause of the coma. UWS is characterized by preserved wakefulness without any signs of awareness or meaningful interactions with the environment. Although individuals in UWS may exhibit sleep-wake cycles and open their eyes, they do not demonstrate purposeful movements or respond to commands. The goals of care for patients in UWS typically involve providing supportive measures, optimizing comfort, and considering potential interventions for rehabilitation. In contrast, the minimally conscious state (MCS) represents a condition where individuals show some level of consciousness but with significantly impaired or inconsistent interactions. Patients in MCS may exhibit intermittent signs of purposeful behavior, such as following simple commands or demonstrating intentional movements. Although the degree of pain perception can vary in MCS, some individuals may demonstrate responses suggesting an awareness of pain as suffering. The goals of care in MCS often involve promoting rehabilitation, optimizing quality of life, and addressing specific needs based on the individual's level

Table 4.5 The coma recovery scale [49]

Auditory	
Consistent movement to command	4
Reproducible movement to command	3
Localization to sound	2
Auditory startle	1
No response	0
Visual function scale	
Object recognition	5
Object localization: Reaching	4
Visual pursuit	3
Visual fixation	2
Visual startle	1
None	0
Motor function scale	
Functional object use	6
Automatic motor response	5
Object manipulation	4
Localization to noxious stimulation	3
Flexion withdrawal	2
Abnormal posturing	1
None/flaccid	0
Oral and verbal function	
Intelligible verbalization	3
Vocalization/oral movement	2
Oral reflexive movement	1
Nothing	0
Communication scale	
Oriented	3
Functional: Accurate	2
Non-functional: Intentional	1
None	0
Arousal scale	
Attention	3
Eyes open without stimulation	2
Eyes open with stimulation	1
Unarousable	0

of responsiveness. Prognostication in these states is a complex task that requires the evaluation of multiple factors by a multidisciplinary team of healthcare professionals. Emergence from a coma or transitioning from UWS to MCS is generally associated with a more favorable prognosis regarding potential recovery of consciousness and functional abilities.

The CRS-R is notable for its use in both acute care and rehabilitation settings. Scores range from 0 to 23, with a score of ≥12 associated with higher chance of emergence from minimally conscious state [50]. CRS-R scores can fluctuate—in one instance, 30% of patients listed as UWS scored as minimally conscious at least once [51], further evidence that there remains a high rate of misdiagnosis (primarily erring in the direction of a *lower* level of consciousness) in DoC [52]. When evaluating patients with DoC, it is crucial to consider and explore confounding factors that may influence the assessment. Two common confounders in the cardiac arrest population are visual and auditory sensory deficits, which are relatively common following cardiac arrest. These deficits can affect the patient's ability to perceive and respond to external stimuli, potentially masking their true level of consciousness. Another important confounding factor to consider in DoC patients is the presence of aphasia and apraxia, particularly in cases where there is a concurrent burden of stroke. Aphasia can make it challenging for patients to understand or express themselves verbally, while apraxia impairs the ability to execute purposeful movements. Both conditions can significantly impact communication and motor responses, making it difficult to accurately assess a patient's level of consciousness solely based on verbal or motor commands. Recognizing the potential confounding effects of visual and auditory sensory deficits, as well as aphasia and apraxia, is essential for obtaining a more accurate understanding of a patient's level of consciousness in DoC cases. Central nervous system (e.g. concurrent focal lesion) and peripheral nervous system (e.g. critical illness neuromyopathy) can also confound CRS-R exam findings.

In the acute care hospital setting, consulting physiatrists are often called upon to evaluate patients with DoC. Assessing the level of consciousness in these patients can be challenging, as it requires a standardized and objective approach that takes into account multiple aspects of the patient's condition. The CRS-R is a widely used tool for assessing the level of consciousness in DoC patients. It consists of subscales that assess motor, communication, visual, oromotor, auditory, and arousal responses, and provides a standardized and reliable assessment of the patient's level of consciousness. The use of the CRS-R by consulting physiatrists can aid in prognostication, inform treatment decisions, and provide valuable information to the patient's care team.

Despite the benefits of using the CRS-R, the time required to administer the scale and the complexity of its subscales can be a challenge for busy clinicians. Reorganizing the subscales, with prioritizing the motor and communication first and stopping once the patient meets criteria for emergence or MCS, may streamline the assessment process [53]. This approach can allow consulting physiatrists to provide efficient and accurate prognostic guidance for patients with DoC, while also reducing the burden on busy clinical teams. However, it is important to note that this approach should not replace the use of the full CRS-R, which provides important information about the patient's level of recovery and can be used to track progress over time. The Coma Recovery Scale-Revised for Accelerated Standardized Assessment (CRSR-FAST) has been recently validated for expedited evaluation of patients with Disorders of Consciousness (DoC). If successful, it could become a valuable tool for acute care [54].

Pittsburgh Cardiac Arrest Category

Specific to ABI, the Pittsburgh Cardiac Arrest Category (PCAC) (Table 4.6) is intended to prognosticate survival and functional outcome at time of discharge from acute hospitalization. The scale was validated on patients within 6 h of ROSC, before any sedation or hypothermia was used [58] and is scored I (awake) to IV (coma with at least 1 absent brainstem reflex). Each PCAC is made up of two additional measurement components: the Four Motor Response (FMR) and Four Brainstem Reflexes (FBR), each of which is graded 0–4 with a higher score corresponding with greater response. Additionally, categories II and III include grading on the Serial Organ Function Assessment (SOFA) [57], which measures any cardiopulmonary end-organ disfunction [55, 59]. PCAC I corresponded with mRS scores of 0–3 and 60% of patients had good outcomes; patients in PCAC IV had only 14% survival rate [55].

These grading systems addressing DoC only assign probabilities, not certainties, and the timing of outcome determination is also very important. Rather than use a 6 month (or less) outcome as dogmatic, one must remember that delayed recovery from DoC even 1-year post-injury is documented [60]. For example, in a longitudinal study of traumatic DoC patients, of 67 patients who did not recover consciousness in inpatient rehabilitation, 66% had become conscious by the 2-year mark; and of the whole cohort, about 20% were able to live unsupervised and/or be eligible for some form of employment [61]. For these reasons, the joint guidelines published by

Table 4.6 The Pittsburgh cardiac arrest categories [55] a focused neurologic exam from the FOUR scoring system [56] plus cardiorespiratory function as defined by the SOFA [57]

Pittsburgh cardiac arrest categories	FOUR motor response (FMR)
I. Awake (FMR + FBR = 8)	4—thumbs up, fist, or peace sign
II. Coma (FMR + FBR = 4–7)	3—localizing to pain
PLUS	2—flexor response to pain
Mild cardiac dysfunction	1—extensor response to pain
(SOFA cardiac + respiratory <4)	0—no response to pain or general myoclonus
III. Coma (as above)	*FOUR brainstem reflexes (FBR)*
PLUS	4—pupil and corneal reflexes present
Moderate-to-severe cardiac dysfunction (SOFA cardiac + respiratory ≥ 4)	3—one pupil wide and fixed
IV. Coma with at least one absent brainstem reflex (FMR + FBR < 4)	2—pupil or corneal reflexes absent
	1—pupil and corneal reflexes absent
	0—absent pupil, corneal, and cough reflexes

the American Academy of Neurologists and American Congress of Rehabilitation Medicine do not recommend making a negative long-term prognostication in the first 4 weeks post-injury [62].

Neurophysiology

The role of electroencephalography in brain injury is twofold: primarily, it is used to detect seizures, especially subclinical seizures that may elude clinical evaluation. Secondly, it can be an adjunct for assessing consciousness and prognosticating a patient's course.

Electroencephalography and Brain Injury Management

Individuals with moderate-to-severe TBI have a high seizure incidence. Within 24 h of injury, 8.9% of patients with moderate-to-severe TBI have "immediate" seizures. While conventional wisdom says these acute seizures have no bearing on future seizures, more recent research found that immediate seizures are a risk factor for late (±7 days post-TBI) seizures, which have a cumulative incidence of 11.9 to 20.5% at 1 and 5 years post-injury, respectively [63]. A person with TBI and poor arousal may benefit from EEG, as non-convulsive status epileptics has been associated with hippocampal injury ipsilateral to the source of the seizure in a small case series, suggesting that faster treatment leads to better outcomes [64].

EEGs are also integral to post-cardiac arrest care. Therapeutic hypothermia protocols typically involve the use of electroencephalograms (EEGs), ideally continuous (cEEG) , for the initial 24 h post-ROSC, as status epilepticus (SE) is not uncommon and is reported to occur in 12% of patients with cardiac arrest [58].

Electroencephalography and Prognostication

In addition to detecting, EEG can be used to help assess consciousness and prognosticate in critically ill, unresponsive patients. Continuous EEG (cEEG) in particular has value in identifying "spindles," which are patterns of neuronal firing associated with sleep. This preservation of a sleep architecture suggests at least some preservation of the reticular activating system and thalamocortical pathways involved in arousal. The presence of sleep architecture may suggest the presence of sleep-wake cycles and that the patient is, strictly speaking, no longer comatose [65]. In both traumatic and nontraumatic brain injury, sleep spindles are associated with improved mortality and functional outcomes (in terms of mRS) at 6 months [66].

Prognostication after cardiac arrest (CA) is an active area of research since 87% of patients with ROSC are comatose in the emergency department (ED), and of the one third that survive hospitalization, ~19% have significant disabilities [15]. While associated with both survival and good neurological outcomes, therapeutic hypothermia for CA patients following ROSC makes prognostication difficult when interpreting electroencephalograms (EEGs) results. The "malignant" EEG findings were largely observed during hypothermia or rewarming. Adequate warming and time to metabolize sedating medications must be employed, along with additional modalities like the clinical examination, MRI, and somatosensory electrical potentials (SSEPs), to obtain the most accurate prognostication [67, 68].

Electric Potentials in Brain Injury

Electrophysiologists may stimulate peripheral somatic nerves or auditory nerves and see if the stimulus evokes a corresponding reaction in the cortex. This can be used to assess cortical function in an unconscious BI patient.

Somatosensory Electric Potentials

When obtaining somatosensory electric potentials (SSEPs), the distal median and/or tibial nerves are stimulated to detect any corresponding neuronal firing in the sensory cortex—lack of such a response signifies cortical dysfunction. In TBI, the presence of SSEPs in the first week of hospitalization was associated with improved cognitive scoring [69], but the number of excluded patients due to peripheral nerve or spinal cord injury is a caution on the use of this modality in the setting of trauma. Among older individuals with TBI, peripheral neuropathy can also confound SSEP results.

Lack of intact SSEPs after a cardiac arrest are associated with a poor prognosis according to a recent meta-analysis, a poor prognosis being death, lack of emergence from DoC or a high degree of dependency for self-care (mRS 4–6 or CPC 3–5), typically at times ranging from discharge from the acute care hospital until about 6 months post-arrest [70]. However, a retrospective case series showed that many "poor-quality" SSEPs were done before the patients had fully rewarmed from therapeutic hypothermia (which can confound the exam by reducing blood flow and potentially affecting the transmission of sensory signals from the periphery to the brain), and of the 11 patients with bilaterally absent SSEPs who died, 7 were from the withdrawal of life sustaining therapy, raising the specter of self-fulfilling prophecy [71]. Moreover, there is a case series of 28 patients with bilateral loss of cortical responses, wherein half of patients later demonstrated recovery of cortical responses after a mean period of about 2 months. These findings corresponded with functional improvements in about half of those with return of SSEP—the recovery, however, recovery was seen primarily in patients with traumatic brain injury [72].

Brainstem Auditory Evoked Potentials

A clicking sound maybe used to induce electrical responses in the brainstem for brainstem auditory evoked potentials (BAEPs). In a review of prognostic modalities, loss of BAEPs is very specific but not sensitive for a poor outcome in post-arrest patients [73]. There is limited evidence that the BAEP may be more useful in traumatic patients [74], but any use of BAEPs must first rule out confounding hearing damage (e.g., from a blast injury or auditory nerve injury after TBI, or somatosensory neuronal ischemia associated with cardiac arrest).

A refinement of the BAEP tracks a cortical response to an unexpected sound within a train of repetitive noises, which is called the mismatch negativity (MMN) [75]. The MMN was found in 7/7 of patients who emerged from coma; 2/10 of those who had no MMN had also emerged. Monitoring the cortical response to patients' hearing their own names being called is another emerging method to find "covert consciousness" in DoC patients [73].

Biomarkers

Serum biomarkers—typically central nervous system (CNS) associated proteins, but also systemic biomarkers like inflammatory markers and also genetic polymorphisms—have attracted attention for detection of injury (such as predicted prolonged symptoms associated mild TBI AKA post-concussive syndrome) or for prognostication and long-term function in moderate-to-severe TBI.

Biomarkers in TBI

For mild TBI (mTBI), the glial fibrillary acidic protein (GFAP) and ubiquitin carboxyl terminal hydroxylase-1 (UCH-L1) proteins have been approved by the FDA to evaluate concussion patients who are increased risk of having an abnormal CT scan [76]. A Scandinavian TBI protocol had previously integrated serum S100B biomarkers to predict the need for CT imaging [77], but the better performance of GFAP for predicting CT abnormalities [78] plus the availability of point of care testing (albeit for serum only at present, not whole blood) for GFAP/UCH-L1 may lead to the latter's greater acceptance. Again, while both biomarkers have good sensitivity and specificity for abnormal CT findings, they are not reliable predictors of impaired functional status 3 months post-TBI as measured by the GOSE [79]. A pediatric study assessing GFAP and UCH-L1 found that neither correlated with Post Concussion Symptom Scale (PCSS), which is far more sensitive to mTBI symptoms than the GOSE [80].

Biomarkers in ABI

Similar to what has been observed in concussion patients, serum GFAP, neuron-specific enolase (NSE), or neurofilament light (NFL), below cutoffs are associated with no evidence of edema on imaging in 77.3–91.7% of unconscious CA patients participating in a hypothermia protocol [81]. Another study, focused on function, found that the combination of GFAP and UCH-L1 were superior to NSE when predicting poor outcome (CPC 3–5) 6 months post-arrest for unconscious CA patients who had received hypothermia [82]. The results did not vary much for blood drawn 24 to 72 h post-arrest, though baseline serum concentrations were altered by the precise temperature used during the protocol, which could be anticipated and corrected in an institutional CA protocol.

Rehabilomics

The use of biomarkers to assess rehabilitation prognosis, and link biology to function, is in its infancy and works to incorporate serum biomarkers and patients' genetic information to assess their potential risks for complications or responses to particular therapies. This personalized medicine approach to rehabilitation has been dubbed "Rehabilomics." [83] One example is the development of an inflammatory load score to inform global outcomes [84] and cognitive deficits [85] after moderate-to-severe TBI. Importantly, this study demonstrated how cognitive deficit associated with inflammatory burden are in the causal pathway linking inflammation to cognition focused activities of daily living and quality of life. Another example are genetic studies analyzing polymorphisms to assess risk for post-traumatic epilepsy (PTE) in patients with TBI [86–91]. While these findings are still very early, they point to an exciting future of using individual genomes to prognosticate and direct therapy.

Case Study

A previously healthy 23-year-old woman was transferred to a regional burn center 4 days after she sustained severe TBI, polytrauma, and 34% total body surface area burns to the face, chest, and extremities in a motor vehicle accident. She had been intubated in the field and transferred to the Level 1 trauma center where she was reported as a GCS 3T. While at the trauma center there was a report of Grade III DAI and thalamic bleed on MRI, and there was concern for a poor neurologic prognosis.

While in the burn unit, she underwent a tracheostomy and PEG placement in addition to multiple debridement procedures and split thickness skin grafts. Dialysis was required temporarily as well. Remarkably, at the end of the second month of hospitalization her mentation was clear enough that the surgeon was able to discuss her injuries, and she was transferred to inpatient rehabilitation 2 weeks later. After 3 weeks of inpatient rehabilitation, she was transferred to a long-term rehabilitation facility due to persistent wound care needs and lack of a wheelchair-accessible home. Her neurological exam showed no focal findings, and her cognition was deemed to be at baseline.

This was a striking example of the pitfalls of attempting to predict a patient's future based on an initial brain scan while still critically ill. Neurological testing, from the GCS at admission onward, was heavily confounded by the need for sedation and intubation. Despite severe burns and multiple organ dysfunction on top of a forboding radiological study, her functional outcome proved excellent, limited more by amputations and burns than the TBI.

Summary

Prognostication tools, while validated in some cases, have course-grained outcomes. The consulting physiatrist must consider the use of a combination of physical exam and clinical as well as radiographic and neurophysiological tools to construct a nuanced picture regarding outcomes. The care team must be prepared to include the patient and caregiver(s) in outcome planning when possible. The consulting physiatrist must be aware of the strengths and weaknesses of these tests and instruments to guide the expectations of the patients, their families, and colleagues in other medical fields who may not be as familiar with the long-term care and outcomes of patients with neurological injuries.

References [1]

1. Salomon EJ, Barfett J, Willems PW, Geibprasert S, Bacigaluppi S, Krings T. Dynamic CT angiography and CT perfusion employing a 320-detector row CT: protocol and current clinical applications. Klin Neuroradiol. 2009;19(3):187–96. https://doi.org/10.1007/s00062-009-9019-7. PubMed PMID: 19705072.
2. Mair G, Wardlaw JM. Imaging of acute stroke prior to treatment: current practice and evolving techniques. Br J Radiol. 2014;87(1040):20140216. https://doi.org/10.1259/bjr.20140216.
3. de Manoel A, Goffi A, Zampieri F, Turkel-Parrella D, Duggal A, Marotta TR, Macdonald LR, Abrahamson S. The critical care management of spontaneous intracranial hemorrhage: a contemporary review. Crit Care. 2016;20(1):272. https://doi.org/10.1186/s13054-016-1432-0.
4. Lindner A, Kunst S, Ianosi BA, Rass V, Schiefecker AJ, Kofler M, Limmert V, Grams AE, Pfausler B, Beer R, Thome C, Helbok R. The location of intraparenchymal bleeding determines functional outcome after spontaneous subarachnoid hemorrhage. Eur J Neurol. 2023;30(2):372–9. https://doi.org/10.1111/ene.15621. PubMed PMID: 36318275.
5. Gentsch A, Storm C, Leithner C, Schroeder T, Ploner CJ, Hamm B, Wiener E, Scheel M. Outcome prediction in patients after cardiac arrest: a simplified method for determination of gray-white matter ratio in cranial computed tomography. Clin Neuroradiol. 2015;25(1):49–54. https://doi.org/10.1007/s00062-013-0281-3. PubMed PMID: 24626778.
6. Scheel M, Storm C, Gentsch A, Nee J, Luckenbach F, Ploner CJ, Leithner C. The prognostic value of gray-white-matter ratio in cardiac arrest patients treated with hypothermia. Scand J Trauma Resusc Emerg Med. 2013;21(1):1–7. https://doi.org/10.1186/1757-7241-21-23.
7. Lang M, Nielsen N, Ullen S, Abul-Kasim K, Johnsson M, Helbok R, Leithner C, Cronberg T, Moseby-Knappe M. A pilot study of methods for prediction of poor outcome by head computed tomography after cardiac arrest. Resuscitation. 2022;179:61–70. https://doi.org/10.1016/j.resuscitation.2022.07.035. PubMed PMID: 35931271.
8. Wintermark M, Li Y, Ding VY, Xu Y, Jiang B, Ball RL, Zeineh M, Gean A, Sanelli P. Neuroimaging radiological interpretation system for acute traumatic brain injury. J Neurotrauma. 2018;35(22):2665–72. https://doi.org/10.1089/neu.2017.5311. PubMed PMID: 29665763.
9. Chen H, Li Y, Jiang B, Zhu G, Rezaii PG, Lu G, Wintermark M. Demographics and clinical characteristics of acute traumatic brain injury patients in the different Neuroimaging Radiological Interpretation System (NIRIS) categories. J Neuroradiol. 2021;48(2):104–11. https://doi.org/10.1016/j.neurad.2019.07.002. PubMed PMID: 31323305.
10. Vert C, Parra-Farinas C, Rovira A. MR imaging in hyperacute ischemic stroke. Eur J Radiol. 2017;96:125–32. https://doi.org/10.1016/j.ejrad.2017.06.013. PubMed PMID: 28652053.
11. Dijkhuizen RM, Knollema S, van der Worp HB, Ter Horst GJ, De Wildt DJ, van der Sprenkel JWB, Tulleken KA, Nicolay K. Dynamics of cerebral tissue injury and perfusion after temporary hypoxia-ischemia in the rat: evidence for region-specific sensitivity and delayed damage. Stroke. 1998;29(3):695–704.
12. Wu O, Sorensen GA, Benner T, Singhal AB, Furie KL, Greer DM. Comatose patients with cardiac arrest: predicting clinical outcome with diffusion-weighted MR Imaging1. Radiology. 2009;252(1):173–81. https://doi.org/10.1148/radiol.2521081232.
13. Heradstveit BE, Larsson EM, Skeidsvoll H, Hammersborg SM, Wentzel-Larsen T, Guttormsen AB, Heltne JK. Repeated magnetic resonance imaging and cerebral performance after cardiac arrest—a pilot study. Resuscitation. 2011;82(5):549–55. https://doi.org/10.1016/j.resuscitation.2011.01.018. PubMed PMID: 21367511.
14. Adams JH, Doyle D, Ford I, Gennarelli TA, Graham DI, McLellan DR. Diffuse axonal injury in head injury: definition, diagnosis and grading. Histopathology. 1989;15(1):49–59. https://doi.org/10.1111/j.1365-2559.1989.tb03040.x.

[1] Key References [49, 50, 59, 67, 82].

15. van Eijck MM, Schoonman GG, van der Naalt J, de Vries J, Roks G. Diffuse axonal injury after traumatic brain injury is a prognostic factor for functional outcome: a systematic review and meta-analysis. Brain Inj. 2018;32(4):395–402. https://doi.org/10.1080/02699052.2018.1429018. PubMed PMID: 29381396.
16. Humble SS, Wilson LD, Wang L, Long DA, Smith MA, Siktberg JC, Mirhoseini MF, Bhatia A, Pruthi S, Day MA, Muehlschlegel S, Patel MB. Prognosis of diffuse axonal injury with traumatic brain injury. J Trauma Acute Care Surg. 2018;85(1):155–9. https://doi.org/10.1097/TA.0000000000001852.
17. Blanco P, Abdo-Cuza A. Transcranial doppler ultrasound in neurocritical care. J Ultrasound. 2018;21(1):1–16. https://doi.org/10.1007/s40477-018-0282-9.
18. Miyake S, Suzuki R, Akimoto T, Iida Y, Shimohigoshi W, Nakai Y, Manaka H, Shimizu N, Yamamoto T. Renal dysfunction is the strongest prognostic factor after carotid artery stenting according to real-world data. J Stroke Cerebrovasc Dis. 2022;31(3):106269. https://doi.org/10.1016/j.jstrokecerebrovasdis.2021.106269. PubMed PMID: 34963079.
19. Tao C, Xu P, Yao Y, Zhu Y, Li R, Li J, Luo W, Hu W. A prospective study to investigate controlling blood pressure under transcranial doppler after endovascular treatment in patients with occlusion of anterior circulation. Front Neurol. 2021;12:735758. https://doi.org/10.3389/fneur.2021.735758.
20. Robba C, Frigieri G, Brasil S, Taccone FS. Early prognostic value of non-invasive intracranial pressure methods in brain-injured patients. Intensive Care Med. 2022;48(12):1812–4. https://doi.org/10.1007/s00134-022-06899-4. PubMed PMID: 36171441.
21. National Institutes of Health. NIH stroke scale. In: NIH_Stroke_Scale_508C, editor. 2003.
22. Brott T, Adams HP, Olinger CP, Marler JR, Barsan WG. Measurements of acute cerebral infarction: a clinical examination scale. Stroke. 1989;20(7):864–70. https://doi.org/10.1161/01.STR.20.7.864.
23. González R. Current state of acute stroke imaging. Stroke. 2013;44(11):3260–4. https://doi.org/10.1161/STROKEAHA.113.003229.
24. Saver JL, Goyal M, Bonafe A, Diener H-C, Levy EI, Pereira VM, Albers GW, Cognard C, Cohen DJ, Hacke W, Jansen O, Jovin TG, Mattle HP, Nogueira RG, Siddiqui AH, Yavagal DR, Baxter BW, Devlin TG, Lopes DK, Reddy VK, du de Rochemont R, Singer OC, Jahan R. Stent-retriever thrombectomy after intravenous t-PA vs. t-PA alone in stroke. N Engl J Med. 2015;372(24):2285–95. https://doi.org/10.1056/NEJMoa1415061.
25. Schaefer PW, Pulli B, Copen WA, Hirsch JA, Leslie-Mazwi T, Schwamm LH, Wu O, González RG, Yoo AJ. Combining MRI with NIHSS thresholds to predict outcome in acute ischemic stroke: value for patient selection. Am J Neuroradiol. 2015;36(2):259–64. https://doi.org/10.3174/ajnr.A4103.
26. Thorpe ER, Garrett KB, Smith AM, Reneker JC, Phillips RS. Outcome measure scores predict discharge destination in patients with acute and subacute stroke: a systematic review and series of meta-analyses. J Neurol Phys Ther. 2018;42(1):2–11. https://doi.org/10.1097/NPT.0000000000000211. PubMed PMID: 29232307.
27. Abdul-Rahim AH, Fulton RL, Sucharew H. National Institutes of Health stroke scale item profiles as predictor of patient outcome. Stroke. 2015;46(10):2779–85. https://doi.org/10.1161/STROKEAHA.115.010380.
28. Kenmuir CL, Hammer M, Jovin T, Reddy V, Wechsler L, Jadhav A. Predictors of outcome in patients presenting with acute ischemic stroke and mild stroke scale scores. J Stroke Cerebrovasc Dis. 2015;24(7):1685–9. https://doi.org/10.1016/j.jstrokecerebrovasdis.2015.03.042. PubMed PMID: 25944544.
29. Rosen DS, Macdonald RL. Subarachnoid hemorrhage grading scales. Neurocrit Care. 2005;2(2):110–8. https://doi.org/10.1385/NCC:2:2:110.
30. Hunt WE, Hess RM. Surgical risk as related to time of intervention in the repair of intracranial aneurysms. J Neurosurg. 1968;28(1):14–20. https://doi.org/10.3171/jns.1968.28.1.0014.
31. de Winkel J, Cras TY, Dammers R, van Doormaal PJ, van der Jagt M, Dippel DWJ, Lingsma HF, Roozenbeek B. Early predictors of functional outcome in poor-grade aneurysmal subarachnoid

hemorrhage: a systematic review and meta-analysis. BMC Neurol. 2022;22(1):239. https://doi.org/10.1186/s12883-022-02734-x.
32. Han Y, Ye F, Long X, Li A, Xu H, Zou L, Yang Y, You C. Ultra-early treatment for poor-grade aneurysmal subarachnoid hemorrhage: a systematic review and meta-analysis. World Neurosurg. 2018;115:e160–e71. https://doi.org/10.1016/j.wneu.2018.03.219. PubMed PMID: 29649648.
33. Teasdale G, Maas A, Lecky F, Manley G, Stocchetti N, Murray G. The Glasgow coma scale at 40 years: standing the test of time. Lancet Neurol. 2014;13(8):844–54. https://doi.org/10.1016/S1474-4422(14)70120-6. PubMed PMID: 25030516.
34. Banks JL, Marotta CA. Outcomes validity and reliability of the modified Rankin scale: implications for stroke clinical trials a literature review and synthesis. Stroke. 2007;38(3):1091–6. https://doi.org/10.1161/01.STR.0000258355.23810.c6.
35. Quinn TJ, Dawson J, Walters MR, Lees KR. Reliability of the modified Rankin scale. Stroke. 2009;40(10):3393–5. https://doi.org/10.1161/STROKEAHA.109.557256.
36. de Berker H, de Berker A, Aung H, Duarte P, Mohammed S, Shetty H, Hughes T. Pre-stroke disability and stroke severity as predictors of discharge destination from an acute stroke ward. Clin Med (Lond). 2021;21(2):e186–e91. https://doi.org/10.7861/clinmed.2020-0834.
37. Huybrechts KF, Caro JJ. The Barthel index and modified Rankin scale as prognostic tools for long-term outcomes after stroke: a qualitative review of the literature. Curr Med Res Opin. 2007;23(7):1627–36. https://doi.org/10.1185/030079907x210444. PubMed PMID: 17559756.
38. Sreekrishnan A, Leasure AC, Shi FD, Hwang DY, Schindler JL, Petersen NH, Gilmore EJ, Kamel H, Sansing LH, Greer DM, Sheth KN. Functional improvement among intracerebral hemorrhage (ICH) survivors up to 12 months post-injury. Neurocrit Care. 2017;27(3):326–33. https://doi.org/10.1007/s12028-017-0425-4.
39. Harrison JK, McArthur KS, Quinn TJ. Assessment scales in stroke: clinimetric and clinical considerations. Clin Interv Aging. 2013;8:201–11. https://doi.org/10.2147/cia.S32405.
40. Wilson L, Boase K, Nelson LD, Temkin NR, Giacino JT, Markowitz AJ, Maas A, Menon DK, Teasdale G, Manley GT. A manual for the Glasgow outcome scale-extended interview. J Neurotrauma. 2021;38(17):2435–46. https://doi.org/10.1089/neu.2020.7527.
41. Wilson JT, Pettigrew LE, Teasdale G. Structured interviews for the Glasgow outcome scale and the extended Glasgow outcome scale: guidelines for their use. J Neurotrauma. 1998;15(8):573–85.
42. Wilson JTL, Pettigrew LEL. Emotional and cognitive consequences of head injury in relation to the Glasgow outcome scale. J Neurol. 2000;69(2):204–9.
43. Gaastra B, Ren D, Alexander S, Awad IA, Blackburn S, Dore S, Hanley D, Nyquist P, Bulters D, Galea I. Evidence-based interconversion of the Glasgow outcome and modified Rankin scales: pitfalls and best practices. J Stroke Cerebrovasc Dis. 2022;31(12):106845. https://doi.org/10.1016/j.jstrokecerebrovasdis.2022.106845. PubMed PMID: 36309002.
44. Raina KD, Callaway C, Rittenberger JC, Holm MB. Neurological and functional status following cardiac arrest: method and tool utility. Resuscitation. 2008;79(2):249–56. https://doi.org/10.1016/j.resuscitation.2008.06.005.
45. Hsu JW, Madsen CD, Callaham ML. Quality-of-life and formal functional testing of survivors of out-of-hospital cardiac arrest correlates poorly with traditional neurologic outcome scales. Ann Emerg Med. 1996;28(6):597–605. https://doi.org/10.1016/s0196-0644(96)70080-x. PubMed PMID: 8953946.
46. Banks JL, Marotta CA. Outcomes validity and reliability of the modified Rankin scale: implications for stroke clinical trials. Stroke. 2007;38(3):1091–6. https://doi.org/10.1161/01.STR.0000258355.23810.c6.
47. Saatman KE, Duhaime A-C, Bullock R, Maas A, Valadka A, Manley GT. Classification of traumatic brain injury for targeted therapies. J Neurotrauma. 2008;25(7):719–38. https://doi.org/10.1089/neu.2008.0586.
48. Balestreri M, Czosnyka M, Chatfield DA. Predictive value of Glasgow coma scale after brain trauma: change in trend over the past ten years. J Neurol. 2004;75(1):161–2.

49. Giacino J, Kalmar K, Whyte J. The JFK coma recovery scale-revised: measurement characteristics and diagnostic utility. Arch Phys Med Rehabil. 2004;85(12):2020–9. https://doi.org/10.1016/j.apmr.2004.02.033.
50. Lucca LF, Lofaro D, Pignolo L, Leto E, Ursino M, Cortese MD, Conforti D, Tonin P, Cerasa A. Outcome prediction in disorders of consciousness: the role of coma recovery scale revised. BMC Neurol. 2019;19(1):68. https://doi.org/10.1186/s12883-019-1293-7.
51. Cortese MD, Riganello F, Arcuri F, Pugliese ME, Lucca LF, Dolce G, Sannita WG. Coma recovery scale-r: variability in the disorder of consciousness. BMC Neurol. 2015;15:186. https://doi.org/10.1186/s12883-015-0455-5.
52. Schnakers C, Vanhaudenhuyse A, Giacino J, Ventura M, Boly M, Majerus S, Moonen G, Laureys S. Diagnostic accuracy of the vegetative and minimally conscious state: clinical consensus versus standardized neurobehavioral assessment. BMC Neurol. 2009;9:35. https://doi.org/10.1186/1471-2377-9-35.
53. Harris K, Linsenmeyer M, Weppner J, Breisinger T, Yukevich AM, Galang G, Wagner AK. "Motor first: a proposed approach to the JFK coma recovery scale-revised for the consulting physician" [Abstract]: abstracts of scientific papers and posters presented at the ISPRM World Congress and Annual Meeting of the Association of Academic Physiatrists, Orlando, Florida March 4–9, 2020. Am J Phys Med Rehabil. 2020;99(3S):a80.
54. Feasibility and Validity of the Coma Recovery Scale-Revised for Accelerated Standardized Testing: A Practical Assessment Tool for Detecting Consciousness in the Intensive Care Unit - PubMed (nih.gov) https://doi.org/10.1002/ana.26740.
55. Nassal MMJ, Nichols D, Demasi S, Rittenberger JC, Panchal AR, Kurz MC, Service UABP-CA. External validation of Pittsburgh cardiac arrest category illness severity score. Resuscitation. 2022;172:32–7. https://doi.org/10.1016/j.resuscitation.2021.12.022. PubMed PMID: 34968531.
56. Wijdicks EF, Bamlet WR, Maramattom BV, Manno EM, McClelland RL. Validation of a new coma scale: the FOUR score. Ann Neurol. 2005;58(4):585–93. https://doi.org/10.1002/ana.20611. PubMed PMID: 16178024.
57. Vincent JL, de Mendonça A, Cantraine F, Moreno R, Takala J, Suter PM, Sprung CL, Colardyn F, Blecher S. Use of the SOFA score to assess the incidence of organ dysfunction/failure in intensive care units: results of a multicenter, prospective study. Working group on "sepsis-related problems" of the European Society of Intensive Care Medicine. Crit Care Med. 1998;26(11):1793–800. https://doi.org/10.1097/00003246-199811000-00016. PubMed PMID: 9824069.
58. Rittenberger JC, Popescu A, Brenner RP, Guyette FX, Callaway CW. Frequency and timing of nonconvulsive status epilepticus in comatose post-cardiac arrest subjects treated with hypothermia. Neurocrit Care. 2012;16(1):114–22. https://doi.org/10.1007/s12028-011-9565-0.
59. Coppler PJ, Elmer J, Calderon L, Sabedra A, Doshi AA, Callaway CW, Rittenberger JC, Dezfulian C. Validation of the Pittsburgh cardiac arrest category illness severity score. Resuscitation. 2015;89:86–92. https://doi.org/10.1016/j.resuscitation.2015.01.020.
60. Whyte J, Nakase-Richardson R, Hammond FM, McNamee S, Giacino JT, Kalmar K, Greenwald B, Yablon SA, Horn LJ. Functional outcomes in traumatic disorders of consciousness: 5-year outcomes from the National Institute on Disability and Rehabilitation Research Traumatic Brain Injury Model Systems. Arch Phys Med Rehabil. 2013;94(10):1855–60.
61. Nakase-Richardson R, Whyte J, Giacino JT, Pavawalla S, Barnett SD, Yablon SA, Sherer M, Kalmar K, Hammond FM, Greenwald B, Horn LJ, Seel R, McCarthy M, Tran J, Walker WC. Longitudinal outcome of patients with disordered consciousness in the NIDRR TBI Model Systems Programs. J Neurotrauma. 2012;29(1):59–65. https://doi.org/10.1089/neu.2011.1829. PubMed PMID: 21663544.
62. Giacino JT, Katz DI, Schiff ND, Whyte J, Ashman EJ, Ashwal S, Barbano R, Hammond FM, Laureys S, GSF L, Nakase-Richardson R, Seel RT, Yablon S, TSD G, Gronseth GS, Armstrong MJ. Practice guideline update recommendations summary: disorders of consciousness: report of the Guideline Development, Dissemination, and Implementation Subcommittee of the

American Academy of Neurology; the American Congress of Rehabilitation Medicine; and the National Institute on Disability, Independent Living, and Rehabilitation Research. Arch Phys Med Rehabil. 2018;99(9):1699–709. https://doi.org/10.1016/j.apmr.2018.07.001. PubMed PMID: 30098791.
63. Ritter AC, Wagner AK, Fabio A, Pugh MJ, Walker WC, Szaflarski JP, Zafonte RD, Brown AW, Hammond FM, Bushnik T, Johnson-Greene D, Shea T, Krellman JW, Rosenthal JA, Dreer LE. Incidence and risk factors of posttraumatic seizures following traumatic brain injury: a traumatic brain injury model systems study. Epilepsia. 2016;57(12):1968–77.
64. Vespa PM, McArthur DL, Xu Y, Eliseo M, Etchepare M, Dinov I, Alger J, Glenn TP, Hovda D. Nonconvulsive seizures after traumatic brain injury are associated with hippocampal atrophy. Neurology. 2010;75(9):792–8. https://doi.org/10.1212/WNL.0b013e3181f07334.
65. Cologan V, Drouot X, Parapatics S, Delorme A, Gruber G, Moonen G, Laureys S. Sleep in the unresponsive wakefulness syndrome and minimally conscious state. J Neurotrauma. 2012;30(5):339–46. https://doi.org/10.1089/neu.2012.2654.
66. Vassallo P, Novy J, Zubler F, Schindler K, Alvarez V, Ruegg S, Rossetti AO. EEG spindles integrity in critical care adults. Analysis of a randomized trial. Acta Neurol Scand. 2021;144(6):655–62. https://doi.org/10.1111/ane.13510.
67. Amorim E, Rittenberger JC, Baldwin ME, Callaway CW, Popescu A. Malignant EEG patterns in cardiac arrest patients treated with targeted temperature management who survive to hospital discharge. Resuscitation. 2015;90:127–32. https://doi.org/10.1016/j.resuscitation.2015.03.005.
68. Greer DM, Rosenthal ES, Wu O. Neuroprognostication of hypoxic-ischaemic coma in the therapeutic hypothermia era. Nat Rev Neurol. 2014;10(4):190–203. https://doi.org/10.1038/nrneurol.2014.36.
69. Houlden DA, Taylor AB, Feinstein A, Midha R, Bethune AJ, Stewart CP, Schwartz ML. Early somatosensory evoked potential grades in comatose traumatic brain injury patients predict cognitive and functional outcome. Crit Care Med. 2010;38(1):167–74. https://doi.org/10.1097/CCM.0b013e3181c031b3. PubMed PMID: 19829103.
70. Sandroni C, D'Arrigo S, Cacciola S, Hoedemaekers CWE, Kamps MJA, Oddo M, Taccone FS, Di Rocco A, Meijer FJA, Westhall E, Antonelli M, Soar J, Nolan JP, Cronberg T. Prediction of poor neurological outcome in comatose survivors of cardiac arrest: a systematic review. Intensive Care Med. 2020;46(10):1803–51. https://doi.org/10.1007/s00134-020-06198-w.
71. Maciel CB, Morawo AO, Tsao CY, Youn TS, Labar DR, Rubens EO, Greer DM. SSEP in therapeutic hypothermia era. J Clin Neurophysiol. 2017;34(5):469–75. https://doi.org/10.1097/wnp.0000000000000392. PubMed PMID: 28557905.
72. Schorl M, Valerius-Kukula SJ, Kemmer TP. Median-evoked somatosensory potentials in severe brain injury: does initial loss of cortical potentials exclude recovery? Clin Neurol Neurosurg. 2014;123:25–33. https://doi.org/10.1016/j.clineuro.2014.05.004. PubMed PMID: 25012007.
73. Benghanem S, Pruvost-Robieux E, Bouchereau E, Gavaret M, Cariou A. Prognostication after cardiac arrest: how EEG and evoked potentials may improve the challenge. Ann Intensive Care. 2022;12(1):111. https://doi.org/10.1186/s13613-022-01083-9.
74. Benghanem S, Mazeraud A, Azabou E, Chhor V, Shinotsuka CR, Claassen J, Rohaut B, Sharshar T. Brainstem dysfunction in critically ill patients. Crit Care. 2020;24(1):5. https://doi.org/10.1186/s13054-019-2718-9.
75. Rodriguez RA, Bussiere M, Froeschl M, Nathan HJ. Auditory-evoked potentials during coma: do they improve our prediction of awakening in comatose patients? J Crit Care. 2014;29(1):93–100. https://doi.org/10.1016/j.jcrc.2013.08.020. PubMed PMID: 24125771.
76. Korley FK, Datwyler SA, Jain S, Sun X, Beligere G, Chandran R, Marino JA, McQuiston B, Zhang H, Caudle KL, Wang KKW, Puccio AM, Okonkwo DO, Yue JK, Taylor SR, Markowitz A, Manley GT, Diaz-Arrastia R. Comparison of GFAP and UCH-L1 measurements from two prototype assays: the Abbott i-STAT and ARCHITECT assays. Neurotrauma Rep. 2021;2(1):193–9. https://doi.org/10.1089/neur.2020.0037.
77. Minkkinen M, Iverson GL, Kotilainen AK, Pauniaho SL, Mattila VM, Lehtimaki T, Berghem K, Posti JP, Luoto TM. Prospective validation of the scandinavian guidelines for

initial management of minimal, mild, and moderate head injuries in adults. J Neurotrauma. 2019;36(20):2904–12. https://doi.org/10.1089/neu.2018.6351. PubMed PMID: 31111795.
78. Czeiter E, Amrein K, Gravesteijn BY, Lecky F, Menon DK, Mondello S, Newcombe VFJ, Richter S, Steyerberg EW, Vyvere TV, Verheyden J, Xu H, Yang Z, Maas AIR, Wang KKW, Buki A, CENTER-TBI Participants and Investigators. Blood biomarkers on admission in acute traumatic brain injury: relations to severity, CT findings and care path in the CENTER-TBI study. EBioMedicine. 2020;56:102785. https://doi.org/10.1016/j.ebiom.2020.102785.
79. Diaz-Arrastia R, Kochanek PM, Bergold P, Kenney K, Marx CE, Grimes CJ, Loh LT, Adam LT, Oskvig D, Curley KC, Salzer W. Pharmacotherapy of traumatic brain injury: state of the science and the road forward: report of the Department of Defense Neurotrauma Pharmacology Workgroup. J Neurotrauma. 2014;31(2):135–58. https://doi.org/10.1089/neu.2013.3019.
80. Rhine T, Babcock L, Zhang N, Leach J, Wade SL. Are UCH-L1 and GFAP promising biomarkers for children with mild traumatic brain injury? Brain Inj. 2016;30(10):1231–8. https://doi.org/10.1080/02699052.2016.1178396.
81. Lagebrant A, Lang M, Nielsen N, Blennow K, Dankiewicz J, Friberg H, Hassager C, Horn J, Kjaergaard J, Kuiper MA, Mattsson-Carlgren N, Pellis T, Rylander C, Sigmund R, Stammet P, Unden J, Zetterberg H, Wise MP, Cronberg T, Moseby-Knappe M. Brain injury markers in blood predict signs of hypoxic ischaemic encephalopathy on head computed tomography after cardiac arrest. Resuscitation. 2023;184:109668. https://doi.org/10.1016/j.resuscitation.2022.12.006. PubMed PMID: 36563954.
82. Ebner F, Moseby-Knappe M, Mattsson-Carlgren N, Lilja G, Dragancea I, Unden J, Friberg H, Erlinge D, Kjaergaard J, Hassager C, Wise MP, Kuiper M, Stammet P, Wanscher M, Horn J, Ullen S, Cronberg T, Nielsen N. Serum GFAP and UCH-L1 for the prediction of neurological outcome in comatose cardiac arrest patients. Resuscitation. 2020;154:61–8. https://doi.org/10.1016/j.resuscitation.2020.05.016. PubMed PMID: 32445783.
83. Wagner AK. A Rehabilomics framework for personalized and translational rehabilitation research and care for individuals with disabilities: perspectives and considerations for spinal cord injury. J Spinal Cord Med. 2014;37(5):493–502. https://doi.org/10.1179/2045772314Y.0000000248.
84. Kumar RG, Boles JA, Wagner AK. Chronic inflammation after severe traumatic brain injury: characterization and associations with outcome at 6 and 12 months Postinjury. J Head Trauma Rehabil. 2015;30(6):369–81. https://doi.org/10.1097/HTR.0000000000000067. PubMed PMID: 24901329.
85. Milleville KA, Awan N, Disanto D, Kumar RG, Wagner AK. Early chronic systemic inflammation and associations with cognitive performance after moderate to severe TBI. Brain Behav Immun Health. 2021;11:100185. https://doi.org/10.1016/j.bbih.2020.100185.
86. Ritter AC, Kammerer CM, Brooks MM, Conley YP, Wagner AK. Genetic variation in neuronal glutamate transport genes and associations with posttraumatic seizure. Epilepsia. 2016;57(6):984–93.
87. Kumar RG, Breslin KB, Ritter AC, Conley YP, Wagner AK. Variability with astroglial glutamate transport genetics is associated with increased risk for post-traumatic seizures. J Neurotrauma. 2019;36(2):230–8. https://doi.org/10.1089/neu.2018.5632.
88. Diamond ML, Ritter AC, Failla MD, Boles JA, Conley YP, Kochanek PM, Wagner AK. IL-1β associations with posttraumatic epilepsy development: a genetics and biomarker cohort study. Epilepsia. 2015;56(7):991–1001. https://doi.org/10.1111/epi.13100. PubMed PMID: 26149793.
89. Darrah SD, Miller MA, Ren D, Hoh NZ, Scanlon JM, Conley YP, Wagner AK. Genetic variability in glutamic acid decarboxylase genes: associations with post-traumatic seizures after severe TBI. Epilepsy Res. 2013;103(2–3):180–94. https://doi.org/10.1016/j.eplepsyres.2012.07.006.
90. Wagner AK, Miller MA, Scanlon J, Ren D, Kochanek PM, Conley YP. Adenosine A1 receptor gene variants associated with post-traumatic seizures after severe TBI. Epilepsy Res. 2010;90(3):259–72. https://doi.org/10.1016/j.eplepsyres.2010.06.001.
91. Diamond ML, Ritter AC, Jackson EK, Conley YP, Kochanek PM, Boison D, Wagner AK. Genetic variation in the adenosine regulatory cycle is associated with posttraumatic epilepsy development. Epilepsia. 2015;56(8):1198–206. https://doi.org/10.1111/epi.13044.

Chapter 5
Arousal and Stimulation

Komal Patel and Amy K. Wagner

Chapter Objectives

1. To review neurotransmitter systems and neuroanatomy relevant to neuropharmacology addressing arousal and cognition.
2. To discuss clinical history and management principles for arousal and cognition after aqcuired brain injury.
3. To understand pharmacological approaches to improve arousal and cognition in the acute care setting.
4. To address sleep in order to facilitate improvements in arousal and cognition.
5. To assess medication effectiveness with regard to improved arousal and cognition.

Introduction

Arousal and cognition are key impairments limiting the initiation of rehabilitation services after an acute acquired brain injury. Naturally, arousal and awareness are necessary to encode and process information as well as react to environmental stimuli; as such, they are key features of cognitive performance that are assessed

K. Patel
James A. Haley Veterans' Hospital and Clinics, U.S. Department of Veterans Affairs, Tampa, FL, USA
e-mail: komal.patel3@va.gov

A. K. Wagner (✉)
Department of Physical Medicine and Rehabilitation, University of Pittsburgh School of Medicine, Pittsburgh, PA, USA
e-mail: wagnerak@upmc.edu

A. K. Wagner, J. Weppner (eds.), *Acute Care Neuroconsultation and Neurorehabilitation Management*, https://doi.org/10.1007/978-3-031-42830-2_5

and addressed in the acute care rehabilitation consultation setting. Additionally, arousal and awareness are foundational for other cognitive features, such as attention, learning, and memory, for which deficits may also be present. Arousal and cognition are based on an interplay between brain regional circuitry and neurotransmitter systems. These features vary based on pattern of injury and regional vulnerability to central nervous system (CNS) insult. Identifying and understanding specific brain regions affected by an injury helps rehabilitation practitioners in the acute care setting successfully improve patient arousal and cognitive abilities, and subsequently, their rehabilitation course.

Primarily managed by the reticular-thalamic, thalamo-cortical, and reticulo-cortical connections, arousal and consciousness are believed to initiate in the brainstem. Diffuse monoaminergic projections target the brain cortex and subcortical regions to influence arousal. The neurotransmitters, dopamine and norepinephrine, play an integral role in supporting the reticular activating system and wakefulness. Changes in dopamine release in the meso-cortico-limbic system, the ventral tegmental area projecting to the prefrontal cortex, amygdala, hippocampus, and nucleus accumbens, affect arousal. Additionally, levels of norepinephrine in the locus coeruleus, along with its connections in the ventrolateral medulla oblongata and hypothalamic-pituitary-adrenal axis, regulate levels of arousal and consciousness. Injuries to different elements along these pathways, and their cortical feedback pathways, can impair arousal and awareness depending on the severity and type of brain injury.

A patient's level of consciousness, whether they are in a coma, unresponsive wakefulness (a.k.a. vegetative), or a minimally conscious state, can vary based on the extent of their brain injury. The features of coma include a lack of a sleep/wake cycle, the patient's eyes remain closed, and there is no purposeful movement or ability to discretely localize noxious stimuli [1]. Comparatively, when a patient is in a state of unresponsive wakefulness, eyes will open, and there is evidence of wakeful cycles; however, there is still no observable self/environmental awareness or purposeful movement [1]. These individuals may respond to visual or auditory startle without tracking or localization. Lastly, a patient who is in a minimally conscious state, will typically display features of eye opening, evidence of a sleep/wake cycle, and will begin to show signs of self and environmental recognition. These individuals may also show evidence of reproducible purposeful and/or functional movements, including following motor commands intermittently [1]. Understanding the disorders of consciousness (DoC) spectrum provides an initial framework for acute care neurorehabilitation consultants to discuss patient prognosis, transition of care possibilities, and early neurostimulation trials for these individuals with severe injuries.

Multiple scales to characterize an individual's level of consciousness after a brain injury are available. In comparison to other scales, the JFK Coma Recovery Scale [2, 3] is recommended with minor reservations by the American Congress of Rehabilitation Medicine, Brain Injury—DoC Task Force, to aid in determining when a patient is emerging through the DoC states. Tracking these scores helps to provide insight into prognosis, as coma lasting less than 2 weeks suggests that severe disability will be unlikely, and coma lasting greater than 4 weeks suggests that good recovery will be unlikely [4].

A trial of neurostimulating medications in the acute care setting can help to improve arousal, awareness, cognition, and potential prognosis after a brain injury. Arousal plays a crucial role in establishing patient rehabilitation goals and determining appropriate transition of care upon acute care discharge. Additionally, neurostimulant use and response during acute care may impact transition of care planning. Determining the most appropriate medication and timing for initiation can be challenging in the context of managing disruptions in circadian rhythms, the sleep-wake cycle, and other medical and neurological comorbidities and complications. An understanding of the key neurotransmitters affecting arousal and cognition, and the impact of neurostimulants on them, may facilitate the integration of these medications into the acute care treatment plan, potentially hastening a patient's recovery after a brain injury. In this context of patients with complex neurological injures—often in the setting of other associated traumas and who require extensive therapy—a primary goal of neurostimulants is to improve participation throughout rehabilitation services. Furthermore, other cognitive abilities that are affected by arousal, including memory, attention, initiation, and processing, may also improve. Importantly, increasing evidence from experimental models of brain injury suggest that early neurostimulation does not exacerbate secondary injury and may have positive early benefits on neurotransmission, plasticity, and repair [5, 6].

Neurotransmitter Systems Relevant to Brain Injury Pharmacology

Table 5.1 summarizes neurotransmitter systems, their critical pathways for arousal and cognition, and key target receptors that are described in more detail below.

Dopamine (DA): Arousal is a redundant brain function primarily involving DA and norepinephrine neurotransmission. The dopaminergic ventral mesencephalic neurons in the substantia nigra and ventral tegmental area extend ascending axonal

Table 5.1 Neurotransmitters with their pathways, actions, and target receptors

Neurotransmitter	Pathway/location	Action	Target receptors
Dopamine	VTA/SN, striatum, hypothalamic, frontal cortex	Arousal, voluntary movements, reward processing	D1, D2, D3, D4, D5
Norepinephrine	Locus coeruleus, pons, cortex	Arousal, alertness, stimulation	Adrenergic—Alpha-1, Alpha-2, Beta-1, Beta-2, Beta-3
Acetylcholine	Meso-pontine tegmentum hippocampus, striatum frontal and temporal cortex	Arousal, memory, attention,	Nicotinic, muscarinic—M1, M2, M3, M4, M5
Serotonin	Raphe nuclei Hippocampus	Arousal, sleep, emotion	5-HT_{1A}, 5-HT_{1B}, 5-HT_{2A}, 5-HT_{2C}
Histamine	Posterior hypothalamus; cortex	Arousal, sleep	H1, H2, H3, H4

projections from the brainstem to basal forebrain, ventral striatum, and cerebral cortex composing the meso-limbo-cortical system [7]. Ventral mesencephalon stimulation promotes arousal via post-synaptic DA receptors. The two primarily studied receptors regarding arousal are D1 and D2 receptors. D1 receptors are more commonly expressed on the post-synaptic pyramidal and non-pyramidal neuronal dendrites within the frontal cortex, hippocampus, and limbic cortex. Both D1 and D2 receptors are highly concentrated on striatal medium spiny neurons, regulating complex globus pallidus GABAergic outflow. D2 receptor isoforms are associated with terminal receptor activation and presynaptic auto-receptor function [8, 9]. DA is also intimately involved with cognitive features related to other areas of the brain, such as working memory, executive function, and attention.

Norepinephrine: Norepinephrine primarily plays a role in the "fight or flight" response via locus coeruleus neurotransmission pathways and its complex interplay with C1 adrenergic neurons in the rostral ventrolateral medulla oblongata and activation of the hypothalamic-pituitary-adrenal axis [7, 10–12]. Locus coeruleus neurons are located in the midpons periventricular gray matter, at the base of the fourth ventricle, sending diffuse axonal projections throughout the brain and spinal cord, including the sympathetic nervous system, which plays a prominent role in modulating immune function [13, 14]. Importantly, locus coeruleus activity varies based on sensory inputs via trigeminal, visceral, and vestibular pathways, which in turn can impact cognition. Locus coeruleus activity also varies based on circadian rhythm physiology, which is often significantly disrupted by brain injuries. Norepinephrine transmission is highest during times of waking and high-vigilance states.

Acetylcholine: Many cognitive features, including arousal, sustained attention, learning, and memory, as well as the promotion of rapid eye movement (REM) sleep, which contributes to the sleep/wake cycle, are dependent on acetylcholine [15, 16]. Acetylcholine neurons project axons into the thalamus, cerebellum, and ascending reticular formation from their origin in the meso-pontine tegmentum region of the brainstem, including the nucleus basalis of Meynert and septal nuclei [7, 11]. Cholinergic neuron stimulation, via the M1 receptor, leads to increased cortical activity, however, the medial temporal lobe, an area rich in cholinergic neurons, is a susceptible area of brain injury. Furthermore, acetylcholine plays a role in modulating DA neurotransmission, and thus, striatal GABAergic outflow in the striatum [17, 18].

Serotonin: The raphe nuclei in the brainstem release serotonin diffusely throughout the brain via projections to the limbic system, neostriatum, thalamus, cerebellum, and cortex, affecting cognitive features like memory, mood, and learning [7, 11]. Serotonin is also crucial in regulating sleep architecture, and medications that are commonly used, such as Trazodone, help modulate serotonin levels to promote sleep. Activity in the raphe nuclei decreases as an individual enters REM sleep, hence decreasing serotonin levels. Addressing sleep can assist in promoting arousal, as the sleep/wake cycle is crucial in differentiating between the stages of coma and unresponsive wakefullness state.

Histamine: Histamine cell bodies, located within the tuberomammillary nuclei in the posterior hypothalamus, send projections to the cortex via the medial forebrain nuclei. The release of histamine promotes arousal by preventing sleep. Its cell bodies increase firing during periods of wakefulness and decrease during times of relaxation. It is believed that these neurons completely stop functioning during REM and non-REM sleep.

Clinical History and Management Considerations for Improving Cognition and Arousal

When considering the use of a neurostimulant in a patient with an acquired brain injury, examining the premorbid brain and the cause/pathophysiology of the injury, may assist in determining the most appropriate agent. Practitioners must also evaluate the medications a patient with a brain injury may already be on for potential sedating effects, including general anesthetics, anti-epileptics, or agents to control agitation or pain. Simply limiting the utilization of these medications can result in improved arousal and cognition.

The Premorbid Brain: In both selecting neurostimulation agents and in assessing treatment response, a key element to consider within the patient's history is the "premorbid brain," and interaction of both age and sex as biological variables. Pre-existing, untreated, or preclinical conditions such as attention deficit, hyperactivity disorder (ADHD), anxiety, depression, Parkinson's disease (PD), dementia, substance abuse, or other psychiatric history may influence current neurotransmitter levels, arousal, and/or cognitive deficits observed in the acute care setting. For example, premorbid conditions such as ADHD and PD may impact both medication choice and dosing strategy for DA stimulants. Individuals with symptom profiles as children and adults consistent with ADHD may respond to a different DA stimulant dosing regimen than others without this history. Older individuals may have underlying mild cognitive impairment, dementia, or preclinical PD, which are unmasked by their brain injury and require additional consideration with regard to neurostimulant selection [19, 20]. The drug abuse literature also suggests that women are more sensitive to the motor activating effects of classic DA stimulants, which again may be relevant when selecting and dosing a neurostimulant [21].

Injury Type: Trauma, Anoxia, Intracranial Hemorrhage Location: The type of brain injury can substantially impact the pharmacological approach chosen for any given patient in the acute care setting. There are key differences in the injury complex associated with brain injury from traumatic versus anoxic causes. Those with traumatic brain injury (TBI) often have evidence of diffuse axonal injury (DAI) affecting the brain stem, midline structures, and cortico-subcortical projections. Cortical contusion, often in the fronto-temporal region, is commonly observed with severe TBI, in combination with DAI. In these injuries, cortical, subcortical, and/or brain stem lesions may contribute to the clinical presentation, depending on the location of the injury.

Older individuals are more likely to have extra-axial lesions associated with their TBI complex, including subdural hematomas. Lesion size, hemisphere laterality, and resultant compression/swelling on other brain areas may impact neurostimulant selection. Those with traumatic injury, as well as those with spontaneous hemorrhage, may have subcortical hemorrhage involving the basal ganglia. Injury in this DA rich region requires thought about whether a DA transmission enhancing agent or a DA replacement agent might be better suited to enhance arousal and participation.

The injury complex associated with anoxic brain injury, including from cardiac arrest, contrasts with TBI presentation in several ways. Global ischemia, which accompanies an anoxic event, often results in tissue damage and dysfunction in multiple regions with low collateral blood flow and watershed areas. Structures often affected include the cortical white matter tracks, hippocampus, basal ganglia, thalamus, superior brainstem, and cerebellum. Also, movement disorders such as chorea, myoclonus, tremors, rigidity, and motor restlessness (e.g., akathisia), are common during acute care hospitalization for this population). Our experience is that these types of associated motor findings indicate that DA modulation, rather than enhancement, can be effective in improving both motor abnormalities and arousal. Clinical and preclinical data suggest that DA enhancing agents may worsen both movement disorders and arousal/cognitive status when initiated in the acute care setting; alternatively, non-dopaminergic agents, including cholinergic and GABAergic agents, can be effective in modulating both movement and arousal during the acute phases of care after global or regional anoxic brain injury [22–24].

Sedating Medications: When considering medications in the acute care setting to improve arousal and/or cognition, several elements of the patient's clinical status must be evaluated. Reviewing the medication(s) a patient is currently receiving will help determine if any of these agents have potential sedating side effects, or if it is otherwise medically appropriate to wean off some medications. Some sedating medications may be necessary in the acute care setting to manage other conditions associated with brain injury, such as paroxysmal sympathetic hyperactivity (PSH), pain, seizures, and/or alcohol withdrawal, among others. Common medication classes with sedating side effects include opiates, benzodiazepines, anticonvulsants, centrally acting anti-hypertensives, and antipsychotics. Initial recommendations focus on reviewing and optimizing sedating medications prior to trialing a neurostimulant, in which the goal would be to promote arousal while avoiding undesired medication side effects. Common neurostimulant medication side effects include restlessness and lowering the seizure threshold.

General Rubric for Pharmacological Treatment Selection

In addition to treatment effects, one must consider whether the anticipated benefits of such medications outweigh the risks, especially in medically complex patients. Patient age, ongoing medical and neurological conditions, and comorbidities must be carefully considered. The timing of medication initiation also poses a difficult question; what is an appropriate timeframe and/or clinical circumstance in which to initiate use of a neurostimulant? How will treatment effects be assessed when

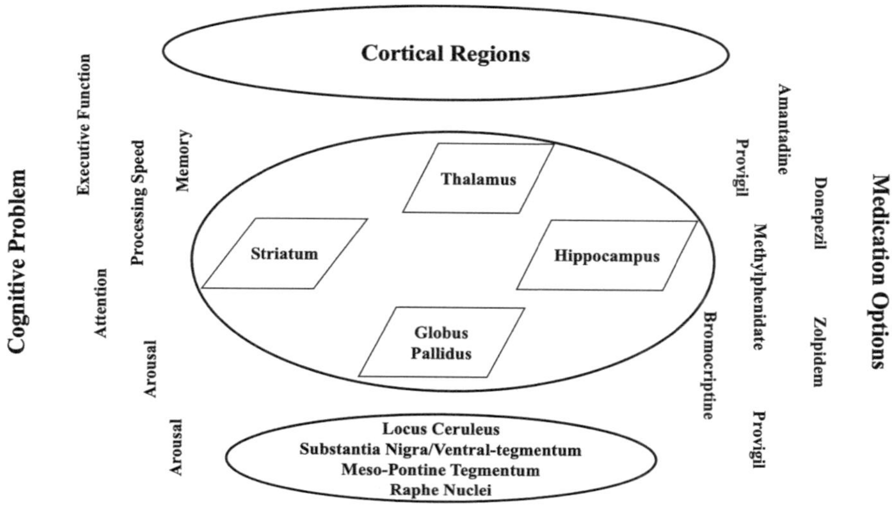

Fig. 5.1 represents a three-tiered schematic rubric for management of arousal and cognition outlining the pertinent anatomy, neurotransmitter systems, symptom profiles, and medications associated with arousal and cognition in the setting of acquired brain injury. The lower oval represents brainstem structures that project to cortical and subcortical structures and play a significant role in arousal and in supporting other areas of cognitive function. The middle oval represents subcortical structures that support the major components of the meso-circuit, and the upper oval represents cortical regions. Though not completely compartmentalized, the available literature suggests that the medications commonly used to improve arousal and cognition can have varied effects in these regions that generate improvements in cognitive features known to be supported by these structures. The figure allows practitioners to assess the level of the primary areas of injury and use the word cloud as a guide to regional correlation with symptomotology and possible effective medications to consider to address arousal and cognitive function in the acute care setting, bearing in mind potential complications and side effects of each medication. Consistent with the meso-circuit hypothesis and cortical/subcortical disconnection, individuals with multicompartment injury (or subcortical/brainstem injury) may require medications that affect brainstem and subcortical regions prior to considering agents that promote cortical activation

considering other critical care and procedures provided? In these regards, practitioners should focus on the goal of beginning a neurostimulant.

When considering the goals of treatment for any given patient, one must consider the brain injury complex including structures affected, based on available imaging, physical exam findings, and integrity of key pathways reflected with electrophysiology studies, where applicable. In reviewing these findings, a useful strategy in selecting an appropriate pharmacological agent is to assess the level of brain structure to be targeted in the context of the cognitive problem to be addressed.

Often, arousal is the initial problem to be addressed and the focus of pharmacological management. Depressed consciousness may result from multiple mechanisms including (1) death of forebrain neurons, (2) deafferentation and disconnection of neurons, and (3) "circuit"-level functional disturbances due to the loss of these neuronal connections [25]. Figure 5.1 outlines these relationships by focusing on

Table 5.2 Medications and their increased or decreased stimulation of neurotransmitters [27–29]

Medications/ neurotransmitter	Dopamine	Norepinephrine	Acetylcholine	Serotonin	Histamine
Stimulation					
Methylphenidate	↑↑	↑↑		↑	↑↑
Atomoxetine	↑	↑↑			
Amantadine	↑↑		↓	↓↓	↓↓
Donepezil	↓		↑↑		↓↓
Bromocriptine	↑↓				↓↓
Provigil	↑↓	↑			↑

the brainstem, subcortical, or cortical symptoms and pharmacology. Particularly early after injury, pharmacological stimulation of arousal centers involved in striatal neurotransmission, and their downstream influence on pallido-thalamic-cortical circuitry supporting the meso-circuit hypothesis of arousal, are critical to early improvements in cognitive functioning [25, 26]. An understanding of the underlying pathophysiology associated with the injury type (e.g., TBI vs. anoxic brain injury) is key to this assessment. Chief among these distinctions regarding injury type includes an understanding of cortical deafferentation and brain stem rotational effects on striatal neurotransmission associated with trauma and well as an understanding of the vulnerability of GABAergic striatal projection neurons to hypoxic conditions associated with anoxic brain injury. When managing higher level cognitive issues, the focus is often on cortical and subcortical structures in selecting appropriate medications and treatment targets.

Medications commonly utilized as neurostimulants include Methylphenidate, Atomoxetine, Amantadine, Donepezil, Bromocriptine, and Modafinil (Table 5.2). Zolpidem has also been used for its paradoxical waking effects among some patients with DoC, however, current studies have primarily trialed this agent at later stages of recovery [30]. Medications that improve sleep architecture and the sleep/wake cycle may also indirectly improve arousal and cognition. While discussed in more detail in Chap. 6, evidence suggests that Trazodone, Seroquel, and neurohormonal supplementation with Melatonin, may improve arousal and cognition when paired with proper sleep hygiene practices and daytime stimulant medication use.

Methylphenidate: More commonly used in ADHD, Methylphenidate has similar effects on cognitive behavioral changes among individuals with acquired brain injury. Fatigue, mental slowing, and distractibility are common to both conditions. Methylphenidate acts primarily at the DA transporter level, blocking the re-uptake of DA and norepinephrine, subsequently increasing extracellular neurotransmitter levels [31, 32]. The striatum and frontal cortex are both pharmacological targets of this medication. Methylphenidate use as an acquired brain injury treatment has been associated with reduced mental fatigue as assessed on the Mental Fatigue Scale, in addition to improving attention, processing speed, and working memory [31]. In more severely impaired individuals, Methylphenidate can improve both arousal and processing speed [32, 33]. Though relatively uncommon, potential side effects of Methylphenidate include aggressive behavior, agitation, arrhythmias, hepatotoxicity, insomnia, nervousness, headaches, palpitations, abdominal pain, and nausea [34–36].

Atomoxetine: Another medication commonly utilized in those with ADHD that has potential to treat patients with brain injury is this selective presynaptic norepinephrine transport inhibitor [37]. As a noradrenaline re-uptake inhibitor, this medication prevents norepinephrine re-uptake, increasing its quantity in the regions of the brain discussed previously [33]. It has also been shown to minimally inhibit DA re-uptake as norepinephrine transporters support dopamine uptake in certain brain regions where there are lower DA transporter densities, such as the frontal cortex [38, 39]. Atomoxetine is believed to have its primary effect in the prefrontal cortex and locus coeruleus, crucial areas in regulating arousal and facilitating neural activity [37, 40]. Atomoxetine has gained attention in treating hypoarousal, initiation disorders, attention impairments, and fatigue [37]. Some research shows that early initiation of low dose Atomoxetine significantly attenuates cognitive deficits in injured animals as well [38]. Potential side effects include insomnia, nausea, vomiting, decreased appetite, weight loss, dyspepsia, dry mouth, and urinary retention [40].

Amantadine: Approved for use as both an anti-viral and an anti-Parkinson drug, Amantadine is a weak NMDA glutamate receptor antagonist that decreases glutamatergic neurotransmission, in addition to indirectly increasing DA release and decreasing DA re-uptake [31]. One large randomized clinical trial showed that Amantadine accelerated functional recovery as measured via the Disability Rating Scale [41]. Overall differences in recovery were not observed with treatment; however, use in the acute recovery stages may help avoid longer immobility periods and other physical, cognitive, and functional impairments that impact post-acute discharge planning. Early improvements may also help clinicians justify disposition to more intensive rehabilitation programs. Side effects include the possibility for over stimulation, particularly among older adults, as well as lowered lower seizure threshold, livedo reticularis, and peripheral edema [35, 42].

Donepezil: Primarily utilized in the dementia population, Donepezil is a centrally acting reversible anti-cholinesterase inhibitor. Although the exact mechanism of action is not well understood, this medication is believed to increase acetylcholine levels in the brain by deactivating acetylcholinesterase, the enzyme that degrades acetylcholine. This neurotransmitter supports multiple cognitive features, but can affect memory and spatial learning particularly after TBI [43]. In rodent research, donepezil facilitates neurogenesis, both in an uninjured and injured brain. With its role in increasing acetylcholine and neurogenesis, Donepezil aids in improving memory and spatial learning. However, Donepezil may also have modulatory effects on DA neurotransmission in the striatum, promoting striato-pallidal GABAergic outflow, particularly in the setting of anoxic brain injury. Although donepezil is generally considered a safe treatment agent, one must consider the risk for adverse events such as hemolytic anemia, Steven-Johnson syndrome, bradycardia, muscle cramps, fatigue, syncope, and urinary frequency and rhabdomyolysis [44–48].

Bromocriptine: This medication is a mixed agonist/antagonist acting at both the pre- and post-synaptic D2 striatum receptors, in addition to the D2 brain stem and hypothalamus auto-receptors. At low doses, Bromocriptine may act as an antagonist at D2 auto-receptors to increase DA release in the midbrain and striatum, which may impact both respiratory drive, arousal, and initiation. Bromocriptine also acts as a D1 antagonist at lower doses, which is also thought to be responsible for cognitive improvements [49, 50]. Post-synaptic D2 receptors, on the other hand, are targeted using higher doses of Bromocriptine. Its action in the striatum and frontal cortex improves cognition while its action in the hypothalamus can modulate hyperthermia and hypertension associated with dysautonomia. Bromocriptine use has been associated with adverse reactions such as hypotension, hallucinations, pulmonary fibrosis, involuntary movements, compulsive behaviors, seizures, and arrhythmias [51].

Modafinil: This medication is believed to work selectively in brain regions that regulate the sleep/wake cycle in helping to improve hypoarousal [52]. Although a DA transporter inhibitor [53] and D2 long receptor agonist [54], some studies suggest it can inhibit midbrain DA neuron firing [55]. Thus, the exact mechanism of action is not well understood. Rodent studies also suggest locus coeruleus activation with Modafinil [27, 28] and can increase histamine release [29]. Also, studies have shown that Modafinil causes posterior hypothalamus and medial pre-optic area gamma amino butyric acid release inhibition [56]. Furthermore, animal models have shown that the anterior hypothalamus, hippocampus, and the amygdala have increased activity after Modafinil administration [52, 57]. When prescribing Modafinil, potential side effects include headaches, nausea, vomiting, nervousness, anxiety, palpitations, chest pain, dyspnea, and insomnia [35, 58, 59].

Facilitating Sleep to Improve Arousal and Cognition (Table 5.3)

Zolpidem: Typically, Zolpidem has been utilized as a sleep aid as it is a non-benzodiazepine sedative-hypnotic agent. Zolpidem, belonging to the imidazoprines drug class, is a highly selective GABA-α1 receptor agonist, which increases total sleep time, and decreases sleep latency and nocturnal awakenings [60, 61]. It may also be useful in the setting of central sleep apnea [62]. Although sleep patterns are crucial to cognitive function, the role of Zolpidem in improving cognition and arousal, for some, goes beyond enhancing sleep habits. Recent studies suggest that pallidal-thalamic GABA receptor binding may increase meso-circuit connectivity after brain injury supporting the pallidal-thalamo-cortical activity needed to increase arousal and other areas of function [25, 26, 63–65]. Even outside of any paradoxical effects on arousal and cognition, restoration of related striato-pallidal outflow can also have a beneficial impact on movement disorders that commonly co-occur with anoxic brain injury [22, 23]. Though generally well tolerated, potential side effects

Table 5.3 Stimulation and sleep promotion medications

Medication practical dosing guide	Treatment indication	Primary mechanism	Starting dose	Dose escalation	Considerations concerns
Stimulation					
Methylphenidate	Arousal, attention, processing speed, working memory, and fatigue	NE and DA re-uptake inhibitor	2.5–5 mg qAM	Increase to BID (AM and noon); increase by 2.5 mg every 2–3 days up to 20 mg BID	Aggression, tachycardia, seizure, anorexia, insomnia
Atomoxetine	Arousal, initiation, attention, and fatigue	Presynaptic norepinephrine transport inhibitor	40 mg qAM	80 mg qAM after 3 days	Insomnia, nausea, vomiting, decreased appetite, weight loss, dyspepsia, dry mouth, urinary retention, suicidal ideation
Amantadine	Arousal, initiation, attention, and fatigue	Weak NMDA glutamate receptor antagonist; increases dopamine pre/post synaptically.	100 mg qAM, 50 in elderly	100 mg BID (AM and noon)	200 mg weekly in dialysis patients Hypotension, lowers seizure threshold, GI effects
Donepezil	Memory and spatial learning; low arousal and delirium particularly in anoxic brain injury	Reversible anti-cholinesterase inhibitor; DA modulation	5 mg qAM or qHS	Increase to 10 mg after 2 weeks	Hemolytic anemia, Steven-Johnson syndrome, bradycardia, muscle cramps, fatigue, syncope, urinary frequency
Bromocriptine	-some evidence for aphasia	D1 antagonist; D2 auto-receptor antagonist (low dose); D2 agonist (high dose)	2.5–5 mg qAM	5–20 mg BID (AM & noon)	Nausea, vomiting, hypotension

(continued)

Table 5.3 (continued)

Medication practical dosing guide	Treatment indication	Primary mechanism	Starting dose	Dose escalation	Considerations concerns
Provigil	Primarily for arousal	Dopamine re-uptake inhibitor	100 mg qAM, 50 in elderly	100 mg BID (AM and noon)	Headaches, nausea, nervousness, diarrhea, insomnia, anxiety
					Insurance coverage
Sleep promotion					
Zolpidem	Sleep initiation and maintenance	Selective GABA A receptor agonist	2.5–5 mg qHS	5–10 mg qHS	Falls. May have paradoxical awakening effects in disorders of consciousness.
Trazodone	Sleep initiation and maintenance	Sedating non-tricyclic anti-depressant	25–50 mg qHS	100–150 mg qHS	Dry mouth, headache, excessive drowsiness, hypotension, rebound insomnia, dizziness, priapism
Quetiapine	Sleep initiation	Atypical antipsychotic	12.5–25 mg qHS	75–100 mg qHS	QTc prolongation
Melatonin	Sleep initiation; circadian rhythm disorders	Exogenous hormone	1.5–3 mg qHS	6–9 mg qHS	Better scheduled than PRN

include hallucinations, amnesia, angioedema, headache, palpitations, and aggressive behavior.

Trazodone: As mentioned earlier, proper sleep patterns are vital to improving arousal and overall cognition. Sleep elements that may be altered after a brain injury include difficulty falling asleep, trouble staying asleep, awaking early, and non-restorative sleep [66]. Trazodone, a non-tricyclic anti-depressant, has sedative properties that facilitate sleep. Studies suggest that Trazodone decreases sleep latency and increases total sleep time [66, 67]. Potential side effects that would caution Trazodone use include dry mouth, headache, excessive drowsiness, hypotension, rebound insomnia, and dizziness [66, 67]. Even though Trazodone has a better cardiac profile than most tricyclic anti-depressants, it can increase QT intervals, which should be properly monitored in individuals with cardiac disease [66, 68] and/or have survived cardiac arrest.

Quetiapine: Agitation is a feature commonly observed after a brain injury. Many medications can help control agitation, however, patients with brain injury tolerate these medications differently than those without a brain injury. One medication commonly used to reduce agitation [69] and support sleep is Quetiapine [70]. This medication affects numerous neurotransmitters, acting as a DA, serotonin, and adrenergic antagonist, in addition to its anti-histamine and anti-cholinergic properties [71]. Quetiapine's role in agitation is discussed in Chap. 7, but this medication has sedating effects that occur via histamine H1 and serotonin 2A receptor antagonism [72]. Although Quetiapine's sedating effects are primarily utilized to assist those with psychiatric disorders sleep better, Quetiapine is notable within its class of medications, as it has a low incidence of extrapyramidal symptoms and may also help with patient's with movement disorders [70]. Potential side effects with Quetiapine use include tardive dyskinesia, dystonia, neuroleptic malignant syndrome, Steven-Johnson syndrome, seizures, QT prolongation, agranulocytosis, rhabdomyolysis, priapism, and pancreatitis [73].

Melatonin: As a natural substance produced in the pineal gland of the brain, Melatonin has both regulatory and protective effects. Most commonly known in its role in regulating the circadian rhythm of the sleep/wake cycle, Melatonin also confers some protection against oxidative stress, modulates the immune system, and regulates energy metabolism [74]. Among individuals with brain injuries, there is reduced evening and overnight levels of Melatonin production [75–77]. This is an important point as Melatonin is secreted diurnally, with its highest secretions occurring between 3 and 4 AM [78]. Evening Melatonin production correlates with REM sleep, hence Melatonin supplementation may assist in improving REM sleep [75]. Improved sleep patterns support better cognitive function, including improved focus and attention. Melatonin improves subjective sleep quality and reduces subjective self-reported anxiety and fatigue, even though it has no role in decreasing daytime sleepiness [75]. Potential side effects of Melatonin include excessive drowsiness [79, 80].

Evaluating Medication Effectiveness in the Context of Treatment Goals and Discharge Planning

With the range of medications to consider for addressing cognition and arousal, it is also essential to evaluate the effects of these medications. Early on, medication effects are difficult to differentiate from what otherwise might occur from natural brain recovery. Thus, a stable neurological and medical exam is essential prior to initiating pharmacotherapy. Moreover, neurorehabilitation consultants must monitor for potential side effects, determining if medication adjustments need to be made to support participation at various levels of care after acute care discharge.

Throughout this process, though, one must determine if the patient is appropriate for further rehabilitation at an acute or subacute level or a DoC care or other program, and if the program can provide an appropriate setting for the patient to improve functionally. Recent studies suggest that individuals with DoC can benefit from daily multidisciplinary rehabilitation program through improved level of arousal and body functions that support transition into regular acute inpatient rehabilitation programs [81]. Also, studies on 5-year outcomes for those with severe TBI and associated DoC suggest that many patients receiving acute inpatient rehabilitation before following commands can recover independent functioning over a 5-year trajectory, particularly if they begin to follow commands prior to inpatient rehabilitation hospital discharge [82]. Together, these studies provide great impetus to support early improvements in cognition and arousal during acute care hospitalization, including those with DoC, through pharmacological intervention. In fact, our own data suggest that doing so improves the chances of emergence from DoC states during acute inpatient rehabilitation compared to standard acute consultative rehabilitation care [83]. Also, early pharmacological intervention may have neuro-restorative capacities that may prevent or mitigate CNS damage and some adverse long-term consequences common to this population. No matter the setting in which the patient transitions after acute care, there is usually functional progress to be made when participating in rehabilitation care, and as the consulting physician, we can greatly influence treatment and discharge disposition goals by advancing patient functional abilities in the acute care setting by advocating for and adopting neuropharmacology modalities to enhance arousal and cognition that have been traditionally reserved for acute rehabilitation.

Case Illustration

Case 1

A 29-year-old male patient was admitted to the hospital following a motor vehicle collision with a Glasgow Coma Scale (GCS) Score on admission of 3T. He was intubated prior to arrival in the trauma bay, and a computed tomography (CT) scan of the brain revealed a left epidural hematoma with significant midline shift requiring emergent decompression and left thalamic intracranial hemorrhage. A magnetic resonance imaging (MRI) scan was performed on hospital day 3 for prognostication, which showed a moderate diffuse axonal injury with gross focal lesions in the corpus callosum. The primary service performed an early tracheostomy and percutaneous endoscopic gastrostomy placement. He was started on Amantadine 100 mg at 7 AM and 1 PM by the primary team, and Physical Medicine & Rehabilitation (PM&R) was consulted on hospital day 7.

Upon entering the room, the patient's eyes were closed, but nursing reported that the patient's eyes were intermittently open throughout the day and night. The patient did not require sedation. On examination, the patient's eyes opened with stimulation, and the patient had a visual and auditory startle, could localize to noxious stimuli, had oral reflexive movements, and had no verbal output or communication. Melatonin was started for sleep-wake cycle regulation. By hospital day 12, the patient's mental status failed to improve on amantadine and was discontinued. Per PM&R recommendation, bromocriptine was started on Day 12 at 1.25 mg at 7 AM and 1PM, with intermittent tracking observed on exam and rapid ventilator wean noted. On Day 16, a zolpidem trial was started, and 10 mg of zolpidem was administered at 8 AM, followed by serial neurologic exams every hour for 4 h. After the administration of zolpidem, there was a sustained behavioral response to visual, auditory, and physical stimuli, and he could engage in limited meaningful conversation. For example, when he was asked to lift his hand, smile, or count to five, he did so. He could also answer simple questions and write his name. From no response before the zolpidem application, there was a limited response to commands at 20–30 min after zolpidem, and maximum arousal was 1 h after administration. The effect lasted for approximately 6 h, and the patient's zolpidem dose was changed to 10 mg twice daily, and the patient was discharged to inpatient rehabilitation by hospital day 16 for further rehabilitation and pharmacological management.

Case 2

A 26-year-old male with a history of Graves' disease post-ablation presented to the emergency department following cardiac arrest secondary to a drug overdose with severe anoxic brain injury MRI performed several days post-admission showed evidence of diffusion restriction involving the basal ganglia and thalamus bilaterally. The patient was not on sedation at the time of PM&R consult examination. On exam, the patient's eyes opened with stimulation. He displayed a visual and auditory startle, flexion posturing to noxious stimuli, oral reflexive movements, and no verbal output or communication. The examination was also notable for myoclonus, with observable fine motor myoclonus affecting intrinsic muscles of hands and feet. On hospital day 6, the patient was started on donepezil 5 mg daily to modulate striatal dopamine release and promote coordinated GABAergic outflow via D1 and D2 type MSN, which are selectively vulnerable to hypoxic ischemic brain injury. The patient progressed with resolution of myoclonus, abilities for spontaneous eye opening with visual pursuit, reproducible command following with object manipulation, and inconsistent vocalization with no functional communication. Seven days after starting donepezil, the patient has a persistently elevated creatinine (2.6). A creatinine phosphokinase (CPK) was ordered and found to be >40,000. Donepezil was stopped, and CPK down trended to 3856 with normal creatinine. An EMG/NCS was performed, which was normal and did not show evidence of myopathy, neuropathy, or neuromuscular disease. It was unclear if the rhabdomyolysis was secondary to myoclonus or donepezil, and donepezil 5 mg was restarted, resulting in CPK trending up from 52 to 373 over 48 h. Donepezil was stopped, and the CPK trended back to normal. Once the donepezil was discontinued, the examination worsened with reduced cognitive function, but myoclonus did not re-emerge. At this point, eye opening was elicited with stimulation, visual and auditory startle were present, flexion posturing to noxious stimuli and oral reflexive movements returned, and no verbal output or communication was noted. The patient was discharged to a DoC program, improving to an emerged, but severely impaired, level of function at the time of inpatient rehabilitation discharge to the community with his family.

References[1]

1. Eapen BC, Georgekutty J, Subbarao B, Bavishi S, Cifu DX. Disorders of consciousness. Phys Med Rehabil Clin N Am. 2017;28(2):245–58.
2. Portaccio E, Morrocchesi A, Romoli AM, et al. Improvement on the coma recovery scale-revised during the first four weeks of hospital stay predicts outcome at discharge in intensive rehabilitation after severe brain injury. Arch Phys Med Rehabil. 2018;99(5):914–9.
3. McDonnell E, Giacino JT, Kolakowsky-Hayner SA. A brief overview of the coma recovery scale-revised: updates from the COMBI. J Head Trauma Rehabil. 2015;30(2):143–5.
4. Kothari S, Flanagan SR, Kwasnica C, Brown AW, Elovic EP. Congenital and acquired brain injury. 5. Emerging concepts in prognostication, evaluation, and treatment. Arch Phys Med Rehabil. 2008;89(3 Suppl 1):S27–31.
5. Wagner AK. Advances in innovative therapies to enhance neural recovery. In: Zasler NK, Katz DI, Zafonte RD, editors. Brain injury medicine: principles and practice. 2nd ed. New York: Demos Medical; 2013.
6. Wagner AK. Research in traumatic brain injury: current concepts and issues. In: Zasler ND, Katz DI, Zafonte RD, editors. Brain injury medicine. 3rd ed. New York: Demos Medical; 2021.
7. Mysiw WJ, Sandel ME. The agitated brain injured patient. Part 2: pathophysiology and treatment. Arch Phys Med Rehabil. 1997;78(2):213–20.
8. Camps M, Cortes R, Gueye B, Probst A, Palacios JM. Dopamine receptors in human brain: autoradiographic distribution of D2 sites. Neuroscience. 1989;28(2):275–90.
9. Booij J, Tissingh G, Winogrodzka A, van Royen EA. Imaging of the dopaminergic neurotransmission system using single-photon emission tomography and positron emission tomography in patients with parkinsonism. Eur J Nucl Med. 1999;26(2):171–82.
10. Abbott SB, Kanbar R, Bochorishvili G, Coates MB, Stornetta RL, Guyenet PG. C1 neurons excite locus coeruleus and A5 noradrenergic neurons along with sympathetic outflow in rats. J Physiol. 2012;590(12):2897–915.
11. Dougall D, Poole N, Agrawal N. Pharmacotherapy for chronic cognitive impairment in traumatic brain injury. Cochrane Database Syst Rev. 2015;12:CD009221.
12. Osier ND, Dixon CE. Catecholaminergic based therapies for functional recovery after TBI. Brain Res. 2016;1640(Pt A):15–35.
13. Schwarz LA, Luo L. Organization of the locus coeruleus-norepinephrine system. Curr Biol. 2015;25(21):R1051–6.
14. De Cicco V, Tramonti Fantozzi MP, Cataldo E, et al. Trigeminal, visceral and vestibular inputs may improve cognitive functions by acting through the locus coeruleus and the ascending reticular activating system: a new hypothesis. Front Neuroanat. 2017;11:130.
15. Gais S, Schonauer M. Untangling a cholinergic pathway from wakefulness to memory. Neuron. 2017;94(4):696–8.
16. Boucetta S, Cisse Y, Mainville L, Morales M, Jones BE. Discharge profiles across the sleep-waking cycle of identified cholinergic, GABAergic, and glutamatergic neurons in the pontomesencephalic tegmentum of the rat. J Neurosci. 2014;34(13):4708–27.
17. Jeon J, Dencker D, Wortwein G, et al. A subpopulation of neuronal M4 muscarinic acetylcholine receptors plays a critical role in modulating dopamine-dependent behaviors. J Neurosci. 2010;30(6):2396–405.
18. Threlfell S, Clements MA, Khodai T, et al. Striatal muscarinic receptors promote activity dependence of dopamine transmission via distinct receptor subtypes on cholinergic interneurons in ventral versus dorsal striatum. J Neurosci. 2010;30(9):3398–408.
19. Kesler SR, Adams HF, Blasey CM, Bigler ED. Premorbid intellectual functioning, education, and brain size in traumatic brain injury: an investigation of the cognitive reserve hypothesis. Appl Neuropsychol. 2003;10(3):153–62.

[1] Key References [1, 5, 7, 11, 25, 31, 33, 64].

20. Crownover J, Galang GNF, Wagner A. Rehabilitation considerations for traumatic brain injury in the geriatric population: epidemiology, neurobiology, prognosis, and management. Cur Translat Geriatr Exp Gerontol Rep. 2012;1(3):149–58.
21. Schindler CW, Carmona GN. Effects of dopamine agonists and antagonists on locomotor activity in male and female rats. Pharmacol Biochem Behav. 2002;72(4):857–63.
22. Pinto S, Kandt J, Ferimer S, Wagner A. Donepezil and zolpidem associated emergence from disordered consciousness after cardiac arrest: implications involving striatal circuitry and dopamine modulation [abstract]. Am J Phys Med Rehabil. 2017;96(3):A46.
23. Sawyer K, Callaway C, Wagner A. Life after death: surviving cardiac arrest—an overview of epidemiology, best acute care practices, and considerations for rehabilitation care. Curr Phys Med Rehabil Rep. 2017;5:30–9.
24. Desmarais LM, Milleville KA, Wagner AK. Postoperative treatment of intracranial hypotension venous congestion-associated brain injury with Zolpidem. Am J Phys Med Rehabil. 2021;100(6):e89–92.
25. Schiff ND. Recovery of consciousness after brain injury: a mesocircuit hypothesis. Trends Neurosci. 2010;33(1):1–9.
26. Giacino JT, Fins JJ, Laureys S, Schiff ND. Disorders of consciousness after acquired brain injury: the state of the science. Nat Rev Neurol. 2014;10(2):99–114.
27. Minzenberg MJ, Watrous AJ, Yoon JH, Ursu S, Carter CS. Modafinil shifts human locus coeruleus to low-tonic, high-phasic activity during functional MRI. Science. 2008;322(5908):1700–2.
28. Hou RH, Freeman C, Langley RW, Szabadi E, Bradshaw CM. Does modafinil activate the locus coeruleus in man? Comparison of modafinil and clonidine on arousal and autonomic functions in human volunteers. Psychopharmacology. 2005;181(3):537–49.
29. Ishizuka T, Murakami M, Yamatodani A. Involvement of central histaminergic systems in modafinil-induced but not methylphenidate-induced increases in locomotor activity in rats. Eur J Pharmacol. 2008;578(2-3):209–15.
30. Thonnard M, Gosseries O, Demertzi A, et al. Effect of zolpidem in chronic disorders of consciousness: a prospective open-label study. Funct Neurol. 2013;28(4):259–64.
31. Liepert J. Update on pharmacotherapy for stroke and traumatic brain injury recovery during rehabilitation. Curr Opin Neurol. 2016;29(6):700–5.
32. Jenkins PO, Mehta MA, Sharp DJ. Catecholamines and cognition after traumatic brain injury. Brain. 2016;139(Pt 9):2345–71.
33. Diaz-Arrastia R, Kochanek PM, Bergold P, et al. Pharmacotherapy of traumatic brain injury: state of the science and the road forward: report of the Department of Defense Neurotrauma Pharmacology Workgroup. J Neurotrauma. 2014;31(2):135–58.
34. Kis B, Lucke C, Abdel-Hamid M, et al. Safety profile of methylphenidate under long-term treatment in adult ADHD patients—results of the COMPAS study. Pharmacopsychiatry. 2020;53(6):263–71.
35. Nourbakhsh B, Revirajan N, Morris B, et al. Safety and efficacy of amantadine, modafinil, and methylphenidate for fatigue in multiple sclerosis: a randomised, placebo-controlled, crossover, double-blind trial. Lancet Neurol. 2021;20(1):38–48.
36. Methylphenidate. 2019. https://medlineplus.gov/druginfo/meds/a682188.html. Accessed 10 Feb 2022.
37. Ripley DL. Atomoxetine for individuals with traumatic brain injury. J Head Trauma Rehabil. 2006;21(1):85–8.
38. Reid WM, Hamm RJ. Post-injury atomoxetine treatment improves cognition following experimental traumatic brain injury. J Neurotrauma. 2008;25(3):248–56.
39. Moron JA, Brockington A, Wise RA, Rocha BA, Hope BT. Dopamine uptake through the norepinephrine transporter in brain regions with low levels of the dopamine transporter: evidence from knock-out mouse lines. J Neurosci. 2002;22(2):389–95.
40. Christman AK, Fermo JD, Markowitz JS. Atomoxetine, a novel treatment for attention-deficit-hyperactivity disorder. Pharmacotherapy. 2004;24(8):1020–36.

41. Giacino JT, Whyte J, Bagiella E, et al. Placebo-controlled trial of amantadine for severe traumatic brain injury. N Engl J Med. 2012;366(9):819–26.
42. Amantadine. 2019. https://medlineplus.gov/druginfo/meds/a682064.html. Accessed 10 Feb 2022.
43. Yu TS, Kim A, Kernie SG. Donepezil rescues spatial learning and memory deficits following traumatic brain injury independent of its effects on neurogenesis. PLoS One. 2015;10(2):e0118793.
44. Jackson S, Ham RJ, Wilkinson D. The safety and tolerability of donepezil in patients with Alzheimer's disease. Br J Clin Pharmacol. 2004;58(Suppl 1):1–8.
45. Malik BH, Hamid P, Khan S, Gupta D, Islam M. Correlation between donepezil and QTc prolongation and Torsades de pointes: a very rare phenomenon. Cureus. 2019;11(12):e6451.
46. Alexander E, Weppner JL. Case report: delayed diagnosis of non-traumatic acute compartment syndrome in an adolescent athlete [abstract]. Am J Phys Med Rehabil. 2021;100(4 Suppl 2):a1–a204.
47. Carrasco MM, Aguera L, Gil P, Morinigo A, Leon T. Safety and effectiveness of donepezil on behavioral symptoms in patients with Alzheimer disease. Alzheimer Dis Assoc Disord. 2011;25(4):333–40.
48. Donepezil. 2019. https://medlineplus.gov/druginfo/meds/a682188.html. Accessed 10 Feb 2022.
49. Goetz CG, Diederich NJ. Dopaminergic agonists in the treatment of Parkinson's disease. Neurol Clin. 1992;10(2):527–40.
50. McDowell S, Whyte J, D'Esposito M. Differential effect of a dopaminergic agonist on prefrontal function in traumatic brain injury patients. Brain. 1998;121(Pt 6):1155–64.
51. Bromocriptine. 2019. https://medlineplus.gov/druginfo/meds/a682079.html. Accessed 10 Feb 2022.
52. Elovic E. Use of provigil for underarousal following TBI. J Head Trauma Rehabil. 2000;15(4):1068–71.
53. Karabacak Y, Sase S, Aher YD, et al. The effect of modafinil on the rat dopamine transporter and dopamine receptors D1-D3 paralleling cognitive enhancement in the radial arm maze. Front Behav Neurosci. 2015;9:215.
54. Seeman P, Guan HC, Hirbec H. Dopamine D2High receptors stimulated by phencyclidines, lysergic acid diethylamide, salvinorin a, and modafinil. Synapse. 2009;63(8):698–704.
55. Korotkova TM, Klyuch BP, Ponomarenko AA, Lin JS, Haas HL, Sergeeva OA. Modafinil inhibits rat midbrain dopaminergic neurons through D2-like receptors. Neuropharmacology. 2007;52(2):626–33.
56. Ferraro L, Antonelli T, Tanganelli S, et al. The vigilance promoting drug modafinil increases extracellular glutamate levels in the medial preoptic area and the posterior hypothalamus of the conscious rat: prevention by local GABAA receptor blockade. Neuropsychopharmacology. 1999;20(4):346–56.
57. Lin JS, Hou Y, Jouvet M. Potential brain neuronal targets for amphetamine-, methylphenidate-, and modafinil-induced wakefulness, evidenced by c-fos immunocytochemistry in the cat. Proc Natl Acad Sci U S A. 1996;93(24):14128–33.
58. Sousa A, Dinis-Oliveira RJ. Pharmacokinetic and pharmacodynamic of the cognitive enhancer modafinil: relevant clinical and forensic aspects. Subst Abus. 2020;41(2):155–73.
59. Modafinil. 2019. https://medlineplus.gov/druginfo/meds/a602016.html. Accessed 10 Feb 2022.
60. Wagner J, Wagner ML. Non-benzodiazepines for the treatment of insomnia. Sleep Med Rev. 2000;4(6):551–81.
61. Whyte J, Rajan R, Rosenbaum A, et al. Zolpidem and restoration of consciousness. Am J Phys Med Rehabil. 2014;93(2):101–13.
62. Quadri S, Drake C, Hudgel DW. Improvement of idiopathic central sleep apnea with zolpidem. J Clin Sleep Med. 2009;5(2):122–9.

63. Sanger DJ. The pharmacology and mechanisms of action of new generation, non-benzodiazepine hypnotic agents. CNS Drugs. 2004;18(Suppl 1):9–15; discussion 41, 43-15.
64. Pistoia F, Mura E, Govoni S, Fini M, Sara M. Awakenings and awareness recovery in disorders of consciousness: is there a role for drugs? CNS Drugs. 2010;24(8):625–38.
65. Noormandi A, Shahrokhi M, Khalili H. Potential benefits of zolpidem in disorders of consciousness. Expert Rev Clin Pharmacol. 2017;10(9):983–92.
66. Flanagan SR, Greenwald B, Wieber S. Pharmacological treatment of insomnia for individuals with brain injury. J Head Trauma Rehabil. 2007;22(1):67–70.
67. Mendelson WB. A review of the evidence for the efficacy and safety of trazodone in insomnia. J Clin Psychiatry. 2005;66(4):469–76.
68. Levenson JL. Prolonged QT interval after trazodone overdose. Am J Psychiatry. 1999;156(6):969–70.
69. Kim E, Bijlani M. A pilot study of quetiapine treatment of aggression due to traumatic brain injury. J Neuropsychiatry Clin Neurosci. 2006;18(4):547–9.
70. Elovic EP, Jasey NN Jr, Eisenberg ME. The use of atypical antipsychotics after traumatic brain injury. J Head Trauma Rehabil. 2008;23(2):132–5.
71. Chew ML, Mulsant BH, Pollock BG, et al. Anticholinergic activity of 107 medications commonly used by older adults. J Am Geriatr Soc. 2008;56(7):1333–41.
72. Anderson SL, Vande Griend JP. Quetiapine for insomnia: a review of the literature. Am J Health Syst Pharm. 2014;71(5):394–402.
73. Quetiapine. 2019. https://medlineplus.gov/druginfo/meds/a698019.html. Accessed 10 Feb 2022.
74. Alghamdi BS. The neuroprotective role of melatonin in neurological disorders. J Neurosci Res. 2018;96:1136–49.
75. Grima NA, Rajaratnam SMW, Mansfield D, Sletten TL, Spitz G, Ponsford JL. Efficacy of melatonin for sleep disturbance following traumatic brain injury: a randomised controlled trial. BMC Med. 2018;16(1):8.
76. Grima NA, Ponsford JL, St Hilaire MA, Mansfield D, Rajaratnam SM. Circadian melatonin rhythm following traumatic brain injury. Neurorehabil Neural Repair. 2016;30(10):972–7.
77. Shekleton JA, Parcell DL, Redman JR, Phipps-Nelson J, Ponsford JL, Rajaratnam SM. Sleep disturbance and melatonin levels following traumatic brain injury. Neurology. 2010;74(21):1732–8.
78. Claustrat B, Leston J. Melatonin: physiological effects in humans. Neurochirurgie. 2015;61(2-3):77–84.
79. Foley HM, Steel AE. Adverse events associated with oral administration of melatonin: a critical systematic review of clinical evidence. Complement Ther Med. 2019;42:65–81.
80. Melatonin. https://medlineplus.gov/druginfo/natural/940.html. Accessed 10 Feb 2022.
81. Seel R, Douglas J, Dennison A, Heaner S, Farris K, Rogers C. Specialized early treatment for persons with disorders of consciousness: program components and outcomes. Arch Phys Med Rehabil. 2013;94(10):1908–23.
82. Whyte J, Nakase-Richardson R, Hammond FM, et al. Functional outcomes in traumatic disorders of consciousness: 5-year outcomes from the National Institute on Disability and Rehabilitation Research Traumatic Brain Injury Model Systems. Arch Phys Med Rehabil. 2013;94(10):1855–60.
83. Weppner JL, Linsenmeyer MA, Wagner AK. Effects of an acute care brain injury medicine continuity consultation service on health care utilization and rehabilitation outcomes. PM R. 2021;13(11):1227–36.

Chapter 6
Sleep Wake Cycle Dysfunction Following Traumatic Brain Injury in the Acute Care Setting

Mary Miller Phillips, Mark Linsenmeyer, and Christian Aponte-Lopez

Chapter Objectives
1. Understand the basic sleep principles and pathophysiology of sleep following traumatic brain injury.
2. Describe the types, prevalence, and effects of sleep wake cycle dysfunction on outcomes in persons with traumatic brain injury.
3. Understand the evaluation of sleep wake cycle dysfunction.
4. Outline non-pharmacological and pharmacological interventions for disordered sleep after traumatic brain injury.

Introduction

Prevalence of SWCD Following TBI

Traumatic brain injury (TBI) survivors experience a greater prevalence of sleep wake cycle dysfunction (SWCD) compared to the general population. In one study, 50% of TBI survivors experienced SWCD, with 25–29% being diagnosed with a formal sleep disorder (insomnia, hypersomnia, sleep-related disordered breathing) [1]. This contrasts with the 9–17% of the general population who report SWCD [2].

M. M. Phillips · C. Aponte-Lopez
Baylor Scott and White Institute for Rehabilitation, Dallas, TX, USA
e-mail: Mary.millerphillips@bswhealth.org; christian.lopez23@upr.edu

M. Linsenmeyer (✉)
Department of Physical Medicine and Rehabilitation, Sunnyview Rehabilitation Hospital, Schenectady, NY, USA
e-mail: mark.linsenmeyer@sphp.com

A. K. Wagner, J. Weppner (eds.), *Acute Care Neuroconsultation and Neurorehabilitation Management*, https://doi.org/10.1007/978-3-031-42830-2_6

Various studies have shown that SWCD prevalence following TBI ranges from 46% to 100% depending on the study's sample selection, time interval from injury, severity of injury, comorbidities, and patient versus examiner assessment of sleep [3]. Sleep disorders are often noted more frequently in mild TBI than in more severe cases, potentially due to increased insight and ability to report symptoms [4]. SWCD after TBI have also been found to be associated with pain, depressive symptoms, and fatigue [2, 4].

Effects of Sleep Wake Cycle Dysfunction on Outcomes

SWCD can have negative effects on TBI survivors' hospital and rehabilitation courses. Naske-Richardson et al. demonstrated high prevalence of SWCD in a prospective study of inpatient rehabilitation (IPR) patients 1-month post-injury. In this population, the severity of sleep wake disturbances predicted duration of post-traumatic amnesia and hospital length of stay (LOS). Given the high prevalence of SWCD in these patients at 1 month post-injury, the authors suggest that sleep disturbances may have been even more prominent earlier in recovery, likely while admitted to acute care settings [5].

SWCD has detrimental effects on mood, cognition, behavior, and pain perception following TBI. TBI patients with concomitant sleep apnea perform worse on neuropsychological testing than their counterparts without SWCD, particularly short-term memory and sustained attention domains [6]. Those with SWCD after chronic TBI also report increased pain, impaired memory, fatigue, and psychological distress with poorer social function and behavioral control [4]. These individuals have reported having more difficulty staying awake during treatment sessions and a higher number of missed outpatient follow-up visits [7, 8]. Finally, among those with acute TBI, individuals with moderate-to-severe OSA (obstructive sleep apnea) demonstrate worse processing speed, working memory, and executive functioning [9].

Sleep Principles

Sleep contributes to brain development and maturation as well as restoration including tissue repair, physical energy, and modulation of psychological functions [10]. Sleep contributes to neurorecovery through growth hormone secretion and cortisol inhibition and also contributes to proper immune system function [11]. A 2015 Joint Consensus Statement of the American Academy of Sleep Medicine and Sleep Research Society recommended that adults sleep for seven or more hours per night on a regular basis and detailed negative effects associated with regularly sleeping fewer hours including weight gain, obesity, diabetes, hypertension, heart disease, stroke, depression, and increased risk of death. Sleeping greater than 9 h was deemed to be appropriate for younger adults and individuals recovering from a sleep debt or illness, with an uncertain health risk in individuals not described by these categories [12].

Sleep regulation is mediated by both the internal circadian clock and homeostatic factors. The circadian clock is influenced by cues in the environment, most importantly the light-dark cycle, while homeostatic factors are influenced most by adenosine accumulation while awake [13]. The term "sleep architecture" refers to the pattern of sleep cycles an individual experiences each night. Most people typically experience 4–5 sleep cycles on average each night; each cycle consists of both non-rapid eye movement sleep (NREM) and rapid eye movement (REM) sleep. NREM sleep lasts approximately 30–90 min followed by 90 min of REM sleep. REM periods increase in duration toward the early morning hours or later sleep cycles. REM sleep accounts for 20–25% of total sleep. Sleep architecture varies greatly depending on age and can be affected by factors such as medical conditions or interventions, neurologic disorders, environment, and genetics [14].

While awake, the brain alternates between alpha and beta activity. Beta waves predominate when an individual is alert and visually scanning the environment. Alpha waves predominate when an individual is inactive and eyes are closed. NREM sleep can be divided into three distinct stages: N1, N2, and N3 with N3 comprised of stage 3 and stage 4 of the previous nomenclature. N1 constitutes 2–5% of sleep and is characterized by intrusion of theta waves and waning of alpha activity—slow rolling eye movements. N2 constitutes 45–55% of sleep and is characterized by multiple frequencies: theta activity, K complexes, and sleep spindles—minimal eye movements. N3, otherwise known as slow wave sleep, is characterized by delta waves increases and dominating. During REM sleep, theta and beta waves return and sleep becomes "paradoxical" as electroencephalography (EEG) appears desynchronized with low voltage fast activity similar to what is seen during wakefulness. Patients demonstrate rapid eye movements with absent muscle activity [15]. After TBI, sleep is more disordered and less deep; there is more N1 and N2 sleep, less REM sleep, and overall, it is more difficult to objectively distinguish between stages of sleep [16].

Pathophysiology of Sleep Wake Cycle Dysfunction Following TBI

Causes of SWCD following TBI are likely multifactorial and include damage to the brain structures, secondary inflammatory factors, predisposing factors, associated symptoms, and environmental factors particularly in hospital and ICU environments.

A primary mechanism by which TBI may affect sleep is direct or indirect damage to sleep center structures or other connections. Damage to the reticular activating system, basal forebrain, or the anterior hypothalamus or their connections can lead to impaired expression of neurohormonal mediators. Damage to the hypothalamus can affect orexin (hypocretin), which plays a key role in sleep regulation; moderate-to-severe TBI can reduce the number orexin-secreting neurons [17] and is associated with abnormally lower hypocretin-1 levels in 95% of patients compared to controls [18]. Damage to the pineal gland, which synthesizes melatonin, a key regulator of sleep wake cycles, can also lead to SWCD [19]. Neurotrauma patients reportedly have significantly lower levels of evening melatonin compared to matched controls [20]. In addition to damage to the pineal gland itself, other factors in the ICU setting can influence melatonin homeostasis, including light exposure, mechanical ventilation, sepsis, or medications. ICU patients without TBI had similarly low levels of serum melatonin compared with those diagnosed with TBI, suggesting that critical illness in isolation may be enough to alter melatonin homeostasis [21]. Cytokine-mediated inflammatory cascades provoked by TBI can negatively impact sleep, particularly with microglial cytokine release, which function as sleep regulatory substances [22]. Interleukin (IL)-6, IL-1β, and tumor necrosis factor (TNF)-α are key cytokines involved in sleep regulation after TBI [23].

Other symptoms associated with TBI can also contribute to SWCD including pain, mood, agitation, and restlessness. The hospital environment, particularly the ICU setting, can also be particularly disruptive to sleep. Patient rooms typically lack windows and have excessive artificial light at night that impact circadian rhythms [24]. Noise levels in ICU settings often exceed Environmental Protection Agency recommendations [25]. Noise sources may include staff conversations, ventilator and other alarms, and neighboring patients. Nighttime vital sign monitoring and phlebotomy draws also affect sleep. Finally, medications such as sedatives, analgesics, and vasoactive drugs, in addition to physical symptoms of critical illness such as dyspnea, anxiety, and pain may also disrupt sleep. Once patients are admitted to an IPR setting, many of the above environmental factors are reduced, however, these deleterious factors should be recognized and controlled. The consulting physiatrist can play a role in reducing these factors in the acute care setting using a collaborative team approach.

Evaluation of Sleep Wake Cycle Dysfunction Following TBI

Sleep can be evaluated both objectively and subjectively. Subjective assessments include sleep diaries, questionnaires, and sleep logs. Sleep assessments in the IPR setting often rely on subjective measures such as self-reports, overnight nurse reports, or nursing sleep logs based on intervals of eye closure throughout the night. In addition, sleep diaries can describe the nature, severity, and frequency of sleep-related problems. Questionnaires, including the Epworth Sleepiness Scale and Pittsburgh Sleep Quality Index, have been partially validated in the TBI population [26]. Other potential questionnaires to consider include the Insomnia Severity Index, Stanford Sleepiness Scale, Morningness-Eveningness Questionnaire, and Sleep Timing Questionnaire.

Objective measures are often more appropriate than the above measures in the TBI population, particularly in the acute setting where patients may exhibit post-traumatic amnesia, impaired short-term memory, or confabulation. Currently, polysomnography (PSG) is the gold standard objective measure of sleep. PSG utilizes EEG, electromyography (EMG), and electrooculography (EOG) to directly measure sleep stages. However, while shown to be feasible, the use of PSG in the acute care or IPR setting is limited. Barriers include cost of equipment, requirement for specialty training for interpretation, and the medical complexity of patients that prevents overnight studies in a traditional sleep laboratory. PSG is also not traditionally used in a serial fashion for tracking intervention-based outcomes [27, 28].

Actigraphy is emerging as an alternative objective measure more suited for sleep measurement in a hospital-based setting. Actigraph devices are typically worn on the wrist but can be placed on any limb. The devices measure movement during sleep. Some actigraph devices are equipped to measure additional parameters that influence sleep such as ambient temperature and light. Importantly, actigraph measurements have been shown to be comparable to PSG measurements for certain variables, not including sleep apnea. A retrospective review of patients receiving concurrent testing with PSG and actigraphy showed that actigraphy is a valid proxy for monitoring total sleep time and sleep efficiency after TBI across injury severity and common comorbidity groups [29]. Prospective evaluation of hospitalized patients with TBI and poor sleep revealed that actigraphy underestimated the level of sleep disruption compared to PSG measurements. Actigraphy to monitor sleep is becoming more common due to is practicality; however, caution is warranted because actigraphy measurements are based on limb movements, which may be influenced by patient characteristics such as severe spasticity, paresis, and disorders of consciousness [30].

While common sleep disorders after TBI include dyssomnias (associated with complaints of insomnia or hypersomnia) or parasomnias (episodic events that occur during sleep), the remainder of our discussion will focus primarily on insomnia, the most common sleep disorder after TBI.

Management of Insomnia

Non-pharmacologic Management

Obtaining a thorough history and physical examination is key to the formulation of an appropriate treatment plan for SWCD. In the acute care setting, this can be limited by the patient's ability to participate, and information may need to be collected from family and staff. It is essential to review the patient's premorbid sleep patterns and medical history as well as any prior sleep medication or continuous or bilevel positive airway pressure (CPAP/BiPAP) use. Inquire about symptoms of SWCD such as snoring, excessive sleepiness, restlessness or agitation, and headache. The sleep environment should also be discussed.

In the acute care setting, a consultant can recommend environmental modifications such as light/temperature adjustments, exposure to daylight, reducing ambient noise, turning off televisions, limiting or rescheduling overnight blood draws and vital sign checks, and placing signs on the patient's door. The timing of neurostimulant medications should be assessed and proper sleep hygiene should be discussed with the patient. A nurse-driven sleep hygiene protocol in the ICU has demonstrated significant improvement in patient-reported sleep disruptions [31]. A few patients may also benefit from pulmonology consultation for sleep disordered breathing in the acute setting, as sleep apnea is a common complication of TBI and can worsen attention and memory if left untreated.

Pharmacologic Management

In addition to the above measures, pharmacologic interventions may be necessary to improve sleep after TBI. Medication categories include melatonin and melatonin receptor agonists, sedating antidepressants, benzodiazepines, non-benzodiazepine-benzodiazepine agonists, antipsychotics, and orexin receptor antagonists. These are described below and detailed in Table 6.1.

Melatonin and Melatonin Receptor Agonists

Melatonin is an endogenous hormone synthesized in the pineal gland and is thought to contribute to sleep initiation and the circadian rhythm. Its production is triggered by darkness. Studies have shown reduced endogenous melatonin secretion in both acute and chronic TBI [20]. The hormone can be taken exogenously. However, there have been few studies on melatonin use after TBI; one study showed shorter sleep latency and improved sleep duration and quality [32]. The medication is generally well-tolerated and may be more effective when scheduled rather than when used as needed.

Ramelteon is a synthetic melatonin MT1 and MT2 receptor agonist. It binds to these receptors with a much higher affinity than melatonin itself does. Limited studies suggest that it decreases sleep latency and increases total sleep time with a favorable side effect profile when compared to benzodiazepines and opioids [33], however, the medication has been prohibited by the European Union for inadequate demonstrated efficacy [34]. It is contraindicated if also taking fluvoxamine, rifampin, or fluconazole. The most common side effects include somnolence, dizziness, nausea, fatigue, and headache. The medication does not appear to be habit forming [35].

Table 6.1 Pharmacologic management of insomnia in the acute care setting

Medication	Description	Starting dose	Higher dose	Pearls
Melatonin and melatonin receptor agonists				
Melatonin	Exogenous hormone	1.5–3 mg qHS	6–9 mg qHS	Better scheduled than PRN
Ramelteon	Synthetic melatonin agonist	8 mg qHS	8 mg qHS	Monitor for somnolence, dizziness, nausea, fatigue, headache Contraindicated if taking fluvoxamine, rifampin, and fluconazole
Sedating antidepressants				
Trazodone	Sedating non-tricyclic antidepressant	25–50 mg qHS	100–150 mg qHS	Black box warning for suicidality Caution in cardiac disease/arrhythmias Risk of serotonin syndrome Monitor for dry mouth, headache, excessive drowsiness, hypotension, rebound insomnia, dizziness, priapism, altered platelet function
Doxepin	Tricyclic antidepressant; more selective H1 blockade	3 mg qHS	6 mg qHS	Approved for elderly; fewer side effects than other TCAs Monitor for sedation, nasopharyngitis, HTN, GI side effects
Amitriptyline	Tricyclic antidepressant	25 mg qHS	150 mg qHS	Avoid in elderly, seizures, or cardiac disease/arrhythmia Monitor for anticholinergic side effects, drowsiness, orthostasis
Mirtazapine	Enhances central noradrenergic and serotonergic activity by inhibiting α2, 5HT2, and 5HT3 receptors	7.5 mg qHS	30 mg qHS	Monitor for drowsiness, dry mouth, weight gain, dizziness, impaired driving performance and daytime arousal May be beneficial in patients trying to gain weight

(continued)

Table 6.1 (continued)

Medication	Description	Starting dose	Higher dose	Pearls
Atypical neuroleptics				
Quetiapine	Atypical neuroleptic	12.5–25 mg qHS	50–100 mg qHS	Black box warning for suicidality
				Monitor for rhabdomyolysis, neutropenia, leukopenia, orthostatic hypotension, tachycardia, and anticholinergic effects
				QTc prolongation
				Not recommended for primary insomnia and use caution
Non-benzodiazepine-benzodiazepine agonists				
Zolpidem	Selective GABA-A receptor agonist	2.5–5 mg qHS	5–10 mg qHS	Monitor for falls, hallucinations, aggression, headache, palpitations, drowsiness
				May have paradoxical effects in unresponsive wakefulness syndrome (UWS, previously known as vegetative state)
Orexin receptor antagonist				
Suvorexant[a]	Orexin receptor antagonist	10 mg qHS (5 mg if taking concomitant CYP3A inhibitor)	15–20 mg qHS	Somnolence (long half-life); avoid driving and heavy machinery on higher doses
				Expense; availability

[a]May not be available in the acute care setting

Sedating Antidepressants

Tricyclic antidepressants (TCAs), mirtazapine, and trazodone are the most commonly prescribed sedating antidepressants.

TCAs, including amitriptyline and doxepin, are attractive choices for use in SWCD due to their sedating antihistaminic and anticholinergic properties. Both medications shorten sleep onset latency, increase total sleep time, decrease awakenings after sleep onset, suppress REM sleep, and improve sleep efficiency [36]. In general, TCAs have significant side effects that are concerning in TBI patients. Side effects include xerostomia, blurred vision, dizziness, hypotension, urinary retention and constipation, worsened cognition, risk of arrhythmias and EKG changes, and lowering of the seizure threshold [37]. Unique among the TCAs, low-dose doxepin has been FDA-approved for the treatment of insomnia and is the only recommended antidepressant medication for sleep maintenance insomnia per AASM clinical practice guidelines. At low doses it is a potent histamine antagonist at H1 receptors but has less action at the other receptors that are responsible for most of the above side effects. Side effects of doxepin may include nasopharyngitis, hypertension, and nausea or diarrhea [38]. TCAs can be considered in patients with insomnia and concurrent pain conditions, such as post-traumatic headache or neuropathic pain, however they should be avoided in patients with known seizure or cardiac conduction histories and those greater than 60. Beers Criteria for Potentially Inappropriate Medications Use in Older Adults classifies all TCAs as inappropriate in patients with delirium, history of falls and syncope, and TCAs are no longer considered first-line agents for older adults.

Mirtazapine is a tetracyclic antidepressant that inhibits presynaptic alpha2, 5-HT2, and 5-HT3 receptors resulting in increases of central noradrenergic and serotonergic activity. It has a long half-life (40 h) that may cause excessive daytime sleepiness, and its effects on sleep have not been studied in non-depressed or TBI populations. The medication can be considered in a patient with concurrent insomnia, depression, and poor appetite.

Trazodone is frequently used as a sleep aid in the acute care setting. It decreases sleep latency and increases total sleep time in depressed patients, however, its mechanism of action is poorly understood. It is thought to block 5-HT2A, alpha-1 adrenergic, and histamine H1 receptors. A 2018 meta-analysis of patients with insomnia demonstrated improved self-reported sleep quality and reduced nighttime awakenings with trazodone use [39]. Side effects include anticholinergic symptoms, rebound insomnia, and rarely priapism. Trazodone has a more favorable cardiac side effect profile when compared to TCAs, however, caution is advised in patients with pre-existing cardiac conditions [40]. At higher doses, trazodone can cause conduction block, arrhythmias, bradycardia, hypotension, and cardiac arrest [41].

Benzodiazepines

Benzodiazepines act as GABA agonists through non-selective binding to the GABA-A receptor [42]. They decrease sleep latency, increase total sleep time, and decrease number of nocturnal awakenings in the general population and may be appropriate agents for acute insomnia in younger patients. However, use in the TBI population is not ideal due to side effects of altered psychomotor skills, decreased alertness and memory, and risk of dizziness and falls [43]. Larson et al. have demonstrated adverse cognitive deficits with long-term use of benzodiazepines in TBI patients [44], and animal studies show interference with neural plasticity, implicating slowing of or decreased functional recovery following TBI [45, 46]. Benzodiazepines carry strong abuse potential and risk of rebound insomnia and paradoxical agitation [4]. In summary, while benzodiazepines are effective for sleep, they should be avoided due to their unfavorable side effect profile, particularly in TBI.

Non-benzodiazepine-benzodiazepine Agonists

Like benzodiazepines, the "non-benzodiazepine-benzodiazepine agonists" act as agonists at the GABA-A receptor. However, they are more selective for the receptor alpha-1 subtype and have shorter half-lives, which reduces hangover effects. Zolpidem can be effective in decreasing sleep latency, increasing total time asleep, and decreasing nocturnal awakenings. Side effects include amnesia, hallucinations, and sleep walking [33]. Zaleplon has a short half-life of 1 h, which is useful for sleep initiation and decreasing daytime side effects, but limits its efficacy for sleep maintenance. Eszopiclone has the longest half-life in its class and is the only sedative-hypnotic approved for long-term use and without evidence of tolerance [33], however, psychomotor speed is reportedly reduced in healthy patients at the time of peak plasma concentration [47]. Neither zolpidem nor eszopiclone have been shown to worsen sleep apnea [48, 49]. Eszopiclone has actually been shown to lower the apnea/hypopnea index in OSA patients with a low arousal threshold [49]. Most research on this class of medications has been primarily performed in non-TBI populations and more investigation is warranted in the TBI population.

Atypical Antipsychotics

Quetiapine, an atypical antipsychotic with sedative properties mediated through blockage of H1 and 5-HT2 receptors, is often used off label to treat SWCD in TBI patients, despite limited evidence for its use in this population. Recently, a review of several large studies and case reports involving TBI concluded that quetiapine should not be used for the treatment of primary insomnia given limited data and safety concerns [50]. In particular, there is concern regarding QTc prolongation with quetiapine use. It should also be noted that use of typical antipsychotics such as haloperidol has been associated with impaired neurologic recovery in animal models [51]. We would recommend against the choice of quetiapine as a first-line agent for SWCD in TBI.

Orexin Receptor Antagonists

Orexin is produced in the lateral thalamus and promotes arousal. Suvorexant, a newer agent for insomnia, blocks the action of orexin at the orexin-1 and -2 receptors. The medication is generally well-tolerated, however, its 12-h half-life may impact daytime arousal, driving performance, and balance. The dose should be limited to 5 mg if taking a concomitant CYP3A inhibitor (i.e., diltiazem, phenytoin, ciprofloxacin, omycins, onazoles). No QTc prolongation has been noted with this medication and the dosing does not need to be adjusted in hepatic or renal failure [52]. Expense and availability may limit prescribing of this medication.

Sleep Wake Cycle Dysfunction in Disorders of Consciousness

Patients with disordered consciousness, a specific subset of TBI, likely require a unique approach when assessing for and treating sleep wake cycle dysfunction. Being able to evaluate and diagnose the sleep patterns of DoC patients will improve clinical care and help determine prognostic outcomes. However, it is difficult to define sleep in this population as both electrophysiological and sleep patterns differ from healthy individuals.

At this time, EEG and PSG remain the only repetitive, safe, non-invasive, and economical methods to assess brain patterns and perform sleep studies in DoC patients [53]. Patients with severe injury show a generalized slowing in the theta or delta range with abnormalities such as epileptiform activity, burst-suppression, and alpha-coma patterns on EEG [54]. For minimally conscious state patients, sleep is similar in appearance to healthy patients with circadian changes on EEG, electrooculogram, and muscle tone while patients in the unresponsive wakefulness state only show EEG/behavioral signs of opening and closing their eyes [55]. For patients in comatose and vegetative states, brain activity resembling standard sleep elements (spindles, phasic arousal activity, and the conservation of sleep stages) seems predictive of better outcomes and the absence of sleep wake cycles seems associated with brainstem or hypothalamus dysfunction. Preliminary evidence suggests this latter case may be associated with a poor outcome, however, more longitudinal sleep studies are needed to determine if this is a reliable outcome marker [56].

Use of these modalities at bedside can be challenging due to both patient and environmental factors. Patients who have severe brain damage have very limited or inconsistent motor responses and are medically fragile. For example, episodes of dysautonomia often encountered during the early stages of recovery may render EEG and PSG data unreliable. Nursing care and medical monitoring equipment may also contribute to artifact on recordings. Finally, PSG signals in DoC patients are often significantly altered and standard sleep criteria cannot be used for sleep stages scoring.

Cacciatore et al. performed a systematic review of sleep treatments in DoC. 2267 articles were assessed with only seven included in the review. Two types of sleep disorder categories were assessed: sleep-related breathing disorders and circadian rhythm dysregulation. Both categories were treated pharmacologically with modafanil and intrathecal baclofen, and also non-pharmacologically with positive airway pressure, bright light stimulation, and central thalamic deep brain stimulation. It was concluded that while the limited number of studies and their heterogeneity did not allow for generalized conclusions, all studies highlighted the effectiveness of treatments on both sleep disorders and levels of awareness [57].

Case Illustration

A 30-year-old male with no significant past medical or psychiatric history presented to the emergency department as a level 1 trauma following helmeted motorcycle accident. On exam, he was disoriented, unable to keep eyes open, and pushed examiner away when painfully stimulated.

Initial imaging revealed a right frontal subdural hemorrhage (SDH) and findings suggestive of diffuse axonal injury. The patient did not require endotracheal intubation; however, he was admitted to the ICU for 48 h for close neurological monitoring.

Further history was taken as the patient's cognitive status improved revealing a history of moderate alcohol use—two beers per day, approximately 14 during the week. In the subsequent days, the patient developed worsening irritability and difficulty engaging during physical and occupational therapies. Routine lab work was drawn, which did not reveal major abnormalities. Repeat brain imaging was ordered and was significant for stable SDH and decreasing brain edema.

When taking a sleep history, the patient and family members reported difficulty falling asleep with multiple interruptions by staff through the night. Environmental modifications such as reducing vital sign monitoring, turning off lights at night, and limiting environmental noise and early AM blood draws were discussed with medical staff. With these modifications, he was noted to perform better with therapies with functional improvement to a modified independent status by discharge from acute care. He was instructed to follow-up with outpatient physiatrist.

At his follow-up visit, he reports ongoing difficulty with sleep, primarily difficulty falling asleep. He reports finally being able to fall asleep around 1:00 AM. He denies using electronic devices close to bedtime, current alcohol consumption, history of past insomnia, snoring, or daytime sleepiness. He has not tried any sleep aids, prescribed or over the counter. His sleep cycle dysfunction is significantly impacting his ability to return to work. Given the patient's complaint and no history of medical comorbidities, trazodone 50 mg at bedtime was prescribed. He was encouraged to continue practicing good sleep hygiene. In a subsequent video visit, the patient stated he was able to fall asleep around 10:00 PM and slept around 7–8 h daily. He denied daytime drowsiness, nausea, vomiting, or associated priapism. Energy levels during the day had improved, and he felt more confident to return to work. Given his good response to medication with no side effects, it was elected to continue this medication with follow-up in 3 months' time for re-evaluation.

Conclusion

Approximately 50% of TBI survivors suffer from some form of SWCD following injury, with 25–29% being diagnosed with a formal sleep disorder (insomnia, hypersomnia, sleep-related disordered breathing), a much higher rate than in the general population. Insomnia is the most common SWCD following TBI (30–50%

of survivors). SWCD has detrimental effects on mood, cognition, behavior, and pain following TBI and is thought to impair neural remodeling. It can also have negative effects on rehabilitation by prolonging duration of post-traumatic amnesia and length of stay. Management of SWCD includes both non-pharmacologic and pharmacologic strategies. It is essential to obtain a thorough history and physical to guide an appropriate treatment plan.

References[1]

1. Mathias JL, Alvaro PK. Prevalence of sleep disturbances, disorders, and problems following traumatic brain injury: a meta-analysis. Sleep Med. 2012;13(7):898–905. https://doi.org/10.1016/j.sleep.2012.04.006.
2. Morin CM, LeBlanc M, Daley M, Gregoire JP, Mérette C. Epidemiology of insomnia: prevalence, self-help treatments, consultations, and determinants of help-seeking behaviors. Sleep Med. 2006;7(2):123–30. https://doi.org/10.1016/j.sleep.2005.08.008.
3. Nakase-Richardson R. Improving the significance and direction of sleep Management in Traumatic Brain Injury. J Head Trauma Rehabil. 2016;31(2):79–81. https://doi.org/10.1097/htr.0000000000000235.
4. Ouellet MC, Beaulieu-Bonneau S, Morin CM. Insomnia in patients with traumatic brain injury: frequency, characteristics, and risk factors. J Head Trauma Rehabil. 2006;21(3):199–212. https://doi.org/10.1097/00001199-200605000-00001.
5. Nakase-Richardson R, Sherer M, Barnett SD, et al. Prospective evaluation of the nature, course, and impact of acute sleep abnormality after traumatic brain injury. Arch Phys Med Rehabil. 2013;94(5):875–82. https://doi.org/10.1016/j.apmr.2013.01.001.
6. Wilde MC, Castriotta RJ, Lai JM, Atanasov S, Masel BE, Kuna ST. Cognitive impairment in patients with traumatic brain injury and obstructive sleep apnea. Arch Phys Med Rehabil. 2007;88(10):1284–8. https://doi.org/10.1016/j.apmr.2007.07.012.
7. Silva MA, Nakase-Richardson R, Sherer M, Barnett SD, Evans CC, Yablon SA. Posttraumatic confusion predicts patient cooperation during traumatic brain injury rehabilitation. Am J Phys Med Rehabil. 2012;91(10):890–3. https://doi.org/10.1097/PHM.0b013e31825a1648.
8. Worthington AD, Melia Y. Rehabilitation is compromised by arousal and sleep disorders: results of a survey of rehabilitation centres. Brain Inj. 2006;20(3):327–32. https://doi.org/10.1080/02699050500488249.
9. Steward KA, Silva MA, Maduri P, et al. Obstructive sleep apnea is associated with worse cognitive outcomes in acute moderate-to-severe traumatic brain injury: a TBI model systems study. Sleep Med. 2022;100:454–61. https://doi.org/10.1016/j.sleep.2022.09.012.
10. Benington JH, Heller HC. Restoration of brain energy metabolism as the function of sleep. Prog Neurobiol. 1995;45(4):347–60. https://doi.org/10.1016/0301-0082(94)00057-o.
11. Van Cauter E, Leproult R, Plat L. Age-related changes in slow wave sleep and REM sleep and relationship with growth hormone and cortisol levels in healthy men. JAMA. 2000;284(7):861–8. https://doi.org/10.1001/jama.284.7.861.
12. Watson NF, Badr MS, Belenky G, et al. Joint Consensus Statement of the American Academy of Sleep Medicine and Sleep Research Society on the recommended amount of sleep for a healthy adult: methodology and discussion. Sleep. 2015;38(8):1161–83. https://doi.org/10.5665/sleep.4886.
13. Ouellet MC, Beaulieu-Bonneau S, Morin CM. Sleep-wake disturbances after traumatic brain injury. Lancet Neurol. 2015;14(7):746–57. https://doi.org/10.1016/s1474-4422(15)00068-x.

[1] Key References [1, 3, 5, 13, 44].

14. Chokroverty S. Overview of sleep & sleep disorders. Indian J Med Res. 2010;131:126–40.
15. Collop NA, Salas RE, Delayo M, Gamaldo C. Normal sleep and circadian processes. Crit Care Clin. 2008;24(3):449–60, v. https://doi.org/10.1016/j.ccc.2008.02.002.
16. Ron S, Algom D, Hary D, Cohen M. Time-related changes in the distribution of sleep stages in brain injured patients. Electroencephalogr Clin Neurophysiol. 1980;48(4):432–41.
17. Baumann CR, Bassetti CL, Valko PO, et al. Loss of hypocretin (orexin) neurons with traumatic brain injury. Ann Neurol. 2009;66(4):555–9. https://doi.org/10.1002/ana.21836.
18. Baumann CR, Stocker R, Imhof HG, et al. Hypocretin-1 (orexin A) deficiency in acute traumatic brain injury. Neurology. 2005;65(1):147–9. https://doi.org/10.1212/01.wnl.0000167605.02541.f2.
19. Mésenge C, Margaill I, Verrecchia C, Allix M, Boulu RG, Plotkine M. Protective effect of melatonin in a model of traumatic brain injury in mice. J Pineal Res. 1998;25(1):41–6. https://doi.org/10.1111/j.1600-079X.1998.tb00384.x.
20. Shekleton JA, Parcell DL, Redman JR, Phipps-Nelson J, Ponsford JL, Rajaratnam SM. Sleep disturbance and melatonin levels following traumatic brain injury. Neurology. 2010;74(21):1732–8. https://doi.org/10.1212/WNL.0b013e3181e0438b.
21. Seifman MA, Gomes K, Nguyen PN, et al. Measurement of serum melatonin in intensive care unit patients: changes in traumatic brain injury, trauma, and medical conditions. Front Neurol. 2014;5:237. https://doi.org/10.3389/fneur.2014.00237.
22. Green TRF, Ortiz JB, Wonnacott S, Williams RJ, Rowe RK. The bidirectional relationship between sleep and inflammation links traumatic brain injury and Alzheimer's disease. Front Neurosci. 2020;14:894. https://doi.org/10.3389/fnins.2020.00894.
23. Krueger JM, Majde JA. Cytokines and sleep. Int Arch Allergy Immunol. 1995;106(2):97–100. https://doi.org/10.1159/000236827.
24. Pulak LM, Jensen L. Sleep in the intensive care unit: a review. J Intensive Care Med. 2016;31(1):14–23. https://doi.org/10.1177/0885066614538749.
25. Freedman NS, Gazendam J, Levan L, Pack AI, Schwab RJ. Abnormal sleep/wake cycles and the effect of environmental noise on sleep disruption in the intensive care unit. Am J Respir Crit Care Med. 2001;163(2):451–7. https://doi.org/10.1164/ajrccm.163.2.9912128.
26. Mollayeva T, Kendzerska T, Colantonio A. Self-report instruments for assessing sleep dysfunction in an adult traumatic brain injury population: a systematic review. Sleep Med Rev. 2013;17(6):411–23. https://doi.org/10.1016/j.smrv.2013.02.001.
27. Wiseman-Hakes C, Duclos C, Blais H, et al. Sleep in the acute phase of severe traumatic brain injury: a snapshot of polysomnography. Neurorehabil Neural Repair. 2016;30(8):713–21. https://doi.org/10.1177/1545968315619697.
28. Wiseman-Hakes C, Gaudreault P, Duclos C, Bernard F, Carrier J, Gosselin N. Examination of polysomnography in hospitalized patients with acute moderate-severe traumatic brain injury. Sleep Med. 2013;14:e305. https://doi.org/10.1016/j.sleep.2013.11.747.
29. Kamper JE, Garofano J, Schwartz DJ, et al. Concordance of actigraphy with polysomnography in traumatic brain injury neurorehabilitation admissions. J Head Trauma Rehabil. 2016;31(2):117–25. https://doi.org/10.1097/htr.0000000000000215.
30. Zeitzer JM, Hon F, Whyte J, et al. Coherence between sleep detection by actigraphy and polysomnography in a multi-center, inpatient cohort of individuals with traumatic brain injury. PM R. 2020;12(12):1205–13. https://doi.org/10.1002/pmrj.12353.
31. Faraklas I, Holt B, Tran S, Lin H, Saffle J, Cochran A. Impact of a nursing-driven sleep hygiene protocol on sleep quality. J Burn Care Res. 2013;34(2):249–54. https://doi.org/10.1097/BCR.0b013e318283d175.
32. Kemp S, Biswas R, Neumann V, Coughlan A. The value of melatonin for sleep disorders occurring post-head injury: a pilot RCT. Brain Inj. 2004;18(9):911–9. https://doi.org/10.1080/02699050410001671892.
33. Flanagan SR, Greenwald B, Wieber S. Pharmacological treatment of insomnia for individuals with brain injury. J Head Trauma Rehabil. 2007;22(1):67–70.

34. Kato K, Hirai K, Nishiyama K, et al. Neurochemical properties of ramelteon (TAK-375), a selective MT1/MT2 receptor agonist. Neuropharmacology. 2005;48(2):301–10. https://doi.org/10.1016/j.neuropharm.2004.09.007.
35. Mayer G, Wang-Weigand S, Roth-Schechter B, Lehmann R, Staner C, Partinen M. Efficacy and safety of 6-month nightly ramelteon administration in adults with chronic primary insomnia. Sleep. 2009;32(3):351–60. https://doi.org/10.1093/sleep/32.3.351.
36. DeMartinis NA, Winokur A. Effects of psychiatric medications on sleep and sleep disorders. CNS Neurol Disord Drug Targets. 2007;6(1):17–29. https://doi.org/10.2174/187152707779940835.
37. Rao V, Rollings P. Sleep disturbances following traumatic brain injury. Curr Treat Options Neurol. 2002;4(1):77–87. https://doi.org/10.1007/s11940-002-0006-4.
38. De Crescenzo F, Foti F, Ciabattini M, et al. Comparative efficacy and acceptability of pharmacological treatments for insomnia in adults: a systematic review and network meta-analysis. Cochrane Database Syst Rev. 2016;2016(9):CD012364. https://doi.org/10.1002/14651858.CD012364.
39. Yi XY, Ni SF, Ghadami MR, et al. Trazodone for the treatment of insomnia: a meta-analysis of randomized placebo-controlled trials. Sleep Med. 2018;45:25–32. https://doi.org/10.1016/j.sleep.2018.01.010.
40. Mendelson WB. A review of the evidence for the efficacy and safety of trazodone in insomnia. J Clin Psychiatry. 2005;66(4):469–76.
41. Bryant SG, Ereshefsky L. Antidepressant properties of trazodone. Clin Pharm. 1982;1(5):406–17.
42. Pagel JF, Parnes BL. Medications for the treatment of sleep disorders: an overview. Prim Care Companion J Clin Psychiatry. 2001;3(3):118–25. https://doi.org/10.4088/pcc.v03n0303.
43. Zeitzer JM, Friedman L, O'Hara R. Insomnia in the context of traumatic brain injury. J Rehabil Res Dev. 2009;46(6):827–36. https://doi.org/10.1682/jrrd.2008.08.0099.
44. Larson EB, Zollman FS. The effect of sleep medications on cognitive recovery from traumatic brain injury. J Head Trauma Rehabil. 2010;25(1):61–7. https://doi.org/10.1097/HTR.0b013e3181c1d1e1.
45. Schallert T, Hernandez TD, Barth TM. Recovery of function after brain damage: severe and chronic disruption by diazepam. Brain Res. 1986;379(1):104–11. https://doi.org/10.1016/0006-8993(86)90261-1.
46. Wan H, Warburton EC, Zhu XO, et al. Benzodiazepine impairment of perirhinal cortical plasticity and recognition memory. Eur J Neurosci. 2004;20(8):2214–24. https://doi.org/10.1111/j.1460-9568.2004.03688.x.
47. Billiard M, Besset A, de Lustrac C, Brissaud L. Dose-response effects of zopiclone on night sleep and on nighttime and daytime functioning. Sleep. 1987;10(Suppl 1):27–34. https://doi.org/10.1093/sleep/10.suppl_1.27.
48. Messineo L, Eckert DJ, Lim R, et al. Zolpidem increases sleep efficiency and the respiratory arousal threshold without changing sleep apnoea severity and pharyngeal muscle activity. J Physiol. 2020;598(20):4681–92. https://doi.org/10.1113/JP280173.
49. Eckert DJ, Owens RL, Kehlmann GB, et al. Eszopiclone increases the respiratory arousal threshold and lowers the apnoea/hypopnoea index in obstructive sleep apnoea patients with a low arousal threshold. Clin Sci (Lond). 2011;120(12):505–14. https://doi.org/10.1042/CS20100588.
50. Coe HV, Hong IS. Safety of low doses of quetiapine when used for insomnia. Ann Pharmacother. 2012;46(5):718–22. https://doi.org/10.1345/aph.1Q697.
51. Hoffman AN, Cheng JP, Zafonte RD, Kline AE. Administration of haloperidol and risperidone after neurobehavioral testing hinders the recovery of traumatic brain injury-induced deficits. Life Sci. 2008;83(17–18):602–7. https://doi.org/10.1016/j.lfs.2008.08.007.
52. Yang LP. Suvorexant: first global approval. Drugs. 2014;74(15):1817–22. https://doi.org/10.1007/s40265-014-0294-5.

53. Bai Y, Xia X, Li X. A review of resting-state electroencephalography analysis in disorders of consciousness. Front Neurol. 2017;8:471. https://doi.org/10.3389/fneur.2017.00471.
54. Brenner RP. The interpretation of the EEG in stupor and coma. Neurologist. 2005;11(5):271–84. https://doi.org/10.1097/01.nrl.0000178756.44055.f6.
55. Raciti L, Raciti G, Militi D, Tonin P, Quartarone A, Calabro RS. Sleep in disorders of consciousness: a brief overview on a still under investigated issue. Brain Sci. 2023;13(2):275. https://doi.org/10.3390/brainsci13020275.
56. Cologan V, Schabus M, Ledoux D, Moonen G, Maquet P, Laureys S. Sleep in disorders of consciousness. Sleep Med Rev. 2010;14(2):97–105. https://doi.org/10.1016/j.smrv.2009.04.003.
57. Cacciatore M, Magnani FG, Leonardi M, Rossi Sebastiano D, Sattin D. Sleep treatments in disorders of consciousness: a systematic review. Diagnostics (Basel). 2021;12(1):88. https://doi.org/10.3390/diagnostics12010088.

Chapter 7
Delirium and Agitation Management

Gerald J. Nora

Chapter Objectives
1. Review the common mechanisms of brain injury related agitation and delirium.
2. Understand the environmental and medical management considerations for agitation and delirium.

Introduction

Acutely hospitalized patients often suffer from cognitive and behavioral disturbances during their inpatient course. Some patients suffer agitation as a direct consequence of a brain injury (BI), traumatic or otherwise. More commonly, metabolic, iatrogenic, infectious, or environmental derangements provoked acute brain dysfunction, termed delirium. In the acute care setting, both impact the patient's functional status and rehabilitation goal-setting, but are clinically and mechanistically distinct entities with their own considerations for diagnosis and management.

Definitions of Agitation and Akathisia

Acute BI patients, classically in the traumatic brain injury (TBI) population but also in anoxic injury, may demonstrate restlessness or agitation. The former is also described as "akathisia"—fidgeting, distractible, high-energy behavior in the

G. J. Nora (✉)
Medrina, Chicago, IL, USA

Department of Physical Medicine and Rehabilitation, Medical College of Wisconsin,
Milwaukee, WI, USA
e-mail: jerry.nora@medrina.com

A. K. Wagner, J. Weppner (eds.), *Acute Care Neuroconsultation and Neurorehabilitation Management*, https://doi.org/10.1007/978-3-031-42830-2_7

absence of aggression [1]. It is important to educate staff and family about the distinction between the nonspecific restlessness seen in BI versus the more dangerous behaviors that require intervention. Agitation is defined as verbally or physically aggressive behavior in the setting of post-traumatic amnesia (PTA), with the period of agitated behavior typically lasting 7 to 10 days [2, 3].

The typical measure of PTA is the Orientation Log (O-Log), which serially tracks how much assistance is required for a patient to correctly identify ten points of orientation (i.e., city, kind of place, hospital name, month, date, year, day of week, clock time, etiology/event, pathology deficits). The O-Log was developed for the daily monitoring of cognitive abilities and may be administered in the acute care setting to assess the duration of PTA. The ten equally weighed items can receive full or partial credit, with a total score ranging from 0 to 30. For example, while correct spontaneous responses receive full credit (3 points), partial credit may be obtained if a correct response is given after the examiner provides a logical cue (2 points), or if the correct answer is recognized when presented in a multiple-choice format (1 point). Emergence from PTA is defined as the first day when a patient obtains two consecutive scores of ≥25 on the O-Log [4]. The O-Log is both simpler than the older Galveston Orientation and Amnesia Test and provides slightly better prognosis for long-term function [5].

Agitation can be quantified as well as PTA, with the preferred instrument being the Agitated Behavior Scale (ABS). A patient observer ranks 14 behaviors (e.g., from distractibility to self-injurious behavior) on a scale of 0 to 4, with 0 denoting "total absence" and 4 denoting "extreme degree" such that the patient cannot be redirected from the given behavior [6]. A score under 21 is "usual behavior"; 22–28 is mild agitation; 29–35 is moderate; 36 and higher is severe.

Mechanisms of Agitation and Akathisia

The sensation of akathisia has been associated with basal ganglia dysfunction in conditions like Parkinson's Disease [7] or the extrapyramidal side effects of antidopaminergic medication [8]. Traumatic and anoxic BI (e.g., due to cardiac arrest) are associated with injury to the basal ganglia [9, 10], and so akathisia is attributed to injuries in those structures.

This inability to orient oneself drives a fight or flight response in the context of a noisy, confusing environment (the hospital), with multiple noxious stimuli (e.g., catheters, restraints, intravenous lines, blood draws), and pain. Agitated behavior has been associated with damage to the limbic system, which classically regulates fight or flight behaviors [11]. Another paradigm involves the balance of serotonin and dopamine in the central nervous system (CNS), with agitation involving a relative deficit of the former and excess of the latter [12].

While the above neurotransmitter derangements predispose the patient to agitation, one must be alert for precipitating factors. Fatigue later in the day and overstimulation are contributing factors. Pain is a consideration for agitation, particularly among patients with polytrauma (e.g., fracture/burn) in addition to BI; therefore, scheduling analgesics in the short term could be valuable. Infection, electrolyte, and drug and/or alcohol withdrawal are also common triggers for agitation [13].

Environmental Management of Agitation

When approaching an agitated BI patient, one should practice empathy with the patient. Consider small tasks or actions that could orient the patient to her/himself and circumstances, such as the presence of loved ones. The number of family and caregivers visiting at one time should be limited to prevent patient overstimulation and agitation. The consultation team and nursing staff should collaborate with family and caregivers to manage visitors by assessing family visiting preferences and providing the family with strategies to manage visitors within the framework of institutional visitation policies [14]. Some restraints are avoidable, such as cardiac monitoring in a patient with a stable cardiopulmonary status, and some may be unavoidable, such as an external fixation for a broken limb. A TBI patient may have pain generators such as occult bone fractures or other wounds, and so scheduled pain medications may be necessary. Infections, dehydration, and metabolic derangements should be methodically considered.

While it is easy to prescribe a medication, a team-based approach can reduce the need for medication and improve the safety of both the patient and staff. It is important to recognize that medications alone are often not sufficient to manage these complex symptoms. A team-based approach that incorporates the expertise of multiple disciplines and caregivers is critical to addressing the multifactorial nature of delirium and agitation. The team-based approach to managing delirium and agitation involves a collaborative effort between medical professionals, nursing staff, therapists, and caregivers. A behavior plan provides a consistent patient-centered method of maintaining a low-stimulation environment, redirection for perseveration or restlessness, and contingencies for escalating behavior. A plan is a dynamic entity and requires communication among the team to adjust it as necessary and learn from any difficulties or successes.

Medical Management of Agitation

While environmental management of agitation and restlessness is paramount, medical management is frequently necessary, and treatment options are summarized in Table 7.1.

Table 7.1 Summary of common agents to treat agitation

Common medications used to treat agitation in TBI and delirium			
Medication	Daily dose range	Important side effects	Special considerations
Antidepressants			
Trazodone	25–150 mg at bedtime; may be scheduled or prn	Dry mouth	Sleep aid
		Constipation	May be a stimulant at 150 mg or higher
		Urinary retention	
		Orthostatic hypotension	
		Priapism	
Antiepileptic agents			
Valproic acid	250–1000 mg q6–12 h	Sedation	Multiple formulations and thus half-lives vary; may have neuroprotective benefit in brain injury. Not recommended for delirium
		Hyperammonemia	
Antipsychotics			
Haloperidol	0.5–10 mg q1–4 h with max dose of 100 mg/day; may be scheduled or prn	Tardive dyskinesia	Relatively contraindicated in TBI
		Neuroleptic malignant syndrome	In delirium may be used for agitation but worse side-effect profile than atypical
		QT prolongation	
		Hyponatremia	
Olanzapine	1–5 mg q24 h–8 h; may be scheduled or prn (max 20 mg/day)	Sedation [15, 16]	IM and PO options
Risperidone	1–6 mg divided daily or q12h; may be scheduled or prn (max 6 mg/day)	Sedation	Consider orthostatic vital signs if hypotension risk
		Increased mortality risk in elderly dementia patients	
Quetiapine	25–150 mg q24h-q6h; may be scheduled or prn	Sedation	Can be scheduled or PRN
		QT prolongation	Primarily antihistaminergic at dosages <300 mg
			While antihistaminergic it is *not* anticholinergic
Aripiprazole	2.5–15 mg qd	Mixed dopamine agonist-antagonist	Not as well-studied in acute care settings for prn use as olanzapine and quetiapine.
Benzodiazepines			
Diazepam		Sedation	Not recommended as first line, rescue or alcohol/benzodiazepine withdrawal only
Lorazepam		Delirium	Diazepam hepatically metabolized
		Paradoxical agitation	
Beta blocker			

(continued)

Table 7.1 (continued)

Common medications used to treat agitation in TBI and delirium			
Medication	Daily dose range	Important side effects	Special considerations
Propranolol	10 mg q8h with rapid titration to 60–420 mg/day [17] divided q6-8h	Hypotension	Associated with reduced mortality in severe TBI; helps with PSH
Neurostimulants			
Amantadine	50–200 mg qd-bid	Anticholinergic effects	If dosed twice a day, amantadine should be timed for morning and mid-day. Avoid administration prior to bedtime
		Livedo reticularis (benign rash)	
Methylphenidate	5–20 mg qd-bid	Tachycardia	Controlled substance
			If dosed twice a day, methylphenidate should be timed for morning and mid-day. Avoid administration prior to bedtime

Some medications are typically given regularly while others may be given "as needed" and so their PRN nature is denoted under dosing. A dosing scheme is not provided for the benzodiazepine exemplars as the dosages can vary wildly according to the use, the tolerance of the patient for the medications, and whether one is also managing withdrawal from benzodiazepines or alcohol

Antipsychotics

Antipsychotics are a common form of chemical restraint used in hospitals. The typical antipsychotics block dopamine receptors, which can blunt agitation (through the limbic system). However, as discussed above, the dopaminergic pathways are already compromised. In addition to increased risk of dyskinesia, typical antipsychotics can cause long-term compromise of motor and cognitive recovery if used daily [18, 19].

Atypical antipsychotics such as quetiapine and olanzapine, however, are relatively safe to use in this population. Although numerous observational studies have reported a reduction in agitation with the use of antipsychotic agents, olanzapine is the only agent that has been elevated in its evidence base with a controlled study [20–24]. Waidele et al. demonstrated the efficiency of olanzapine in their controlled study to decrease irritability, aggression, and insomnia following severe TBI [25].

Beta Blockers

A secondary driver of agitation is the catecholamine surge frequently observed with BI. In addition to purely autonomic symptoms, this adrenergic stimulation drives a fight or flight response. Beta blockers, typically propranolol, can help defervesce agitation [26]. Propranolol has been shown to significantly reduce agitation in the acute care population with severe nonpenetrating TBI at doses of 60–420 mg/day [27]. It should be noted that Propranolol is well tolerated up to 420 mg/day [27]. Still, in another study, most patients developed bradycardia or hypotension with dosing up to 529 mg/day [28]. There is evidence that propranolol can reduce mortality in BI patients, though the precise mechanism is unclear [29].

Benzodiazepines

Benzodiazepines work by GABAergic activity and can have a sedating effect. They have the advantage of rapid onset and the ability to be given parenterally. The brain, however, has multiple classes of GABA receptors in both the cortex and subcortical structures, and these receptors are differentially blocked. Systemic reviews of agitation in brain injury were unable to identify evidence supporting the efficacy of benzodiazepines in managing agitation [13, 26, 30–38]. There are uncontrolled studies reporting worsening of agitation with benzodiazepine administration in the setting of brain injury [34]. Benzodiazepines can slow functional recovery following brain injury in animal models [39–42], and they are believed to have a comparable effect on human brain recovery [43–46]. Until benzodiazepines are further investigated in brain injury, they generally should be reserved for patients requiring treatment for seizures or alcohol or benzodiazepine withdrawal.

Antiepileptic Drugs (AEDs)

AEDs work according to multiple pathways. The most employed AED, valproic acid, is thought to upregulate GABA pathways in postsynaptic neurons, though the precise mechanism is unclear. There is limited investigation exploring AEDs for agitation regulation in brain injury in the acute hospital setting, but valproic acid has been shown to reduce agitation among chronic TBI survivors with comorbid alcohol use disorder [47, 48]. Oxcarbazepine has also been shown in a controlled study to decrease agitation in a heterogeneous cohort of subjects, including those with TBI [49]. There are additional uncontrolled studies supporting carbamazepine use to treat agitation in BI [13, 26, 30, 31, 34].

Neurostimulants

While counterintuitive, neurostimulants may reduce restlessness by increasing dopamine levels in neural circuits involved with attention and working memory, palliating sensitivity to stimulus overload and cognitive fatigue. Amantadine, an NMDA antagonist which indirectly affects dopamine, has been long used in

Parkinson's Disease, and this agent has randomized controlled trials showing efficacy in BI [50, 51]. Dopamine reuptake inhibitors such as methylphenidate and dextroamphetamine are also used, with one study demonstrating a significant reduction in anger and aggression with methylphenidate use [52].

Antidepressants

As selective serotonin reuptake inhibitors take weeks to have an effect, they are of limited use in acute care BI patients. However, trazodone, while rarely used for depression, has use for promoting sleep maintenance at lower doses. It is of more limited use for sleep initiation, for which melatonin, or in more restless patients, quetiapine may be considered.

Definition of Delirium

Delirium is defined as a disorder of consciousness and attention with an acute onset and waxing and waning clinical course [53]. Approximately 11–14% of hospitalized patients may develop delirium, which is associated with increases in hospital length of stay and mortality [54]. While previously thought to be a transient condition brought about by an underlying illness, delirium is increasingly recognized to be a form of non-traumatic BI, with cognitive sequelae in patients lasting months or years after the resolution of the original delirium [55, 56]. The overarching mechanism of delirium seems to be diffuse dysfunction of inter-neuron and glial communication and function [53, 57].

Mechanisms and Management of Delirium

Environment and Circadian Rhythm

Delirium may stem from the patient's surroundings, or in deficits of a patient's ability to perceive their surroundings. One potential mechanism of delirium is an imbalance between the limbic ("fight or flight") brain systems versus the inhibitory personality-drive role of the frontal lobes [58]. Restraints, noxious stimuli, pain, and other disruptions trigger limbically-mediated agitation; suppression of the frontal lobe inhibition—whether through drug side effects (see below) or underlying dementia or other brain disorder—could then precipitate agitated delirium. In the elderly, restraints alone can more than quadruple the relative risk of delirium [59]. In addition to environmental disturbances, a patient with impaired sight or vision may be at risk for developing delirium even in a relatively benign hospital environment. Thus, getting hearing aids and glasses from a caregiver may be of prime importance [59]. A management program (Hospital Elder Life Program) targeting six delirium risk factors in the elderly (nutrition, hydration, sleep, immobility, hearing, and vision) [60] reduced delirium by over 50% versus the baseline, lowered the average length of stay by 2.15 days, and saved a large academic hospital an estimated $7.3 million annually [61].

The neurotransmitter melatonin is the keystone of regulating the circadian rhythm that influences acetylcholine, cortisol, and catecholamine activity in the brain. Disruption in the circadian cycle can also promote delirium, with low serum levels of melatonin found in delirious patients in some studies [62]. A randomized trial of melatonin in 452 patients with hip fracture, however, found no protective effect against delirium with melatonin [63]. A significant limitation of this study, however, was that there was no accounting for the types of home medications those patients were on, and thus, no control for the confounding effect of deliriogenic drugs.

Iatrogenic

Unfortunately, a significant percentage of delirium is accountable to side effects of medication [59]. Many commonly implicated medications are those that have antagonize acetylcholine receptors, such as tricyclic antidepressants, antihistamines, and H2-antagonists [64]. The anticholinergic effects of these medications suppresses modulation of attention and emotional regulation in the frontal lobes [58].

The use of benzodiazepines causes diffuse suppression of cortical activity [65], and in one study, lorazepam was found to be a dose-dependent predictor of delirium in hospitalized patients [66]. Withdrawal from benzodiazepines, just like alcohol withdrawal, however, is another cause for delirium, and thus, any delirium work-up of a patient should consider any history of drug use or abuse.

Delirium management lies more in the removal of offending drugs rather than adding new ones as initiating three or more medications is itself a risk factor for delirium [59]. The Beers criteria were developed to organize medications according to their risks for the elderly [64]. It can also be a valuable resource for finding offending agents affecting a patient's cognition regardless of age, as even a young BI patient will be more vulnerable to sedating or anticholinergic medications (Table 7.2).

For agitated medical delirium—not traumatic or anoxic BI—typical and atypical antipsychotics can relieve some symptoms by dampening the limbically-mediate "fight or flight" response, with the atypical antipsychotics causing fewer side effects [53, 67, 68]. "Hypoactive" delirium, however, with a patient who is not restless but whose mentation is compromised, a sedating antipsychotic will not necessarily improve things, and quite possibly makes things worse. Since a patient with

Table 7.2 Medications with adverse side effects

Medications with adverse cognitive side effects	
Medication class	Notes
Early antihistamines	Anticholinergic side effects
For example, diphenhydramine, hydroxyzine	Consider topical agents for pruritus
	Second generation agents like loratadine better tolerated
Tricyclic antidepressants	Orthostatic hypotension, sedation, anticholinergic side effects.
For example, amitriptyline, imipramine	
Typical antipsychotics	Extrapyramidal side effects (EPS)
For example, haloperidol	Oversedation
Atypical antipsychotics	While less likely to cause EPS, still can cause oversedation
For example, quetiapine, olanzapine	
Benzodiazepines	May need to gradual taper due to withdrawal risk
For example, alprazolam, clonazepam	
Muscle relaxants	Anticholinergic side effects, some also have sedating metabolites
For example, cyclobenzaprine, methocarbamol	
Antiemetics	Sedating (antihistamine), anticholinergic
For example, promethazine, doxylamine, metoclopramide	Typical antipsychotic; sedating, extrapyramidal effects
Diabetes	Assess diabetes medications for hypoglycemia risk
For example, insulin, sulfonylureas	Metformin can be complicated by lactic acidosis and renal injury
Z-drugs	Can cause "hangover" effects day after use
For example, zolpidem, eszopiclone	Parasomnias

This list is adapted in part from the Beers Criteria [64] but is not an exhaustive list

hypoactive delirium is "behaving," they will not attract as much attention from the staff as one who is restless or aggressive, and this form of delirium is underdiagnosed [69].

Infection and Toxic-Metabolic

Metabolic derangements or sepsis can provoke neural-glial dysfunction and thus delirium. In sepsis, the systemic inflammatory response syndrome (SIRS) may trigger activation of the microglia in the CNS, which when activated behave similarly to macrophages. This pathologic activation of the microglia can damage the CNS. A recent study found that statins had a protective role against delirium, particularly in septic patients, which is attributed to the drug's anti-inflammatory properties [70]. Conversely, the cessation of statins seemed to increase delirium risk as a sort of "rebound" or withdrawal effect. As such, a patient with a home statin should have this started in the hospital promptly, barring any other patient specific contraindications.

Any electrolytic, acid-base, infectious, or toxic derangement can cause delirium [71]. Appropriate monitoring and correction of infection or electrolyte abnormality is the best prevention or treatment. In the case of diabetes, one should avoid overly strict glycemic control [72].

Case Illustrations

Case 1

A 40-year-old woman with history of neuropathy, diabetes, and chronic kidney disease was admitted for altered mental status. Her exam was noted for somnolence and myoclonus without any focal neurologic findings. Physiatry was consulted as a second opinion on the cause for symptoms that had no overt infectious or metabolic etiology. The consultant noted that the patient was on 600 mg of gabapentin 3 times a day. Her glomerular filtrate rate (GFR), however, had showed a slight decrement from about 60 mL/min (which had been obtained in a previous clinical encounter a month or more prior) to about 56 mL/min at the present admission, with a maximum daily dosage of no more than 1400 mg recommended for the latter GFR. There was no obvious acute renal insult, and it was thought that the patient's baseline GFR was at the margin of safety for her original gabapentin dosage. The dose of gabapentin was cut in half, and the patient's myoclonus and hypoactive delirium resolved within about 24 h. She was discharged home and fully independent again.

Case 2

A 43-year-old previously healthy patient was admitted for an out of the hospital cardiac arrest. The etiology for the arrest was an arrhythmia, and a long QTc interval was noted. Due to the resulting anoxic BI, the patient was oriented only to himself and very restless, pacing around the floor with upwards of three staff to help redirect him to his room. Due to his long QT interval, antipsychotics were largely contraindicated, as was use of a cholinergic agent like donepezil. Rather, staff on the acute care hospital went to extended efforts to redirect him and allowed him to work out his psychomotor restlessness by walking with him around the floor. Valproic acid was used as a mood-stabilizing adjunct starting at 250 mg 4 times daily. The patient began to respond to valproic acid over the course of the following few days, with a reduction in their agitated behavior observed. While there was initially discussion of a "LifeVest" for treating future arrythmia, it was clear that the patient would not be able to safely operate the device. An implantable cardiac defibrillator was placed prior to transfer to a locked brain injury unit for rehabilitation.

Summary and Key Points

A consulting physiatrist may encounter a range of neurobehavioral abnormalities, which barring psychiatric concerns, can be very broadly grouped into the syndromes of acquired BI (e.g., anoxic and traumatic) and delirium. While there are distinctions between the underlying mechanisms for the two broad syndromes, many of the underlying principles of management are similar. A team-based approach incorporating medical, nursing, and therapy staff members, as well as caregivers, is critical to management of the environmental factors that often precipitate or aggravate delirium and agitation. Pharmacologic management of these syndromes is most efficacious in conjunction with nonpharmacologic measures, in addition to avoiding medications contraindicated in BI and delirium.

References[1]

1. Lombard LA, Zafonte RD. Agitation after traumatic brain injury: considerations and treatment options. Am J Phys Med Rehabil. 2005;84(10):797–812. https://doi.org/10.1097/01.phm.0000179438.22235.08.
2. Brooke MM, Questad KA, Patterson DR, Bashak KJ. Agitation and restlessness after closed head injury: a prospective study of 100 consecutive admissions. Arch Phys Med Rehabil. 1992;73(4):320–3. https://doi.org/10.1016/0003-9993(92)90003-f.
3. Kadyan V, Mysiw WJ, Bogner JA, Corrigan JD, Fugate LP, Clinchot DM. Gender differences in agitation after traumatic brain injury. Am J Phys Med Rehabil. 2004;83(10):747–52. https://doi.org/10.1097/01.phm.0000140790.30468.f4.
4. Novack TA, Dowler RN, Bush BA, Glen T, Schneider JJ. Validity of the orientation log, relative to the Galveston orientation and amnesia test. J Head Trauma Rehabil. 2000;15(3):957–61. https://doi.org/10.1097/00001199-200006000-00008.
5. Frey KL, Rojas DC, Anderson CA, Arciniegas DB. Comparison of the O-Log and GOAT as measures of posttraumatic amnesia. Brain Inj. 2007;21(5):513–20. https://doi.org/10.1080/02699050701311026.
6. Bogner JA, Corrigan JD, Stange M, Rabold D. Reliability of the agitated behavior scale. J Head Trauma Rehabil. 1999;14(1):91–6. https://doi.org/10.1097/00001199-199902000-00012.
7. Patel N, Jankovic J, Hallett M. Sensory aspects of movement disorders. Lancet Neurol. 2014;13(1):100–12. https://doi.org/10.1016/s1474-4422(13)70213-8.
8. Guehl D, Cuny E, Ghorayeb I, Michelet T, Bioulac B, Burbaud P. Primate models of dystonia. Prog Neurobiol. 2009;87(2):118–31. https://doi.org/10.1016/j.pneurobio.2008.10.003.
9. Bales JW, Wagner AK, Kline AE, Dixon CE. Persistent cognitive dysfunction after traumatic brain injury: a dopamine hypothesis. Neurosci Biobehav Rev. 2009;33(7):981–1003. https://doi.org/10.1016/j.neubiorev.2009.03.011.

[1] Key References [1, 53, 56, 61, 64].

10. Wu X, Drabek T, Kochanek PM, et al. Induction of profound hypothermia for emergency preservation and resuscitation allows intact survival after cardiac arrest resulting from prolonged lethal hemorrhage and trauma in dogs. Circulation. 2006;113(16):1974–82. https://doi.org/10.1161/circulationaha.105.587204.
11. Siegel A, Schubert KL, Shaikh MB. Neurotransmitters regulating defensive rage behavior in the cat. Neurosci Biobehav Rev. 1997;21(6):733–42. https://doi.org/10.1016/s0149-7634(96)00056-5.
12. van Erp AM, Miczek KA. Aggressive behavior, increased accumbal dopamine, and decreased cortical serotonin in rats. J Neurosci. 2000;20(24):9320–5. https://doi.org/10.1523/jneurosci.20-24-09320.2000.
13. Luauté J, Plantier D, Wiart L, Tell L. Care management of the agitation or aggressiveness crisis in patients with TBI. Systematic review of the literature and practice recommendations. Ann Phys Rehabil Med. 2016;59(1):58–67. https://doi.org/10.1016/j.rehab.2015.11.001.
14. Oyesanya TO, Bowers B. Managing visitors during the hospital stay: the experience of family caregivers of patients with traumatic brain injury. J Fam Nurs. 2017;23(2):273–98. https://doi.org/10.1177/1074840717697673.
15. Czekalla J, Beasley CM Jr, Dellva MA, Berg PH, Grundy S. Analysis of the QTc interval during olanzapine treatment of patients with schizophrenia and related psychosis. J Clin Psychiatry. 2001;62(3):191–8. https://doi.org/10.4088/jcp.v62n0310.
16. Shoja Shafti S, Fallah Jahromi P. Olanzapine induced Q-Tc shortening. Ther Adv Psychopharmacol. 2014;4(6):240–6. https://doi.org/10.1177/2045125314546484.
17. Brooke MM, Patterson DR, Questad KA, et al. The treatment of agitation during initial hospitalization after traumatic brain injury. Arch Phys Med Rehabil. 1992;73:917–21.
18. Free KE, Greene AM, Bondi CO, Lajud N, de la Tremblaye PB, Kline AE. Comparable impediment of cognitive function in female and male rats subsequent to daily administration of haloperidol after traumatic brain injury. Exp Neurol. 2017;296:62–8. https://doi.org/10.1016/j.expneurol.2017.07.004.
19. Bao GC, Bleimeister IH, Zimmerman LA, et al. Intermittent administration of haloperidol after cortical impact injury neither impedes spontaneous recovery nor attenuates the efficacy of environmental enrichment. J Neurotrauma. 2019;36(10):1606–14. https://doi.org/10.1089/neu.2018.6212.
20. Kim E, Bijlani M. A pilot study of quetiapine treatment of aggression due to traumatic brain injury. J Neuropsychiatr Clin Neurosci. 2006;18(4):547–9.
21. Maryniak O, Manchanda R, Velani A. Methotrimeprazine in the treatment of agitation in acquired brain injury patients. Brain Inj. 2001;15(2):167–74. https://doi.org/10.1080/026990501458399.
22. Ponsford J, Janzen S, McIntyre A, Bayley M, Velikonja D, Tate R. INCOG recommendations for management of cognition following traumatic brain injury, part I: posttraumatic amnesia/delirium. J Head Trauma Rehabil. 2014;29(4):307–20. https://doi.org/10.1097/htr.0000000000000074.
23. Stanislav SW, Childs A. Evaluating the usage of droperidol in acutely agitated persons with brain injury. Brain Inj. 2000;14(3):261–5. https://doi.org/10.1080/026990500120736.
24. Wilson MS, Gibson CJ, Hamm RJ. Haloperidol, but not olanzapine, impairs cognitive performance after traumatic brain injury in rats. Am J Phys Med Rehabil. 2003;82(11):871–9.
25. Maturana Waidele R, Maturana Rodillo R. Control de la agresividad con olanzapina en pacientes post tec/aggressiveness control using olanzapine in post tbi patients. Cienc Trab. 2009;11(31):22–4.
26. Plantier D, Luaute J, SOFMER Group. Drugs for behavior disorders after traumatic brain injury: systematic review and expert consensus leading to French recommendations for good practice. Ann Phys Rehabil Med. 2016;59(1):42–57. https://doi.org/10.1016/j.rehab.2015.10.003.
27. Brooke MM, Patterson DR, Questad KA, Cardenas D, Farrel-Roberts L. The treatment of agitation during initial hospitalization after traumatic brain injury. Arch Phys Med Rehabil. 1992;73(10):917–21.

28. Greendyke RM, Kanter DR, Schuster DB, Verstreate S, Wootton J. Propranolol treatment of assaultive patients with organic brain disease. A double-blind crossover, placebo-controlled study. J Nerv Ment Dis. 1986;174(5):290–4. https://doi.org/10.1097/00005053-198605000-00005.
29. Ley EJ, Leonard SD, Barmparas G, et al. Beta blockers in critically ill patients with traumatic brain injury: results from a multicenter, prospective, observational American Association for the Surgery of Trauma study. J Trauma Acute Care Surg. 2018;84(2):234–44. https://doi.org/10.1097/TA.0000000000001747.
30. Hicks AJ, Clay FJ, Hopwood M, et al. The efficacy and harms of pharmacological interventions for aggression after traumatic brain injury-systematic review. Front Neurol. 2019;10:1169. https://doi.org/10.3389/fneur.2019.01169.
31. Mehta S, McIntyre A, Janzen S, Iruthayarajah J, Bateman A, Teasell R. Pharmacological management of agitation among individuals with moderate to severe acquired brain injury: a systematic review. Brain Inj. 2018;32(3):287–96. https://doi.org/10.1080/02699052.2017.1419377.
32. Mohamed Ali O, Faruqui RA. Efficacy and tolerability of antipsychotics in treatment of agitation and aggression following traumatic brain injury (TBI): systematic review of clinical trials. Eur Psychiatry. 2015;30(1):28–31.
33. Ter Mors BJ, Backx APM, Spauwen P, Ponds RWHM, Van Harten PN, Van Heugten CM. Efficacy of amantadine on behavioural problems due to acquired brain injury: a systematic review. Brain Inj. 2019;33(9):1137–50. https://doi.org/10.1080/02699052.2019.1631482.
34. Nash RP, Weinberg MS, Laughon SL, McCall RC, Bateman JR, Rosenstein DL. Acute pharmacological management of behavioral and emotional dysregulation following a traumatic brain injury: a systematic review of the literature. Psychosomatics. 2019;60(2):139–52. https://doi.org/10.1016/j.psym.2018.11.009.
35. Sami MB, Faruqui R. The effectiveness of dopamine agonists for treatment of neuropsychiatric symptoms post brain injury and stroke. Acta Neuropsychiatr. 2015;27(6):317–26. https://doi.org/10.1017/neu.2015.17.
36. Stelmaschuk S, Will MC, Meyers T. Amantadine to treat cognitive dysfunction in moderate to severe traumatic brain injury. J Trauma Nurs. 2015;22(4):194–203; quiz E1–2. https://doi.org/10.1097/jtn.0000000000000138.
37. Wheaton P, Mathias JL, Vink R. Impact of pharmacological treatments on cognitive and behavioral outcome in the postacute stages of adult traumatic brain injury: a meta-analysis. J Clin Psychopharmacol. 2011;31(6):745–57. https://doi.org/10.1097/JCP.0b013e318235f4ac.
38. Williamson D, Frenette AJ, Burry LD, et al. Pharmacological interventions for agitated behaviours in patients with traumatic brain injury: a systematic review. BMJ Open. 2019;9(7):e029604. https://doi.org/10.1136/bmjopen-2019-029604.
39. Villasana LE, Peters A, McCallum R, Liu C, Schnell E. Diazepam inhibits post-traumatic neurogenesis and blocks aberrant dendritic development. J Neurotrauma. 2019;36(16):2454–67. https://doi.org/10.1089/neu.2018.6162.
40. Goldstein LB. Effects of amphetamines and small related molecules on recovery after stroke in animals and man. Neuropharmacology. 2000;39(5):852–9. https://doi.org/10.1016/s0028-3908(99)00249-x.
41. Hasselt PV. Effect of butyrophenones on motor function in rats after recovery from brain damage. Neuropharmacology. 1973;12(3):245–7. https://doi.org/10.1016/0028-3908(73)90109-3.
42. Ochalski PG, Fellows-Mayle W, Hsieh LB, et al. Flumazenil administration attenuates cognitive impairment in immature rats after controlled cortical impact. J Neurotrauma. 2010;27(3):647–51. https://doi.org/10.1089/neu.2009.1142.
43. Perna R. Brain injury. J Head Trauma Rehabil. 2006;21(1):82–4.
44. Larson EB, Zollman FS. The effect of sleep medications on cognitive recovery from traumatic brain injury. J Head Trauma Rehabil. 2010;25(1):61–7. https://doi.org/10.1097/HTR.0b013e3181c1d1e1.

45. Goldstein LB, Matchar DB, Morgenlander JC, Davis JN. Influence of drugs on the recovery of sensorimotor function after stroke. J Neurol Rehabil. 1990;4(3):137–44. https://doi.org/10.1177/136140969000400303.
46. Goldstein LB. Common drugs may influence motor recovery after stroke. The Sygen in acute stroke study investigators. Neurology. 1995;45(5):865–71. https://doi.org/10.1212/wnl.45.5.865.
47. Beresford (Principal Investigator) TP. A double blind trial of divalproex sodium for affective lability and alcohol use following traumatic brain injury [Annual Report]. Prepared for U.S. Army Medical Research and Material Command. 2010. https://apps.dtic.mil/sti/pdfs/ADA549156.pdf
48. Beresford T, Ronan PJ, Hipp D, et al. A double-blind placebo-controlled, randomized trial of divalproex sodium for posttraumatic irritability greater than 1 year after mild to moderate traumatic brain injury. J Neuropsychiatry Clin Neurosci Summer. 2022;34(3):224–32. https://doi.org/10.1176/appi.neuropsych.19070159.
49. Mattes JA. Oxcarbazepine in patients with impulsive aggression: a double-blind, placebo-controlled trial. J Clin Psychopharmacol. 2005;25(6):575–9. https://doi.org/10.1097/01.jcp.0000186739.22395.6b.
50. Giacino JT, Whyte J, Bagiella E, et al. Placebo-controlled trial of amantadine for severe traumatic brain injury. N Engl J Med. 2012;366(9):819–26.
51. Reddy CC, Collins M, Lovell M, Kontos AP. Efficacy of amantadine treatment on symptoms and neurocognitive performance among adolescents following sports-related concussion. J Head Trauma Rehabil. 2013;28(4):260–5.
52. Mooney GF, Haas LJ. Effect of methylphenidate on brain injury-related anger. Arch Phys Med Rehabil. 1993;74(2):153–60. https://doi.org/10.5555/uri:pii:000399939390355E.
53. Fong TG, Tulebaev SR, Inouye SK. Delirium in elderly adults: diagnosis, prevention and treatment. Nat Rev Neurol. 2009;5(4):210–20. https://doi.org/10.1038/nrneurol.2009.24.
54. Inouye SK, Westendorp RG, Saczynski JS. Delirium in elderly people. Lancet. 2014;383(9920):911–22. https://doi.org/10.1016/s0140-6736(13)60688-1.
55. Hopkins RO, Jackson JC. Long-term neurocognitive function after critical illness. Chest. 2006;130(3):869–78. https://doi.org/10.1378/chest.130.3.869.
56. Pandharipande PP, Girard TD, Ely EW. Long-term cognitive impairment after critical illness. N Engl J Med. 2014;370(2):185–6. https://doi.org/10.1056/NEJMc1313886.
57. Gofton TE, Young GB. Sepsis-associated encephalopathy. Nat Rev Neurol. 2012;8(10):557–66. https://doi.org/10.1038/nrneurol.2012.183.
58. Hshieh TT, Fong TG, Marcantonio ER, Inouye SK. Cholinergic deficiency hypothesis in delirium: a synthesis of current evidence. J Gerontol A Biol Sci Med Sci. 2008;63(7):764–72. https://doi.org/10.1093/gerona/63.7.764.
59. Inouye SK, Charpentier PA. Precipitating factors for delirium in hospitalized elderly persons. Predictive model and interrelationship with baseline vulnerability. JAMA. 1996;275(11):852–7.
60. Gross AL, Jones RN, Habtemariam DA, et al. Delirium and long-term cognitive trajectory among persons with dementia. Arch Intern Med. 2012;172(17):1324–31. https://doi.org/10.1001/archinternmed.2012.3203.
61. Rubin FH, Neal K, Fenlon K, Hassan S, Inouye SK. Sustainability and scalability of the hospital elder life program at a community hospital. J Am Geriatr Soc. 2011;59(2):359–65. https://doi.org/10.1111/j.1532-5415.2010.03243.x.
62. Fitzgerald JM, Adamis D, Trzepacz PT, et al. Delirium: a disturbance of circadian integrity? Med Hypotheses. 2013;81(4):568–76. https://doi.org/10.1016/j.mehy.2013.06.032.
63. de Jonghe A, van Munster BC, Goslings JC, et al. Effect of melatonin on incidence of delirium among patients with hip fracture: a multicentre, double-blind randomized controlled trial. CMAJ. 2014;186(14):E547–56. https://doi.org/10.1503/cmaj.140495.
64. American Geriatrics Society 2015 Beers Criteria Update Expert Panel. American Geriatrics Society 2015 updated beers criteria for potentially inappropriate medication use in older adults. J Am Geriatr Soc. 2015;63(11):2227–46. https://doi.org/10.1111/jgs.13702.

65. Brown EN, Purdon PL, Van Dort CJ. General anesthesia and altered states of arousal: a systems neuroscience analysis. Annu Rev Neurosci. 2011;34:601–28. https://doi.org/10.1146/annurev-neuro-060909-153200.
66. Pandharipande P, Shintani A, Peterson J, et al. Lorazepam is an independent risk factor for transitioning to delirium in intensive care unit patients. Anesthesiology. 2006;104(1):21–6. https://doi.org/10.1097/00000542-200601000-00005.
67. Breitbart W, Marotta R, Platt MM, et al. A double-blind trial of haloperidol, chlorpromazine, and lorazepam in the treatment of delirium in hospitalized AIDS patients. Am J Psychiatry. 1996;153(2):231–7. https://doi.org/10.1176/ajp.153.2.231.
68. Han CS, Kim YK. A double-blind trial of risperidone and haloperidol for the treatment of delirium. Psychosomatics. 2004;45(4):297–301. https://doi.org/10.1016/s0033-3182(04)70170-x.
69. de la Cruz M, Fan J, Yennu S, et al. The frequency of missed delirium in patients referred to palliative care in a comprehensive cancer center. Support Care Cancer. 2015;23(8):2427–33. https://doi.org/10.1007/s00520-015-2610-3.
70. Morandi A, Hughes CG, Thompson JL, et al. Statins and delirium during critical illness: a multicenter, prospective cohort study. Crit Care Med. 2014;42(8):1899–909. https://doi.org/10.1097/ccm.0000000000000398.
71. Brummel NE, Girard TD. Preventing delirium in the intensive care unit. Crit Care Clin. 2013;29(1):51–65. https://doi.org/10.1016/j.ccc.2012.10.007.
72. Duning T, van den Heuvel I, Dickmann A, et al. Hypoglycemia aggravates critical illness-induced neurocognitive dysfunction. Diabetes Care. 2010;33(3):639–44. https://doi.org/10.2337/dc09-1740.

Chapter 8
Spasticity Management

Gary Galang, Mark Linsenmeyer, Justin Weppner, and Amy K. Wagner

Chapter Objectives
1. Define spasticity and discuss its impact on function and quality of life.
2. Discuss tools to measure spasticity.
3. Delineate common pharmacologic and non-pharmacologic treatment approaches for spasticity with an emphasis on inpatient and consultant management.

Introduction

Spasticity is a major health problem for many individuals following neurologic injury and can markedly impair mobility, positioning, and independence. The acute care rehabilitation consultant has the opportunity and responsibility to identify spasticity and expedite treatment in order to improve outcomes. Physiatry's multimodal approach to patient care is uniquely suited to assess and treat spasticity and its complications in the acute care setting. This chapter will address key concepts in the rehabilitative approach to early spasticity development.

G. Galang A. K. Wagner
Department of Physical Medicine and Rehabilitation, University of Pittsburgh School of Medicine, Pittsburgh, PA, USA
e-mail: galangg@upmc.edu; wagnerak@upmc.edu

M. Linsenmeyer (✉)
Department of Physical Medicine and Rehabilitation, Sunnyview Rehabilitation Hospital, Schenectady, NY, USA
e-mail: mark.linsenmeyer@sphp.com

J. Weppner
Virginia Tech Carilion School of Medicine, Edward Via College of Osteopathic Medicine, Roanoke, VA, USA
e-mail: jlweppner@carilionclinic.org

A. K. Wagner, J. Weppner (eds.), *Acute Care Neuroconsultation and Neurorehabilitation Management*, https://doi.org/10.1007/978-3-031-42830-2_8

Background and Clinical Features

Spasticity is a secondary condition frequently experienced by individuals with upper motor neuron damage following central nervous system (CNS) trauma or disease. It is traditionally defined as velocity-dependent increase in the tonic stretch reflex (muscle tone) with exaggerated stretch reflexes (tendon jerks, clonus, spasms) resulting from hyperexcitability of the stretch reflex [1]. More recently, this definition has been expanded, and spasticity has been categorized as part of upper motor neuron syndrome (UMNS). Signs and symptoms of UMNS are broadly classified as positive phenomena (increased levels of involuntary motor activity) or negative phenomena (decreased levels of voluntary motor activity). Examples of positive features include increased tendon reflexes, spasms, clonus, dystonia, and dyssynergia patterns of co-contraction during movement. Negative features include loss of dexterity, weakness, fatigue, and pain [2]. Taken together, these features of UMNS can adversely affect independence, quality of life (QOL), and the amount of required caregiver assistance needed to support impairment and disability related to an individual's UMNS. Potential complications of severe spasticity include contracture, long bone fracture, and chronic skin ulceration and pain [3]. Management of spasticity should focus on all elements of UMNS to improve function and relieve pain.

The prevalence of spasticity varies by causative etiology. Problematic spasticity affects an estimated 30% of those with stroke, 33% of those with spinal cord injury (SCI), at least 25% of those with traumatic brain injury (TBI), and 38% of those with multiple sclerosis [4]. Spasticity may manifest at a single joint, multiple joints within a single limb, multiple limbs, the neck or trunk, or may be generalized and manifest throughout the body. The distribution of muscle groups affected by spasticity often follows typical patterns based on the underlying lesion. For example, upper extremity flexor spasticity is common after stroke, while lower extremity extensor spasms are more common after SCI [5]. Lesions above the foramen magnum (including TBI, stroke, and cerebral palsy) produce central spasticity due to a loss of descending neuron inhibition, while lesions below the foramen magnum (such as SCI, amyotrophic lateral sclerosis, and multiple sclerosis) produce spinal spasticity, which results from increased excitability of motor neurons due to the removal of supraspinal control [6].

Clinical Assessment

Multiple scales have been developed to assess spasticity, including but not limited to the Ashworth Scale, Modified Ashworth Scale (MAS), Spinal Cord Assessment Tool for Spasticity (SCATS), Penn Spasm Frequency Score, and Tardieu Scale [7–10]. There is no universally preferred scale as all scales have different uses and limitations [11, 12]. The Ashworth and Modified Ashworth scales are among the most recognized measures of spasticity and are commonly used clinically and in research studies. The Ashworth Scale was first published in 1964 and the MAS was later developed to add an additional measure to the scale (the 1+ grade; Table 8.1). In both scales, the examiner passively ranges the extremity at a joint and grades the amount of resistance perceived, with a score of 0 representing no tone and a score of 4 representing rigidity at the affected joint [13]. MAS use is widespread and is easy to learn and perform, however, inter-rater reliability is limited [14]. Inter- and intra-rater reliability may be better when measuring the upper extremities compared to when measuring the lower [15]. The Tardieu and Modified Tardieu scales are separate bedside measures of spasticity involving passive range of motion at a joint (Table 8.2). Unlike the Ashworth scales, the Tardieu scales incorporate different velocities into their assessment. There has not been any evidence showing that the scale is superior to the MAS, and the current literature does not provide firm conclusions on the validity or reliability of the scale [13, 16].

One difficulty in developing clinical scales for spasticity is that spasticity measurement and functional assessment may not go hand-in-hand. Regardless of which scale is used, overall assessment of well-being and function should be a major component of the larger clinical evaluation of spasticity. Clinicians may incorporate additional tools such as FIM scores, the pain Visual Analogue Scale, and range of motion assessments in conjunction with the above scales to obtain a more complete understanding of spasticity's impact [17]. Electrophysiologic studies can also quantify spasticity, however, these are primarily used in research rather than clinical settings [18].

Differentiating Spasticity from Paratonia and Other Forms of Hypertonia

In contrast to velocity dependent increases in muscle tone associated with spasticity, other forms of hypertonia may be present on physical exam that need to be appreciated as distinct from spasticity.

Table 8.1 Modified Ashworth Scale [7]

Grade	Description
0	No increase in muscle tone
1	Slight increase in muscle tone, manifested by a catch and release or by minimal resistance at the end of the range of motion when the affected part(s) is moved in flexion or extension
1+	Slight increase in muscle tone, manifested by a catch, followed by minimal resistance throughout the remainder (less than half) of the ROM
2	More marked increase in muscle tone through most of the ROM, but affected part(s) easily moved
3	Considerable increase in muscle tone, passive movement difficult
4	Affected part(s) rigid in flexion or extension

Table 8.2 Tardieu scale [10]

Principles	Grading always performed:
	• On a muscle at rest before the stretch maneuver
	• At a reproducible velocity of stretch. Once the fast velocity is selected for a muscle, it remains the same for all subsequent tests
	• At the same time of the day
	• In a constant body position for a given limb
	• Other joints, particularly the neck, must also remain in a constant position throughout the assessment and for all other assessments
	Velocity of Stretch
	• SLOW = V1: As slow as possible (slower than the rate of natural drop of the limb segment under gravity)
	• FAST = Either V2 or V3
	– V2: Speed of the limb segment falling under gravity
	– V3: As fast as possible (faster than the rate of natural drop of the limb segment under gravity)
Grading	X = Spasticity angle (threshold) = angle of arrest at slow speed X_{V1} *minus* angle of catch at fast speed X_{V3}
	Y = spasticity grade (gain)
	0 No resistance throughout passive movement
	1 Slight resistance throughout passive movement
	2 Clear catch at precise angle, interrupting passive movement, followed by release
	3 Fatigable clonus (<10 s when maintaining pressure) occurring at a precise angle, followed by release
	4 Unfatigable clonus (>10 s when maintaining pressure) occurring at a precise angle
	• Catch without release: Graded 0 if $X_{V1} = X_{V3}$; "unratable" spasticity otherwise
	• Catch with "minimal" release: Graded 2 if X_{V3} is consistent and consistently less than X_{V1}
	• Angle 0° = position of minimal stretch of the tested muscle
	• For grades 0 and 1, spasticity angle X = 0° by definition

- *Paratonia* is considered the inability to relax muscles during passive range of motion examination. For some, involuntary physical resistance, or opposition, can occur in response to passive limb movements attempted by the examiner (gegenhalten), while others may involuntarily assist with passive limb movements attempted by the examiner (mitgehen). Paratonia may be more often observed in older patients, particularly those with underlying dementia various forms of frontal lobe dysfunction. Paratonia may be appreciated at times as velocity dependent.
- *Rigidity* is typically appreciated as velocity independent increase in hypertonic resistance to passive movements. It can be linked to diseases associated with dopamine system dysfunction, such as Parkinson's Disease (Parkinsonian rigidity) and Schizophrenia (catatonic rigidity). Cogwheeling, or a sense of ratcheting during passive range of motion, may accompany Parkinsonian rigidity as muscles contract and relax during passive range of motion. Rigidity noted on physical

exam may accompany changes in dopamine systems associated with both brain injury and medication trials addressing brain injury deficits and/or behaviors.

Spasticity Treatment

A multidisciplinary and multimodal approach is essential to optimally treat spasticity. Rather than following a simple algorithmic approach, treatment plans should be individualized and reassessed frequently. All medical interventions are adjunctive to a program of physical and occupational therapy, removal of exacerbating stimuli, and caregiver education in the acute hospital phase of treatment. Pharmacological interventions can be broadly grouped into those for the relief of generalized spasticity with oral medication, those for the relief of regional spasticity problems with intrathecal baclofen, and those for the focal and multi-focal spasticity problems with chemodenervation with botulinum toxin or phenol/alcohol induced nerve blockade. Oral medication used for managing spasticity has been well-established, extensively researched, and found to be effective. However, oral medications should be used cautiously during acute hospitalization as they can cause unwanted adverse effects, including sedation and changes in cognition and mood that may impact therapy participation and tolerance for higher intensity rehabilitation programs available for post-acute care. The risks of sedation and reduced arousal should be weighed against the benefits of spasticity treatment during acute hospitalization.

Sudden worsening of spasticity is often a sign of an underlying noxious stimulus in an area where the individual no longer has sensation or voluntary motor control. Thus, after an initial patient assessment, the first step in spasticity treatment is to identify and treat any modifiable pathologic stimuli. Such stimuli may include pain, tight clothing or orthoses, urinary retention or kinked catheters, urinary tract infection, other infection or abscesses, pressure sores, constipation, heterotopic ossification, or occult injury [19]. Prior to initiating treatment, clinicians should consider the potential functional benefits of spasticity in a given patient, as complete elimination of hypertonicity could potentially result in more harm than benefit. For example, lower extremity spasticity may sometimes compensate for weakness and allow an individual to stand or transfer [3]. Spasticity may also improve ability to cough, maintain muscle bulk, assist in preventing deep vein thromboses (DVTs) by increasing venous return, and protect against osteoporosis [18]. In deciding to initiate therapy for spasticity, appropriate goals of treatment may include improvement in range of motion, mobility, and dexterity, improvement in uncomfortable body positioning or poor orthotic fit, facilitation of therapy, prevention of contracture, and reduction of caregiver assistance to maximize independence [20].

The role of the physical (PT) or occupational therapist (OT) in non-pharmacological spasticity management cannot be overstated. Spastic muscles remain shortened, which can lead to contracture and joint deformation. Daily passive stretching and strengthening of both spastic and synergistic muscles can reduce muscle tone, increase joint ROM, and prevent contractures [5]. For the acute care physiatry consultant, special attention should be paid to the fact that therapy

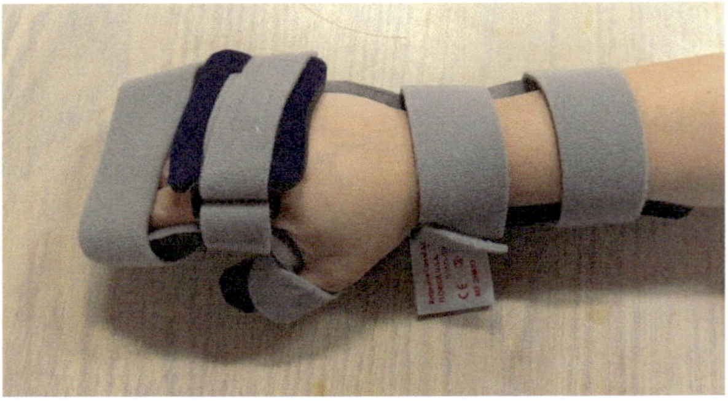

Fig. 8.1 Resting hand splint

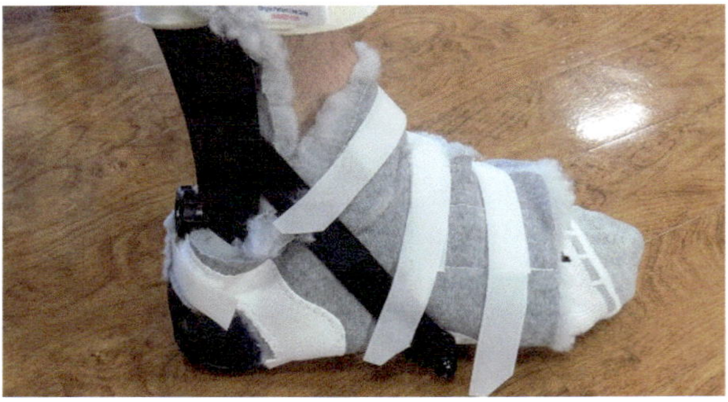

Fig. 8.2 PRAFO boot

services often cannot provide daily treatment for extended periods of time. Thus, nursing and family training on appropriate ROM exercises may be helpful to support joint function. Splints and orthoses can prevent improper positioning and provide prolonged stretch outside of therapy hours. In general, orthotic intervention should focus on realigning limb segments to normal anatomical positions [21]. The choice of an appropriate orthosis should be individualized and done in consultation with therapists. Common choices in the initial management of spasticity include resting hand splints (Fig. 8.1) and pressure relief ankle foot orthoses (PRAFOs) (Fig. 8.2).

If troublesome tone persists despite removal of noxious stimuli and initiation of therapeutic modalities, pharmacologic treatment should be considered. Targeted injections alone may be a sufficient treatment for localized spasticity, while oral medications should be considered for generalized spasticity. This chapter will next discuss oral medications that have been systematically reviewed, including centrally acting muscle relaxants (baclofen, benzodiazepines, and tizanidine) and peripherally-acting muscle relaxants (dantrolene). Oral agent selection in the acute care setting may be impacted by factors such as age, renal function, liver function, medical stability. Both chemodenervation and oral agents have utility when managing other conditions such as PSH (Chap. 9). Side effects associated with centrally acting agents, such as sedation, may create challenges with accurate neurological and functional assessment in patients with impaired arousal, which may impact important decisions regarding next level of care and should be considered carefully by the acute care consultant when establishing a spasticity management plan.

Baclofen

Baclofen is a frequently prescribed medication for spasticity. As an analog of the inhibitory neurotransmitter GABA, it selectively binds to GABA-B receptors in the brain and spinal cord. This binding inhibits pre-synaptic calcium influx, thus suppressing release of excitatory neurotransmitters [18]. Its efficacy is approximately equivalent to that of tizanidine and diazepam, with less of a sedative effect [22]. The typical starting dose for baclofen is 5 mg 3 times per day. It can be titrated slowly by increasing the total daily dose by 15 mg every 3 days up to 80 mg per day in divided doses [6]. However, dosing in the setting of renal dysfunction should be reduced, and dosing selected in consultation with the team pharmacist and/or renal replacement consultants [23]. Common side effects typically include sedation, weakness, nausea, vertigo or ataxia, and confusion. Signs of sudden withdrawal include seizures, hallucinations, anxiety, psychosis, confusion, and rebound spasticity [24]. Intrathecal baclofen will be discussed later in this chapter.

Tizanidine

The efficacy of tizanidine in multiple sclerosis and stroke is comparable to that of diazepam and baclofen [22]. Tizanidine is a centrally acting alpha-2 adrenergic agonist. It decreases the release of excitatory amino acids (glutamate and aspartate) at spinal and supraspinal levels, thus decreasing muscle tone [25]. Due to its alpha-2 adrenergic activity, cardiovascular side effects can also occur, such as hypotension, lightheadedness, bradycardia, or rarely syncope. Other common side effects include dry mouth, dizziness, and somnolence. About 5% of individuals experience an increase in hepatic transaminase levels, which typically resolves after tizanidine is stopped. Liver function tests should be monitored regularly for the first 6 months of treatment and then periodically afterwards [26]. However, dosing in geriatric patients and in the setting of renal dysfunction should be reduced, and dosing selected in consultation with the team pharmacist and/or renal replacement consultants [27]. Dosing typically starts at 2–4 mg per day and can be titrated over 2–4 weeks to up to 36 mg per day, typically in three divided doses [6]. Since it is extensively metabolized by cytochrome P450 (CYP) 1A2, using tizanidine is contraindicated in patients also taking CYP1A2 inhibitors, such as ciprofloxacin or fluvoxamine as well as some oral contraceptives, to prevent toxic plasma tizanidine accumulation [28–31].

Dantrolene Sodium

Dantrolene sodium is the only oral anti-spasticity medication that works peripherally on muscle fibers. It suppresses the release of calcium from the sarcoplasmic reticulum of muscle fibers, which decreases the force produced by excitation-contraction coupling during muscle contraction [32]. Due to its peripheral action, its immediate side effect profile is generally better tolerated than that of the other oral medications, with less drowsiness and cognitive impairment. Accordingly, it is a compelling option for individuals with reduced arousal [20]. This point is particularly important in the acute care setting; for acute care neurorehabilitation consultants, level of arousal is a key area of functional assessment as is evaluating capacity to tolerate inpatient rehabilitation. Its most common side effects are typically mild and include weakness, lightheadedness, paresthesias, and rare gastrointestinal upset. Classically, its most serious side effect is hepatotoxicity; liver function tests (LFTs) should be monitored before initiating the drug, during titration, and on a regular basis during prolonged use of the medication. It should be noted that some clinical and animal studies have not been able to reproduce hepatotoxicity with prolonged dantrolene sodium use [33, 34]. Dosing typically starts at 25 mg per day and can be increased by 25–50 mg every 4–7 days to a max dose of 400 mg per day, typically in three to four divided doses [6].

Benzodiazepines

Benzodiazepines such as diazepam and clonazepam are used primarily in spinal rather than central spasticity. They amplify the inhibitory action of GABA-A by binding to GABA-A receptors, which facilitates the post-synaptic effects of GABA and inhibits pre-synaptic excitatory release. They act diffusely throughout the brain and spinal cord [18]. This central action commonly leads to sedation; therefore, alternative agents should be considered for those with impairments in arousal or attention. Additionally, animal studies have shown that continued use of GABAergic medications can impair neural recovery and cognition after a brain injury [19, 35–37]. Benzodiazepines also carry a potential for abuse and dependency. Muscle hypotonicity and decreased reflexes are side effects that are potentially clinically useful in the treatment of painful spasms. Diazepam can be initiated at 2–5 mg twice per day and up-titrated to 30 mg total per day. If shorter acting effects are desired, such as in the control of occasional painful spasms, clonazepam may be utilized, typically starting at 0.5 mg at night and slowly increasing to a maximum of 4 mg per day in 3–4 divided doses [6]. Special attention should be paid to dosing in older adults, and those at risk for respiratory depression and worsening of COPD and sleep apnea [38].

Other Oral Medications

The above medications are the current mainstays in oral spasticity treatment. Additional medications such as gabapentin, cyrproheptadine, opioids, tricyclic antidepressants, and cannabis have been used as adjunctive treatments for spasticity, although they have not been extensively investigated. A randomized control trial of a small number of subjects showed good efficacy and safety of gabapentin at 2700–3600 mg/day in divided doses [39]. Further research is needed to illuminate the role of these medications as a part of a comprehensive approach to spasticity, particularly in the acute care hospital setting.

Chemodenervation in the Treatment of Spasticity

If spasticity is focal or localized, as opposed to generalized spasticity affecting multiple body areas, local injections can be effectively used with a much smaller risk of systemic side effects compared to oral medications [40]. Injections target spastic muscles with chemical neurolysis or botulinum toxin [5]. Injections can be used in conjunction with therapeutic modalities and oral medications as part of a comprehensive approach to spasticity [41].

Chemical neurolysis with alcohol or phenol causes axonal destruction and demyelination. The agents penetrate nerve tissue and coagulate protein, which results in nerve tissue destruction. Wallerian degeneration follows and shows its maximal effect after 2 weeks. Partial nerve regeneration begins a few weeks after the neurolysis and regeneration is almost complete after approximately 14 weeks. The obturator, medial popliteal, sciatic, and musculocutaneous nerves are common targets for chemical neurolysis. Nerve blocks in the upper extremities may be more likely to cause loss of skin sensation and vascular damage [42]. Chemical neurolysis is more time consuming than botulinum toxin injections, which are increasingly used, and reimbursed, in the acute care setting.

Botulinum toxin (BoNT) is the most common injectate for localized spasticity. It is a neurotoxin produced by *Clostridium botulinum* bacteria. Of the seven serotypes of BoNT, labeled A to G, serotypes A and B are the toxins used most frequently in the clinical setting. The toxin acts by inhibiting acetylcholine release from presynaptic nerve terminals in the neuromuscular junction. This leads to chemical denervation and a reduction in spasticity. There is typically at least a 2–4 day delay between injection of the toxin and perceptible clinical effects, and maximum benefit is usually observed by 2–3 weeks post-injection. The duration of effect is usually approximately 3 months, at which time injections can be repeated. Electromyography

(EMG) and ultrasound guidance can be helpful in localizing smaller muscles for injection. Approximately 3% of individuals develop neutralizing antibodies to the toxin, which manifests as a decreased clinical response to increased doses of the toxin [43]. Otherwise, side effects are typically very mild and include weakness, flu-like symptoms, and pain or hemorrhage around the injection site. Acute illnesses such as pneumonia, urinary tract infections, and systemic inflammatory response syndrome should be considered when timing botulinum toxin administration in the acute care setting. Botulinum toxin injection should be avoided when the patient is medically unstable with an untreated illness. There are no known CNS or systemic side effects associated with long-term use. Long-term use of the toxin has been shown to reduce muscle tone in spastic muscle and to improve function [44]. Cost and insurance reimbursement can be limiting factors, especially in the inpatient setting, and should be considered prior to the procedure. In certain situations, however, effective use of botulinum toxin in the acute care setting can significantly impact function and recovery and should strongly be considered. For example, injections treating noxious spasticity could improve paroxysmal sympathetic hyperactivity, bruxism, or uncomfortable focal limb spasticity [45, 46]. When planning botulinum toxin injections in the acute phase of care, areas of emerging spasticity should also be considered in the overall injection plan, given that botulinum toxin can only be administered every 3 months.

Surgical Options

A number of surgical options are available for those with spasticity that is not responsive to the above interventions. Intrathecal baclofen pumps and orthopedic surgical procedures can be helpful when used as part of a multimodal approach to spasticity.

Intrathecal baclofen (ITB) pumps may be indicated for patients with persistent spasticity despite maximal dosing of oral medications or for patients with intolerable adverse effects to these medications. Baclofen is administered via an implanted programmable pump and an intrathecal catheter. An ITB screening procedure is performed prior to pump placement [47]. Intrathecal delivery is generally tolerated well with few adverse effects. However, ensuring good patient compliance and follow-up for pump refills is a prerequisite, as withdrawal from the medication can be fatal. Acute care neurorehabilitation consultants should be aware that withdrawal typically progresses and evolves over 1–3 days, starting with rebound spasticity and then leading to hallucinations, generalized seizures, tachycardia, blood pressure lability, itching or paresthesias, rhabdomyolysis, dysphoria, decreased responsiveness, and death. If withdrawal is suspected, the pump's manufacturer should be contacted for pump interrogation. Oral baclofen or intravenous benzodiazepines should be titrated to achieve reduction in symptoms until intrathecal supply is reestablished [48].

Some patients encountered by acute care consultants may have chronic spasticity that has failed the above interventions or that has led to fixed contractures or significant skin breakdown. For these individuals, surgical procedures may be indicated to control pain, improve function, and prevent contracture. Common procedures include tendon releases or transfers [25]. Alternative options include peripheral neurotomies, which involve distal sectioning of individual nerves, or dorsal rhizotomies that are primarily used in spastic cerebral palsy [49, 50].

Case Illustration

As the physiatry consultant, you are asked to evaluate a 32-year-old man in the intensive care unit with a TBI status-post assault. When you arrive at the unit, the primary team alerts you that the patient has recently become more somnolent. Recent complete blood count, urinalysis, and chest x-ray are unremarkable and vital signs are stable. Upon evaluation, you immediately notice that the patient's elbows, wrists, and fingers are flexed. His legs are extended at the hip and knee, with plantar flexion and inversion at both ankles. His foley catheter appears to be draining well, and examination reveals no pressure sores, tight braces, or clothing. A medication review shows that the patient was recently started on baclofen 5 mg 3 times daily, and baclofen is discontinued as a potential source of sedation. However, recognizing that these synergy patterns may represent signs of underlying pathology, you recommend a computerized tomography (CT) of the head. CT shows acute hydrocephalus, and a ventriculoperitoneal shunt is placed with subsequent improvement in arousal and posturing. There is still some spasticity on physical examination: Modified Ashworth Scale is 2 in the upper extremities and 1 in the lower extremities. At your recommendation, the primary team obtains normal liver enzymes and starts dantrolene 25 mg daily. A stretching and strengthening program is initiated with physical and occupational therapy in the intensive care unit. After a week of dantrolene treatment, repeat liver enzymes are obtained and normal. Dantrolene is increased to 25 mg 3 times a day with a recommendation to continue to assess weekly liver enzymes before further titration of dantrolene. You follow the patient through admission to inpatient rehabilitation, where his function and mobility continue to improve with therapeutic modalities and titration of his dantrolene dose.

Summary

Spasticity, a consequence of upper motor neuron disease or injury, can significantly impair function and QOL. Optimal management of spasticity involves early detection and contributions from multiple disciplines including physicians, nurses, and therapists. Clinical assessment should include consideration of the impact spasticity has on pain and function. Early treatment starts with stretching and muscle strengthening, and can incorporate braces, splinting, oral medications, and localized injections.

References[1]

1. Lance JW. The control of muscle tone, reflexes, and movement: Robert Wartenberg lecture. Neurology. 1980;30(12):1303–13. https://doi.org/10.1212/wnl.30.12.1303.
2. Pandyan AD, Gregoric M, Barnes MP, et al. Spasticity: clinical perceptions, neurological realities and meaningful measurement. Disabil Rehabil. 2005;27(1–2):2–6. https://doi.org/10.1080/09638280400014576.
3. Nance PW, Satkunam L, Ethans K. Spasticity management. In: Braddom RL, Chan L, Harrast MA, et al., editors. Physical medicine & rehabilitation. 4th ed. Philadelphia: Elsevier Saunders; 2011. p. 641–59.
4. McGuire JR. Epidemiology of spasticity in the adult and child. In: Brashear A, Elovic EP, editors. Spasticity: diagnosis and management. New York: Demos Medical Publishing; 2010. p. 5–16.
5. Elbasiouny SM, Moroz D, Bakr MM, Mushahwar VK. Management of spasticity after spinal cord injury: current techniques and future directions. Neurorehabil Neural Repair. 2010;24(1):23–33. https://doi.org/10.1177/1545968309343213.
6. Lapeyre E, Kuks JB, Meijler WJ. Spasticity: revisiting the role and the individual value of several pharmacological treatments. NeuroRehabilitation. 2010;27(2):193–200. https://doi.org/10.3233/nre-2010-0596.
7. Bohannon RW, Smith MB. Interrater reliability of a modified Ashworth scale of muscle spasticity. Phys Ther. 1987;67(2):206–7. https://doi.org/10.1093/ptj/67.2.206.
8. Benz EN, Hornby TG, Bode RK, Scheidt RA, Schmit BD. A physiologically based clinical measure for spastic reflexes in spinal cord injury. Arch Phys Med Rehabil. 2005;86(1):52–9. https://doi.org/10.1016/j.apmr.2004.01.033.
9. Sköld C. Spasticity in spinal cord injury: self- and clinically rated intrinsic fluctuations and intervention-induced changes. Arch Phys Med Rehabil. 2000;81(2):144–9. https://doi.org/10.1016/s0003-9993(00)90132-1.
10. Gracies JM, Burke K, Clegg NJ, et al. Reliability of the Tardieu scale for assessing spasticity in children with cerebral palsy. Arch Phys Med Rehabil. 2010;91(3):421–8. https://doi.org/10.1016/j.apmr.2009.11.017.
11. Hsieh JT, Wolfe DL, Miller WC, Curt A. Spasticity outcome measures in spinal cord injury: psychometric properties and clinical utility. Spinal Cord. 2008;46(2):86–95. https://doi.org/10.1038/sj.sc.3102125.
12. Priebe MM, Sherwood AM, Thornby JI, Kharas NF, Markowski J. Clinical assessment of spasticity in spinal cord injury: a multidimensional problem. Arch Phys Med Rehabil. 1996;77(7):713–6. https://doi.org/10.1016/s0003-9993(96)90014-3.
13. Gomez-Medina O, Elovic EP. Measurement tools and treatment outcomes in patients with spasticity. In: Brashear A, Elovic EP, editors. Spasticity: diagnosis and management. New York: Demos Medical Publishing; 2010. p. 51–70.
14. Ansari NN, Naghdi S, Arab TK, Jalaie S. The interrater and intrarater reliability of the modified Ashworth scale in the assessment of muscle spasticity: limb and muscle group effect. NeuroRehabilitation. 2008;23(3):231–7.

[1] Key References [2, 3, 5, 6, 17].

15. Meseguer-Henarejos AB, Sanchez-Meca J, Lopez-Pina JA, Carles-Hernandez R. Inter- and intra-rater reliability of the modified ashworth scale: a systematic review and meta-analysis. Eur J Phys Rehabil Med. 2018;54(4):576–90. https://doi.org/10.23736/S1973-9087.17.04796-7.
16. Haugh AB, Pandyan AD, Johnson GR. A systematic review of the Tardieu Scale for the measurement of spasticity. Disabil Rehabil. 2006;28(15):899–907. https://doi.org/10.1080/09638280500404305.
17. Taricco M, Adone R, Pagliacci C, Telaro E. Pharmacological interventions for spasticity following spinal cord injury. Cochrane Database Syst Rev. 2000;2000(2):CD001131. https://doi.org/10.1002/14651858.Cd001131.
18. Elovic E, Baerga E, Escaldi SV, Reyna M. Associated topics in physical medicine and rehabilitation: spasticity. In: Cuccurullo SJ, editor. Physical medicine and rehabilitation board review. 3rd ed. New York: Demos Medical Publishing; 2015. p. 861–73.
19. Zafonte R, Elovic EP, Lombard L. Acute care management of post-TBI spasticity. J Head Trauma Rehabil. 2004;19(2):89–100.
20. Ward AB, Javaid S. Pharmacological management of spasticity. In: Barnes MP, Johnson GR, editors. Upper motor neurone syndrome and spasticity: clinical management and neurophysiology. 2nd ed. Cambridge: Cambridge University Press; 2008. p. 130–49.
21. Charlton PT, Ferguson DWN. Orthoses, splints, and casts. In: Barnes MP, Johnson GR, editors. Upper motor neurone syndrome and spasticity: clinical management and neurophysiology. 2nd ed. Cambridge: Cambridge University Press; 2008. p. 113–30.
22. Chou R, Peterson K, Helfand M. Comparative efficacy and safety of skeletal muscle relaxants for spasticity and musculoskeletal conditions: a systematic review. J Pain Symptom Manag. 2004;28(2):140–75. https://doi.org/10.1016/j.jpainsymman.2004.05.002.
23. Prescribers' Digital Reference LLC. Baclofen—drug summary. https://www.pdr.net/drug-summary/Baclofen-baclofen-1058#topPage. Accessed 9 Jan 2023.
24. Rivas DA, Chancellor MB, Hill K, Freedman MK. Neurological manifestations of baclofen withdrawal. J Urol. 1993;150(6):1903–5. https://doi.org/10.1016/s0022-5347(17)35930-x.
25. Pinto SM, Galang G. Concurrent SCI and TBI: epidemiology, shared pathophysiology, assessment, and prognostication. Curr Phys Med Rehabil Rep. 2016;4(1):71–9. https://doi.org/10.1007/s40141-016-0109-6.
26. Wagstaff AJ, Bryson HM. Tizanidine. A review of its pharmacology, clinical efficacy and tolerability in the management of spasticity associated with cerebral and spinal disorders. Drugs. 1997;53(3):435–52. https://doi.org/10.2165/00003495-199753030-00007.
27. Prescribers' Digital Reference LLC. Tizanidine—drug summary. https://www.pdr.net/drug-summary/Tizanidine-tizanidine-3138. Accessed 9 Jan 2023.
28. Granfors MT, Backman JT, Neuvonen M, Ahonen J, Neuvonen PJ. Fluvoxamine drastically increases concentrations and effects of tizanidine: a potentially hazardous interaction. Clin Pharmacol Ther. 2004;75(4):331–41. https://doi.org/10.1016/j.clpt.2003.12.005.
29. Granfors MT, Backman JT, Neuvonen M, Neuvonen PJ. Ciprofloxacin greatly increases concentrations and hypotensive effect of tizanidine by inhibiting its cytochrome P450 1A2-mediated presystemic metabolism. Clin Pharmacol Ther. 2004;76(6):598–606. https://doi.org/10.1016/j.clpt.2004.08.018.
30. Granfors MT, Backman JT, Laitila J, Neuvonen PJ. Oral contraceptives containing ethinyl estradiol and gestodene markedly increase plasma concentrations and effects of tizanidine by inhibiting cytochrome P450 1A2. Clin Pharmacol Ther. 2005;78(4):400–11. https://doi.org/10.1016/j.clpt.2005.06.009.
31. Rudolph A, Dahmke H, Kupferschmidt H, Burden A, Weiler S. Coadministration of tizanidine and ciprofloxacin: a retrospective analysis of the WHO pharmacovigilance database. Eur J Clin Pharmacol. 2021;77(6):895–902. https://doi.org/10.1007/s00228-020-02981-2.
32. Krause T, Gerbershagen MU, Fiege M, Weisshorn R, Wappler F. Dantrolene—a review of its pharmacology, therapeutic use and new developments. Anaesthesia. 2004;59(4):364–73. https://doi.org/10.1111/j.1365-2044.2004.03658.x.
33. Kim JY, Chun S, Bang MS, Shin HI, Lee SU. Safety of low-dose oral dantrolene sodium on hepatic function. Arch Phys Med Rehabil. 2011;92(9):1359–63. https://doi.org/10.1016/j.apmr.2011.04.012.

34. Muehlschlegel S, Sims JR. Dantrolene: mechanisms of neuroprotection and possible clinical applications in the neurointensive care unit. Neurocrit Care. 2009;10(1):103–15. https://doi.org/10.1007/s12028-008-9133-4.
35. Goldstein LB. Neuropharmacology of TBI-induced plasticity. Brain Inj. 2003;17(8):685–94. https://doi.org/10.1080/0269905031000107179.
36. O'Dell DM, Gibson CJ, Wilson MS, DeFord SM, Hamm RJ. Positive and negative modulation of the GABA(a) receptor and outcome after traumatic brain injury in rats. Brain Res. 2000;861(2):325–32.
37. Goldstein LB. Prescribing of potentially harmful drugs to patients admitted to hospital after head injury. J Neurol Neurosurg Psychiatry. 1995;58(6):753–5. https://doi.org/10.1136/jnnp.58.6.753.
38. Prescribers' Digital Reference LLC. Clonazepam—drug summary. https://www.pdr.net/drug-summary/Clonazepam-Orally-Disintegrating-Tablets-clonazepam-703. Accessed 9 Jan 2023.
39. Formica A, Verger K, Sol JM, Morralla C. Gabapentin for spasticity: a randomized, double-blind, placebo-controlled trial. Med Clin (Barc). 2005;124(3):81–5. https://doi.org/10.1157/13070862.
40. Nalysnyk L, Papapetropoulos S, Rotella P, Simeone JC, Alter KE, Esquenazi A. OnabotulinumtoxinA muscle injection patterns in adult spasticity: a systematic literature review. BMC Neurol. 2013;13:118. https://doi.org/10.1186/1471-2377-13-118.
41. Ward AB. A summary of spasticity management—a treatment algorithm. Eur J Neurol. 2002;9(Suppl 1):48–52; dicussion 53–61. https://doi.org/10.1046/j.1468-1331.2002.0090s1048.x.
42. Bakheit AMO. Chemical neurolysis in the management of muscle spasticity. In: Barnes MP, Johnson GR, editors. Upper motor neurone syndrome and spasticity: clinical management and neurophysiology. 2nd ed. Cambridge: Cambridge University Press; 2008. p. 150–64.
43. Barnes MP, Davis EC. Spasticity and botulinum toxin. In: Barnes MP, Johnson GR, editors. Upper motor neurone syndrome and spasticity: clinical management and neurophysiology. 2nd ed. Cambridge: Cambridge University Press; 2008. p. 165–80.
44. Gordon MF, Brashear A, Elovic E, et al. Repeated dosing of botulinum toxin type A for upper limb spasticity following stroke. Neurology. 2004;63(10):1971–3. https://doi.org/10.1212/01.wnl.0000144349.95487.91.
45. Micham B, Munin MC, Wagner AK, Galang GN. Early chemodeneryation for malignant tone improving long-term outcomes in anoxic brain injury. Am J Phys Med Rehabil. 2019;98(3 Suppl 1):a1–a158.
46. Weppner J, Meriggi J, Franzese K. Severe traumatic brain injury complicated by bruxism: effective management with Onabotulinumtoxina. Am J Phys Med Rehabil. 2020;99(3):a107.
47. Dario A, Tomei G. A benefit-risk assessment of baclofen in severe spinal spasticity. Drug Saf. 2004;27(11):799–818. https://doi.org/10.2165/00002018-200427110-00004.
48. Coffey RJ, Edgar TS, Francisco GE, et al. Abrupt withdrawal from intrathecal baclofen: recognition and management of a potentially life-threatening syndrome. Arch Phys Med Rehabil. 2002;83(6):735–41. https://doi.org/10.1053/apmr.2002.32820.
49. Lazorthes Y, Sol JC, Sallerin B, Verdie JC. The surgical management of spasticity. Eur J Neurol. 2002;9(Suppl 1):35–41; dicussion 53–61. https://doi.org/10.1046/j.1468-1331.2002.0090s1035.x.
50. Steinbok P. Selective dorsal rhizotomy for spastic cerebral palsy: a review. Childs Nerv Syst. 2007;23(9):981–90. https://doi.org/10.1007/s00381-007-0379-5.

Chapter 9
Paroxysmal Sympathetic Hyperactivity

Gary Galang, Anne Tita, Justin Weppner, and Amy K. Wagner

Chapter Objectives

1. Discuss the epidemiology and incidence of PSH.
2. Review current understanding of the pathophysiology of PSH.
3. Review the diagnostic criteria and clinical evaluation of PSH.
4. Discuss recommended treatment strategies for management of PSH.
5. Illustrate practical application of diagnostic and treatment principles via a case illustration.
6. Summarize key educational points.

Introduction

Paroxysmal sympathetic hyperactivity (PSH) is a clinical syndrome associated with many types of acquired brain injuries characterized by episodic uncontrolled physiologic surges of sympathetic activity. The syndrome features varying combinations and degrees of hyperthermia, diaphoresis, tachycardia, hypertension, tachypnea,

G. Galang (✉) · A. K. Wagner
Department of Physical Medicine and Rehabilitation, University of Pittsburgh School of Medicine, Pittsburgh, PA, USA
e-mail: galangg@upmc.edu; wagnerak@upmc.edu

A. Tita
Allina Health, Minneapolis, MN, USA
e-mail: anne.tita@allina.com

J. Weppner
Virginia Tech Carilion School of Medicine, Edward Via College of Osteopathic Medicine, Roanoke, VA, USA
e-mail: jlweppner@carilionclinic.org

A. K. Wagner, J. Weppner (eds.), *Acute Care Neuroconsultation and Neurorehabilitation Management*, https://doi.org/10.1007/978-3-031-42830-2_9

and dystonic posturing. The absolute incidence of PSH is unclear, as clinicians often fail to recognize it or misdiagnose it as another process entirely due to its similar clinical appearance to several other conditions [1]. Its estimated incidence ranges from 7.7% to 33% of patients with brain injury admitted to the intensive care unit (ICU) [2–9] with the wide range attributed to variations in study populations, diagnostic criteria, and exam timing [1, 10]. It appears that the higher end of this range tends to represent short duration PSH, lasting for hours to days [3, 9], with longer duration PSH (lasting weeks to months) being relatively less common [1] but associated with significantly worse outcomes following rehabilitation [3, 6, 7, 10, 11]. Development of PSH of any duration is associated with longer hospital stays, higher rates of complications, and increased costs of care [3, 4, 6–8, 11–14]. Furthermore, delayed recognition and treatment can result in higher morbidity in the form of secondary brain injury from prolonged hypertension and hyperthermia [15–18], contracture formation, development of heterotopic ossification [8], weight loss [3, 14], cardiac damage [19], and even death.

To streamline understanding and recognition of the syndrome, an international, multidisciplinary steering committee published a consensus paper in 2014, which concluded it should officially be called "paroxysmal sympathetic hyperactivity," as this name is specific and accurate without preempting an underlying pathophysiology [20]. Additionally, a conceptual definition of PSH was developed stating that PSH is "a syndrome, recognized in a subgroup of survivors of severe acquired brain injury, of simultaneous, paroxysmal transient increases in sympathetic (elevated heart rate, blood pressure, respiratory rate, temperature, sweating) and motor (posturing) activity" [20].

Background

Epidemiology

Among the cases of PSH reported in the literature, the majority developed because of traumatic brain injury (TBI) (79.4%), followed distantly by hypoxic brain injury (9.7%) and stroke (5.4%)—with hemorrhagic strokes more often associated than ischemic strokes [1]. PSH has also been reported in other diagnostic groups including encephalitis, perhaps with even higher prevalence than in traumatic brain injury (TBI) [21, 22], however, due to their relative rarity, these diagnoses account for a much smaller proportion of PSH cases overall [23]. Regardless of the underlying causative etiology, the clinical features of PSH do not appear to differ [1]. The most significant risk factor for developing PSH following acute brain injury is the severity of the brain injury itself [23]. Additionally cited risk factors are evidence of diffuse axonal injury on imaging studies [13, 24], younger age at the time of injury and male gender [1]—although these characteristics may simply reflect the population most likely to sustain a TBI in general [2, 6, 24].

Pathophysiology

The excitatory–inhibitory ratio (EIR) model is the current widely accepted framework for explaining the pathophysiology of PSH. This model proposes that different regions of the central nervous system (CNS) are responsible for maintaining balance between parasympathetic and sympathetic outflow within the body. While numerous discrete CNS regions have been implicated in the pathogenesis of PSH [25, 26], the current consensus is that a lesion anywhere along the pathway can result in unbalanced activation of the sympathetic and parasympathetic nervous systems, producing the clinical syndrome of PSH [23, 27]. More specifically, research suggests that the cortex, diencephalon, and upper brain stem exert a tonic inhibitory drive over the rest of the CNS, while other areas such as the lower brain stem and spinal cord have an allodynic, excitatory tendency. When the tonic inhibitory pathways are injured, the allodynic tendency predominates, resulting in an amplification of the sensory afferents from the spinal cord through a positive feedback loop that produces an unchecked sympathetic response to any stimulus [28, 29]. This model effectively explains the observation that PHS episodes are often triggered by relatively benign actions such as patient repositioning or airway suctioning [23].

It is also important to note that while increased levels of plasma catecholamines have been observed in acute TBI [30] and non-traumatic subarachnoid hemorrhage [31, 32], absolute plasma catecholamine levels do not appear to directly correlate with sympathetic outflow severity [28]. As such, using plasma catecholamines as a potential diagnostic marker for PSH is felt to be impractical [23].

In the setting of severe acquired brain injury, there is an overlap between PSH, cytokine storm, and severe inflammatory response [33–35]. Systemic inflammatory response syndrome (SIRS) may occur following severe acquired brain injury with or without infection, with trauma being a recognized non-infectious precipitant for systemic inflammation [34]. The presence of inflammation complicates PSH diagnosis as three of the four clinical parameters for SIRS—elevated heart rate, respiratory rate, and temperature—are also characteristics of PSH diagnostic criteria. While systemic inflammation and PSH may overlap and be present simultaneously, hypotension in sepsis may provide a practical discriminator between SIRS and PSH, since hypotension is considered incompatible with current conceptual definitions of PSH [1].

Propranolol, a medication commonly prescribed for PSH, may treat both systemic inflammation and PSH symptoms, as propranolol has been shown to decrease catecholamine levels with correlated improvements in Glasgow Coma Scale (GCS) scores for persons with TBI [36]. Beta-blockers improve neurological and histological outcomes following focal cerebral ischemia, attenuate cerebral glucose metabolism, and increase motor performance in animal models [37, 38]. For persons with moderate-to-severe TBI, β-blockers can address both PSH itself and the associated systemic inflammation response commonly observed. Reduced acute care hospital length of stay and mortality rate with early (acute care) β-blocker usage was seen in some observational and randomized clinical trial studies [39]. Beta-blockers such as propranolol are particularly effective in reducing catecholamine levels and PSH symptoms in severe acquired brain injury. They have anti-inflammatory, neuroprotective, and glucose regulation mechanisms that combine to improve outcomes for persons with TBI [36–40].

Diagnostic Criteria and Assessments

Perhaps the most important consideration in the diagnosis of PSH is recognition that it remains a diagnosis of exclusion at this time [10], as no pathognomonic signs or biomarkers have yet been identified [20]. It necessitates consideration and workup of many alternative diagnoses including, but not limited to, infection or sepsis, seizure, venous thromboembolism, occult fracture, heterotopic ossification, pressure injury, pain (especially from spasticity or dystonia), withdrawal (especially from opiates, alcohol, or sedative medications), and similar or overlapping syndromes such as neuroleptic malignant syndrome or autonomic dysreflexia [20]. It is also important to note that detection of any of the above diagnoses does not necessarily exclude the possibility of PSH, as multiple conditions can co-exist.

The 2014 PSH consensus paper detailed a novel assessment tool consisting of two parts to aid in better recognition and treatment of this syndrome, together referred to as the PSH Assessment Measure (PSH-AM, Table 9.1). The first part, the Diagnosis Likelihood Tool (DLT), serves to determine the probability of PSH based on 11 diagnostic criteria. Since few patients with PSH display all features of the syndrome [3, 7, 8, 41], the absence of any given symptom does not preclude a diagnosis of PSH, but rather decreases the overall probability [20]. The second part, the Clinical Feature Scale, functions to help assess the severity of PSH in a given patient by assigning value to the measurable data associated with the syndrome. The PSH-AM was designed for use as a serial assessment tool to monitor the symptoms of PSH over time, and to help determine the effectiveness of treatment. It is suggested that the PSH-AM be administered daily in the intensive care setting to enable early recognition of the syndrome and to avoid treatment delays [20]. Its use should be continued into the rehabilitation setting in cases where symptoms persist through this phase of care. Preliminary data indicates that serial recordings of the PSH-AM allow the monitoring of clinical trends to assess the treatment effects of interventions, which provide helpful information for making decisions in the pharmacologic management of PSH. The PSH-AM promises to be a valuable guide for not only the diagnosis of PSH but also for management through serial assessments [42].

Treatment Strategies

Due to the complexity and poorly understood pathophysiology of PSH, treatment options at this time are limited to focusing on symptom management using both pharmacologic and nonpharmacologic modalities. Nonpharmacologic treatment

Table 9.1 PSH-AM [20]

Diagnosis likelihood tool (score 1 point for each feature present)					Score
Clinical features occur simultaneously					
Episodes are paroxysmal in nature					
Sympathetic over-reactivity to normal non-painful stimuli					
Features persist at least 3 consecutive days					
Features persist at least 2 weeks post-brain injury					
Features persist despite treatment of alternative diagnoses					
Medication administered to decrease sympathetic features					
At least two episodes daily					
Absence of parasympathetic features during episodes					
Absence of other presumed causes of features					
Antecedent acquired brain injury					
DLT subtotal					
Clinical feature scale					
	0	1	2	3	Score
Heart rate	<100	100–119	120–139	≥140	
Respiratory rate	<18	18–23	24–29	≥30	
Systolic blood pressure	<140	140–159	160–179	≥180	
Temperature	<37	37–37.9	38–38.9	≥39.0	
Sweating[a]	None	Mild	Moderate	Severe	
Posturing during episodes[b]	None	Mild	Moderate	Severe	
CFS subtotal					

PSH diagnostic likelihood = DLT subtotal + CFS subtotal
<8 Unlikely, 8–16 Possible, >17 Probable
Clinical feature severity: Mild 1–6, Moderate 7–12, Severe ≥13
[a]Sweating: Mild refers to moist or glistening skin, moderate refers to visible beads of sweat, and severe refers to profuse, drenching sweat
[b]Posturing: Mild refers to increased tone during episodes with limbs that are movable with modest force, moderate refers to increased tone during episodes that is hard to overcome and requires medication to address, and severe refers to tone that is rigid and refractory to treatment measures

strategies include identifying and limiting, when possible, physical triggers that predictably bring on episodes of PSH in a given patient such as touching, positioning, airway suctioning, dressing, or bathing. Additionally, manual efforts should be made to normalize body temperature when appropriate [27]. Pharmacologic treatment of PSH, on the other hand, has several aims: preventing symptoms by decreasing the frequency and intensity of episodes; aborting discrete breakthrough episodes when they occur; and escalating care when symptoms are refractory to first line treatments. While numerous medications are often required to effectively control PSH symptoms, clinicians should be cautious of over medicating patients or using medications that may unintentionally worsen symptoms. For details on specific medications and doses recommended in the treatment of PSH (Table 9.2).

The primary goal of pharmacologic treatments aimed at PSH symptom prevention is to decrease the frequency and intensity of sympathetic episodes. This goal is best achieved by using regularly scheduled medications from a combination of classes with varied mechanisms of action and physiologic targets [23, 27]. The

Table 9.2 Pharmacologic treatment of PSH

Medication	Mechanism of action	Dosing	Symptoms targeted	Notes
Propranolol	Lipophilic nonselective beta-blocker	*Preventative:* Start at 10 mg PO Q6H *Abortive:* 1–3 mg IV Q2–5 min as needed	Tachycardia, hypertension, hyperthermia, diaphoresis, dystonic posturing	– Most common beta-blocker used in PSH – Reduces length of stay and mortality in TBI patients with PSH [39]
Labetalol	Nonselective beta-blocker with additional alpha-1 blocking effects	*Preventative:* Start at 100 mg PO Q8H *Abortive:* 10–20 mg IV Q1-2H as needed	Tachycardia, hypertension, hyperthermia, diaphoresis, dystonic posturing	– Less literature to support use compared to propranolol [43–46] – Vasodilator properties resulting from alpha-1 blockade which reduce peripheral vascular resistance, blood pressure, and coronary vascular resistance, a potential advantage over other beta-blockers [47]
Bromocriptine	Synthetic dopamine agonist	Start at 2.5 mg PO BID at 7 am and noon Max dose: 10 mg BID	Dystonic posturing, hyperthermia	– May also enhance arousal in TBI [48]
Baclofen	GABA-B agonist	Start: 10 mg TID Max dose: 20 mg QID	Pain, spasticity, clonus	– Consider when patient has spasticity
Dantrolene	Inhibit release of calcium from skeletal muscle sarcoplasmic reticulum	Start at 25 mg PO TID Max dose: 400 mg/day	Spasticity, muscle rigidity, posturing	– Consider when patient has spasticity – Check liver function studies prior to initiating dantrolene and routinely during treatment course
Clonidine	Alpha-2 receptor agonist	Start at 0.1 mg PO BID Max dose: 0.3 mg TID	Hypertension	– Clonidine may impair motor recovery following acquired brain [49] – Avoid prolonged use and consider risks versus benefits

(continued)

Table 9.2 (continued)

Medication	Mechanism of action	Dosing	Symptoms targeted	Notes
Gabapentin	GABA analog	Start at 300 mg PO TID Max dose: 3600 mg/day	Pain, spasticity	– Pain adjuvant in multi-trauma – Consider when patient is at risk for alcohol withdrawal [50, 51] – Gabapentin enhances the analgesic effect of opioids
Clonazepam	Long-acting GABA—A agonist	Start at 0.5 mg PO BID	Agitation, hypertension, tachycardia, dystonic posturing	– Benzodiazepines have a negative effect on cognitive function, visuospatial ability, and sustained attention [52–54]
Diazepam	Long-acting GABA-A agonist	Start at 5 mg PO Q8H	Agitation, hypertension, tachycardia, dystonic posturing	– Consider if alcohol withdrawal is suspected and patient is not responding to benzodiazepine sparing CIWA protocol
Lorazepam	Intermediate acting GABA-A agonist	*Preventative:* Start at 2 mg PO Q8H *Abortive:* 0.5–2 mg IV Q4H as needed	Agitation, hypertension, tachycardia, dystonic posturing	
Midazolam	Short acting GABA-A agonist	*Abortive:* 1–2 mg IV Q4H as needed	Agitation, hypertension, tachycardia, dystonic posturing	

Table 9.2 (continued)

Medication	Mechanism of action	Dosing	Symptoms targeted	Notes
Oxycodone	Mu-opiate receptor agonist	IR formulation: Start at 5–10 mg PO Q6-8H	Pain, tachycardia, hypertension	– Monitor for opioid induced constipation
		ER formulation: Start at 10 mg PO Q12H		
Morphine	Mu-opioid receptor agonist	*Abortive:* 2–5 mg IV Q1-2H as needed	Pain, tachycardia, hypertension	
Fentanyl	Mu-opioid receptor agonist	*Abortive:* 25–50 mcg IV Q30–60 min as needed	Pain, tachycardia, hypertension	
Dexmedetomidine	Alpha-2 receptor agonist	*Refractory:* 0.2–0.7 mcg/kg/hr. IV infusion	Tachycardia, hypertension, agitation	– Prevents PSH in severe TBI patients who have undergone surgery [55]
				– Can effectively control the onset of PSH symptoms and shorten its course
				– Does not improve the long-term prognosis of patients

GABA gamma aminobutyric acid, *CIWA* clinical institute withdrawal assessment, *TBI* traumatic brain injury, *PSH* paroxysmal sympathetic hyperactivity objective is to simultaneously inhibit central sympathetic outflow while also inhibiting afferent sensory processing to prevent the development of allodynia. Medication timing and dosing should be optimized to limit undesirable side effects such as sedation [27].

The medications recommended for symptom prevention include nonselective β-blockers (propranolol, labetalol), α-2 agonists (clonidine), bromocriptine, dantrolene, baclofen, gabapentin, and long-acting benzodiazepines (clonazepam, lorazepam, diazepam). Enterally administered medications are favored in PSH symptom prevention, as these can continue to be administered safely in lower acuity care settings such as inpatient rehabilitation. It is also worth mentioning that dopamine antagonists such as chlorpromazine and haloperidol are not recommended for use in PSH because they may worsen cognitive symptoms [23, 27, 56, 57]. The risks versus benefits of benzodiazepines and α-2 agonists such as clonidine need to be considered, especially if given in the acute period following acquired brain injury or for a prolonged period. There is a concern that clonidine may impair motor recovery following acquired brain injury and benzodiazepines have a negative effect on cognitive function, visuospatial ability, and sustained attention [49, 52–54]. Once preventative medications are on board, the second goal of treatment is to stop breakthrough episodes when they occur. The medications utilized for abortive therapy are ideally those that have a rapid onset of action to enable immediate resolution of pathologic symptoms, and a short half-life to limit the likelihood and duration of side effects. To achieve this end, intravenous (IV) formulations of medications are often favored in abortive therapy. Medication selection should be specific to address the predominant symptoms displayed during a given breakthrough episode, i.e., hyperthermia should be treated with antipyretics, agitation with sedation, and hypertension with antihypertensive agents [27]. Morphine is a powerful μ-opioid receptor agonist that is considered first line treatment of breakthrough episodes due to its broad effect on PSH symptoms including analgesia, bradycardia, and peripheral vasodilation [58–60]. Shorter-acting benzodiazepines such as midazolam or lorazepam are similarly efficacious; in addition, benzodiazepines have the benefit of addressing issues with dystonic posturing and spasticity [27].

Sometimes, even with regularly scheduled medications for prevention and as-needed medications for breakthrough episodes, certain patients continue to have uncontrolled sympathetic activity. In these cases, it may be appropriate to escalate to more potent IV medications, or continuous infusions, as uncontrolled PSH symptoms can lead to secondary brain injury [15–18]. In treating refractory PSH, one should consider use of IV or drip benzodiazepines, propofol, opioids, or dexmedetomidine for symptom management. In this setting, there is relatively less concern for medication side effects such as sedation given the goal is prevention of progressive morbidity or even death. Dexmedetomidine, in particular, is recommended highly for treatment of refractory PSH since it demonstrates favorable effects on heart rate, blood pressure and agitation, and is available for use in patients not requiring mechanical ventilation [27, 61]. Treatment of refractory PSH symptoms should be continued until the frequency and intensity of the episodes diminish significantly, and prevention therapy should be initiated prior to stopping continuous infusions [27].

Case Illustration

A 33-year-old male with a past medical history of ankylosing spondylitis presented to the acute hospital following an unhelmeted motorcycle crash. GCS on arrival was 3T. Head computerized tomography (CT) demonstrated diffuse subarachnoid hemorrhage, bilateral frontal contusions, and large right temporal lobe contusion. Additional traumatic injuries included facial and scalp lacerations, multiple spinal fractures without cord compression, and bilateral ankle fractures. He underwent right hemicraniectomy and temporal lobectomy on hospital day 2 due to rapidly increasing intracranial swelling. On the following day, sedation was weaned to enable spontaneous breathing trials, and an examination off sedation was consistent with a UWS. He was noted to be profusely diaphoretic, tachycardic, and hypertensive with systolic pressures near 200 mmHg. The symptoms appeared to resolve with administration of IV fentanyl. Due to concern for developing sepsis, a comprehensive infectious workup was ordered including blood cultures, cerebral spinal fluid culture, urinalysis, chest X-ray, and bronchoscopy with bronchoalveolar lavage. All these tests returned negative; however, the patient began spiking several fevers per day so antibiotic treatment for presumed hospital acquired pneumonia was initiated, and antipyretics were scheduled around the clock. Physiatry was consulted for medical management of "autonomic storming."

After reviewing the case in detail and discussing with staff, the consultant recommended an electroencephalograph (EEG) to rule out seizure since the patient had been displaying myoclonic movements. Additionally, skin wounds were examined closely for any signs of infection, and bilateral lower extremity venous duplex scans were completed to evaluate for venous thromboembolism. When these additional tests returned negative, the patient was initiated on therapy to address suspected PSH: propranolol 10 mg every 6 h, gabapentin 300 mg every 8 h, and scheduled oxycodone 5 mg every 4 h. IV fentanyl remained available as needed for acute episodes. Over the next several days, propranolol was increased gradually to 40 mg every 6 h due to persistent tachycardia and hypertension, and clonidine 0.1 mg every 8 h was also added. While the episodes became somewhat less frequent and intense on this regimen, the patient was noted to have increasing leukocytosis and diarrhea, so *Clostridium difficile* testing was completed and returned positive. He was started on appropriate antibiotic treatment for *C. difficile* colitis, but nursing staff continued to report persistent episodes of sweating and dystonic posturing with certain types of physical stimulation such as tracheostomy suctioning. After ensuring normal baseline hepatic function levels, dantrolene 25 mg three times daily and bromocriptine 2.5 mg at 7 am and 12 pm were added. With these changes, the episodes decreased significantly in frequency and intensity. The patient was subsequently weaned to room air and transferred out of the ICU. Within several days he was deemed medically stable for transfer to acute inpatient rehabilitation.

On the proposed day of discharge to rehabilitation, he was noted to have new persistent tachycardia, fever, and hypotension. The primary service reported that the symptoms were consistent with PSH. Re-evaluatioin by the physiatry consultation service was requested for medical stability before discharge to acute inpatient rehabilitation. Initial evaluation was concerning for severe SIRS, given symptoms of persistent fevers and tachycardia associated with hypotension. Laboratory analysis revealed a worsening leukocytosis, and urinalysis was consistent with acute cystitis. The patient was started on intravenous fluids, ceftriaxone, and blood pressure-lowering medications were held. His condition improved over the next 24 h with the normalization of vital signs. He later was deemed medically stable for transfer to acute inpatient rehabilitation, where the above PSH medicines were gradually weaned as the patient's consciousness improved.

Summary

- According to the PSH consensus committee position, the correct nomenclature for this syndrome is paroxysmal sympathetic hyperactivity. It is conceptually defined as "a syndrome, recognized in a subgroup of survivors of severe acquired brain injury, of simultaneous, paroxysmal transient increases in sympathetic (elevated heart rate, blood pressure, respiratory rate, temperature, sweating) and motor (posturing) activity" [20].
- Most cases result from traumatic brain injury (79.4%), followed distantly by hypoxic brain injury (9.7%), and stroke (5.4%) [1]. Other causes are considered rare. Risk factors for developing PSH include increased severity of brain injury, evidence of diffuse axonal injury on imaging studies [13, 24], younger age and male gender [1].
- Researchers currently believe that PSH pathophysiology follows an excitatory–inhibitory ratio model. PSH results when there is unbalanced parasympathetic and sympathetic activation due to a functional disconnection within the central nervous system [23, 28, 29].
- The diagnosis of PSH remains one of exclusion and necessitates consideration of many other potentially confounding diagnoses. The PSH-AM is a two-part scale designed for serial assessment of patients with PSH to monitor their symptoms over time [20]. Exclusion and
- A generally recommended strategy for treatment is to have regularly scheduled medications (e.g., long-acting benzodiazepines, nonselective β-blockers, α2-agonists, opiates, and gabapentin) to limit the frequency and severity of episodes, accompanied by as-needed medications (e.g., morphine or short acting benzodiazepines) available for use during breakthrough episodes [23, 27]. Nonpharmacologic measures should also be implemented to avoid triggering PSH episodes [27].

References[1]

1. Perkes I, Baguley IJ, Nott MT, Menon DK. A review of paroxysmal sympathetic hyperactivity after acquired brain injury. Ann Neurol. 2010;68(2):126–35. https://doi.org/10.1002/ana.22066.
2. Perkes IE, Menon DK, Nott MT, Baguley IJ. Paroxysmal sympathetic hyperactivity after acquired brain injury: a review of diagnostic criteria. Brain Inj. 2011;25(10):925–32. https://doi.org/10.3109/02699052.2011.589797.
3. Baguley IJ, Slewa-Younan S, Heriseanu RE, Nott MT, Mudaliar Y, Nayyar V. The incidence of dysautonomia and its relationship with autonomic arousal following traumatic brain injury. Brain Inj. 2007;21(11):1175–81. https://doi.org/10.1080/02699050701687375.
4. Dolce G, Quintieri M, Leto E, et al. Dysautonomia and clinical outcome in vegetative state. J Neurotrauma. 2021;38(10):1441–4. https://doi.org/10.1089/neu.2008.0536.
5. Fearnside MR, Cook RJ, McDougall P, McNeil RJ. The Westmead head injury project outcome in severe head injury. A comparative analysis of pre-hospital, clinical and CT variables. Br J Neurosurg. 1993;7(3):267–79. https://doi.org/10.3109/02688699309023809.
6. Fernandez-Ortega JF, Prieto-Palomino MA, Garcia-Caballero M, Galeas-Lopez JL, Quesada-Garcia G, Baguley IJ. Paroxysmal sympathetic hyperactivity after traumatic brain injury: clinical and prognostic implications. J Neurotrauma. 2012;29(7):1364–70. https://doi.org/10.1089/neu.2011.2033.
7. Fernandez-Ortega JF, Prieto-Palomino MA, Munoz-Lopez A, Lebron-Gallardo M, Cabrera-Ortiz H, Quesada-Garcia G. Prognostic influence and computed tomography findings in dysautonomic crises after traumatic brain injury. J Trauma. 2006;61(5):1129–33. https://doi.org/10.1097/01.ta.0000197634.83217.80.
8. Hendricks HT, Geurts AC, van Ginneken BC, Heeren AJ, Vos PE. Brain injury severity and autonomic dysregulation accurately predict heterotopic ossification in patients with traumatic brain injury. Clin Rehabil. 2007;21(6):545–53.
9. Rabinstein AA. Paroxysmal sympathetic hyperactivity in the neurological intensive care unit. Neurol Res. 2007;29(7):680–2. https://doi.org/10.1179/016164107X240071.
10. Baguley IJ. Autonomic complications following central nervous system injury. Semin Neurol. 2008;28(5):716–25. https://doi.org/10.1055/s-0028-1105971.
11. Baguley IJ, Nicholls JL, Felmingham KL, Crooks J, Gurka JA, Wade LD. Dysautonomia after traumatic brain injury: a forgotten syndrome? J Neurol Neurosurg Psychiatry. 1999;67(1):39–43. https://doi.org/10.1136/jnnp.67.1.39.
12. Hinson HE, Sheth KN. Manifestations of the hyperadrenergic state after acute brain injury. Curr Opin Crit Care. 2012;18(2):139–45. https://doi.org/10.1097/MCC.0b013e3283513290.
13. Lv LQ, Hou LJ, Yu MK, et al. Prognostic influence and magnetic resonance imaging findings in paroxysmal sympathetic hyperactivity after severe traumatic brain injury. J Neurotrauma. 2010;27(11):1945–50. https://doi.org/10.1089/neu.2010.1391.
14. Mehta NM, Bechard LJ, Leavitt K, Duggan C. Severe weight loss and hypermetabolic paroxysmal dysautonomia following hypoxic ischemic brain injury: the role of indirect calorimetry in the intensive care unit. JPEN J Parenter Enteral Nutr. 2008;32(3):281–4. https://doi.org/10.1177/0148607108316196.
15. Baena RC, Busto R, Dietrich WD, Globus MY, Ginsberg MD. Hyperthermia delayed by 24 hours aggravates neuronal damage in rat hippocampus following global ischemia. Neurology. 1997;48(3):768–73. https://doi.org/10.1212/wnl.48.3.768.
16. Hickey RW, Kochanek PM, Ferimer H, Alexander HL, Garman RH, Graham SH. Induced hyperthermia exacerbates neurologic neuronal histologic damage after asphyxial cardiac arrest in rats. Crit Care Med. 2003;31(2):531–5. https://doi.org/10.1097/01.CCM.0000050323.84293.11.

[1] Key References [1, 20, 23, 27].

17. Fernandez A, Schmidt JM, Claassen J, et al. Fever after subarachnoid hemorrhage: risk factors and impact on outcome. Neurology. 2007;68(13):1013–9. https://doi.org/10.1212/01.wnl.0000258543.45879.f5.
18. Greer DM, Funk SE, Reaven NL, Ouzounelli M, Uman GC. Impact of fever on outcome in patients with stroke and neurologic injury: a comprehensive meta-analysis. Stroke. 2008;39(11):3029–35. https://doi.org/10.1161/STROKEAHA.108.521583.
19. Ryan JB, Hicks M, Cropper JR, et al. Functional evidence of reversible ischemic injury immediately after the sympathetic storm associated with experimental brain death. J Heart Lung Transplant. 2003;22(8):922–8. https://doi.org/10.1016/s1053-2498(02)00558-2.
20. Baguley IJ, Perkes IE, Fernandez-Ortega J-F, et al. Paroxysmal sympathetic hyperactivity after acquired brain injury: consensus on conceptual definition, nomenclature, and diagnostic criteria. J Neurotrauma. 2014;31(17):1515–20. https://doi.org/10.1089/neu.2013.3301.
21. Dalmau J, Gleichman AJ, Hughes EG, et al. Anti-NMDA-receptor encephalitis: case series and analysis of the effects of antibodies. Lancet Neurol. 2008;7(12):1091–8. https://doi.org/10.1016/S1474-4422(08)70224-2.
22. Nazif TM, Vazquez J, Honig LS, Dizon JM. Anti-N-methyl-D-aspartate receptor encephalitis: an emerging cause of centrally mediated sinus node dysfunction. Europace. 2012;14(8):1188–94. https://doi.org/10.1093/europace/eus014.
23. Choi HA, Jeon SB, Samuel S, Allison T, Lee K. Paroxysmal sympathetic hyperactivity after acute brain injury. Curr Neurol Neurosci Rep. 2013;13(8):370. https://doi.org/10.1007/s11910-013-0370-3.
24. Lv LQ, Hou LJ, Yu MK, et al. Risk factors related to dysautonomia after severe traumatic brain injury. J Trauma. 2011;71(3):538–42. https://doi.org/10.1097/TA.0b013e31820ebee1.
25. Carmel PW. Vegetative dysfunctions of the hypothalamus. Acta Neurochir. 1985;75(1–4):113–21. https://doi.org/10.1007/BF01406331.
26. Pranzatelli MR, Pavlakis SG, Gould RJ, De Vivo DC. Hypothalamic-midbrain dysregulation syndrome: hypertension, hyperthermia, hyperventilation, and decerebration. J Child Neurol. 1991;6(2):115–22. https://doi.org/10.1177/088307389100600204.
27. Samuel S, Allison TA, Lee K, Choi HA. Pharmacologic management of paroxysmal sympathetic hyperactivity after brain injury. J Neurosci Nurs. 2016;48(2):82–9. https://doi.org/10.1097/JNN.0000000000000207.
28. Baguley IJ. The excitatory:inhibitory ratio model (EIR model): an integrative explanation of acute autonomic overactivity syndromes. Med Hypotheses. 2008;70(1):26–35. https://doi.org/10.1016/j.mehy.2007.04.037.
29. Baguley IJ, Nott MT, Slewa-Younan S, Heriseanu RE, Perkes IE. Diagnosing dysautonomia after acute traumatic brain injury: evidence for overresponsiveness to afferent stimuli. Arch Phys Med Rehabil. 2009;90(4):580–6. https://doi.org/10.1016/j.apmr.2008.10.020.
30. Wang VY, Manley G. Recognition of paroxysmal autonomic instability with dystonia (PAID) in a patient with traumatic brain injury. J Trauma. 2008;64(2):500–2. https://doi.org/10.1097/TA.0b013e31804a5738.
31. Naredi S, Lambert G, Eden E, et al. Increased sympathetic nervous activity in patients with nontraumatic subarachnoid hemorrhage. Stroke. 2000;31(4):901–6. https://doi.org/10.1161/01.str.31.4.901.
32. Naredi S, Lambert G, Friberg P, et al. Sympathetic activation and inflammatory response in patients with subarachnoid haemorrhage. Intensive Care Med. 2006;32(12):1955–61. https://doi.org/10.1007/s00134-006-0408-y.
33. Mehta P, McAuley DF, Brown M, Sanchez E, Tattersall RS, Manson JJ. COVID-19: consider cytokine storm syndromes and immunosuppression. Lancet. 2020;395(10229):1033–4. https://doi.org/10.1016/S0140-6736(20)30628-0.
34. Bone RC, Balk RA, Cerra FB, et al. Definitions for sepsis and organ failure and guidelines for the use of innovative therapies in sepsis. The ACCP/SCCM Consensus Conference Committee. American College of Chest Physicians/Society of Critical Care Medicine. Chest. 1992;101(6):1644–55. https://doi.org/10.1378/chest.101.6.1644.

35. Singh K, Kumar N, Kumar A, Kumar A, Shaju AR. Sympathetic storm or cytokine storm: a diagnostic dilemma in patient of traumatic brain injury with COVID 19. Acta Neurol Taiwanica. 2021;30(2):78–80.
36. Ammar MA, Hussein NS. Using propranolol in traumatic brain injury to reduce sympathetic storm phenomenon: a prospective randomized clinical trial. Saudi J Anaesth. 2018;12(4):514–20. https://doi.org/10.4103/sja.SJA_33_18.
37. Goyagi T, Kimura T, Nishikawa T, Tobe Y, Masaki Y. Beta-adrenoreceptor antagonists attenuate brain injury after transient focal ischemia in rats. Anesth Analg. 2006;103(3):658–63. https://doi.org/10.1213/01.ane.0000228859.95126.69.
38. Ley EJ, Clond MA, Bukur M, et al. β-Adrenergic receptor inhibition affects cerebral glucose metabolism, motor performance, and inflammatory response after traumatic brain injury. J Trauma Acute Care Surg. 2012;73(1):33–40. https://doi.org/10.1097/TA.0b013e31825a769b.
39. Nguembu S, Meloni M, Endalle G, et al. Paroxysmal sympathetic hyperactivity in moderate-to-severe traumatic brain injury and the role of beta-blockers: a scoping review. Emerg Med Int. 2021;2021:5589239. https://doi.org/10.1155/2021/5589239.
40. Rabinstein AA. Paroxysmal autonomic instability after brain injury. Arch Neurol. 2004;61(10):1625.; author reply 1625. https://doi.org/10.1001/archneur.61.10.1625-a.
41. Godo S, Irino S, Nakagawa A, et al. Diagnosis and management of patients with paroxysmal sympathetic hyperactivity following acute brain injuries using a consensus-based diagnostic tool: a single institutional case series. Tohoku J Exp Med. 2017;243(1):11–8. https://doi.org/10.1620/tjem.243.11.
42. Sandel ME, Olive DA, Rader MA. Chlorpromazine-induced psychosis after brain injury. Brain Inj. 1993;7(1):77–83. https://doi.org/10.3109/02699059309008159.
43. Feng Y, Zheng X, Fang Z. Treatment Progress of paroxysmal sympathetic hyperactivity after acquired brain injury. Pediatr Neurosurg. 2015;50(6):301–9. https://doi.org/10.1159/000439282.
44. Monteiro FB, Fonseca RC, Mendes R. Paroxysmal sympathetic hyperactivity: an old but unrecognized condition. Eur J Case Rep Intern Med. 2017;4(3):000562. https://doi.org/10.12890/2017_000562.
45. Zheng RZ, Lei ZQ, Yang RZ, Huang GH, Zhang GM. Identification and management of paroxysmal sympathetic hyperactivity after traumatic brain injury. Front Neurol. 2020;11:81. https://doi.org/10.3389/fneur.2020.00081.
46. Do D, Sheen VL, Bromfield E. Treatment of paroxysmal sympathetic storm with labetalol. J Neurol Neurosurg Psychiatry. 2000;69(6):832–3. https://doi.org/10.1136/jnnp.69.6.832.
47. Munakomi S, Bhattarai B, Mohan Kumar B. Role of bromocriptine in multi-spectral manifestations of traumatic brain injury. Chin J Traumatol. 2017;20(2):84–6. https://doi.org/10.1016/j.cjtee.2016.04.009.
48. Anton RF, Latham P, Voronin K, et al. Efficacy of gabapentin for the treatment of alcohol use disorder in patients with alcohol withdrawal symptoms: a randomized clinical trial. JAMA Intern Med. 2020;180(5):728–36. https://doi.org/10.1001/jamainternmed.2020.0249.
49. Mintzer MZ, Griffiths RR. Drugs, memory, and metamemory: a dose-effect study with lorazepam and scopolamine. Exp Clin Psychopharmacol. 2005;13(4):336–47. https://doi.org/10.1037/1064-1297.13.4.336.
50. Myrick H, Malcolm R, Randall PK, et al. A double-blind trial of gabapentin versus lorazepam in the treatment of alcohol withdrawal. Alcohol Clin Exp Res. 2009;33(9):1582–8. https://doi.org/10.1111/j.1530-0277.2009.00986.x.
51. Tang Q, Wu X, Weng W, et al. The preventive effect of dexmedetomidine on paroxysmal sympathetic hyperactivity in severe traumatic brain injury patients who have undergone surgery: a retrospective study. PeerJ. 2017;5:e2986. https://doi.org/10.7717/peerj.2986.
52. Stewart SA. The effects of benzodiazepines on cognition. J Clin Psychiatry. 2005;66(Suppl 2):9–13.

53. Goldstein LB. Common drugs may influence motor recovery after stroke. The Sygen in acute stroke study investigators. Neurology. 1995;45(5):865–71. https://doi.org/10.1212/wnl.45.5.865.
54. Bullard DE. Diencephalic seizures: responsiveness to bromocriptine and morphine. Ann Neurol. 1987;21(6):609–11. https://doi.org/10.1002/ana.410210617.
55. Peng Y, Zhu H, Chen H, et al. Dexmedetomidine attenuates acute paroxysmal sympathetic hyperactivity. Oncotarget. 2017;8(40):69012–9. https://doi.org/10.18632/oncotarget.16920.
56. Wilkinson R, Meythaler JM, Guin-Renfroe S. Case study Neuroleptic malignant syndrome induced by haloperidol following traumatic brain injury. Brain Injury. 1999;13(12):1025–31. https://doi.org/10.1080/026990599121034.
57. Golombok S, Moodley P, Lader M. Cognitive impairment in long-term benzodiazepine users. Psychol Med. 1988;18(2):365–74. https://doi.org/10.1017/s0033291700007911.
58. Boeve BF, Wijdicks EF, Benarroch EE, Schmidt KD. Paroxysmal sympathetic storms ("diencephalic seizures") after severe diffuse axonal head injury. Mayo Clin Proc. 1998;73(2):148–52. https://doi.org/10.1016/s0025-6196(11)63647-1.
59. Ko SB, Kim CK, Lee SH, Bae HJ, Yoon BW. Morphine-sensitive paroxysmal sympathetic storm in pontine intracerebral hemorrhage. Neurologist. 2010;16(6):384–5. https://doi.org/10.1097/NRL.0b013e3181b1cdff.
60. Goddeau RP Jr, Silverman SB, Sims JR. Dexmedetomidine for the treatment of paroxysmal autonomic instability with dystonia. Neurocrit Care. 2007;7(3):217–20. https://doi.org/10.1007/s12028-007-0066-0.
61. Diamond AL, Callison RC, Shokri J, Cruz-Flores S, Kinsella LJ. Paroxysmal sympathetic storm. Neurocrit Care. 2005;2(3):288–91. https://doi.org/10.1385/ncc:2:3:288.

Chapter 10
Acute Care Cardiovascular Abnormalities and Autonomic Dysreflexia After SCI

William Ide, Aileen Giordano, Heather Asthagiri, and Geoffrey Smith

Chapter Objectives

1. Summarize the incidence, etiology, and pathophysiology of AD in acute spinal cord injury.
2. Review risk factors for AD relevant to the acute care setting.
3. Review impact of AD on recovery and functional status
4. Discuss pharmacologic and non-pharmacologic interventions for the management and prevention of AD.

W. Ide (✉)
Department of Physical Medicine and Rehabilitation, University of Virginia, Charlottesville, VA, USA

Kennedy Krieger Institute, Baltimore, MD, USA

Department of Physical Medicine and Rehabilitation, Johns Hopkins University School of Medicine, University of Virginia, Baltimore, MD, USA
e-mail: ide@kennedykrieger.org

A. Giordano
Parham Doctors Hospital, Richmond, VA, USA
e-mail: alg8e@virginia.edu

H. Asthagiri
Department of Physical Medicine and Rehabilitation, University of Virginia, Charlottesville, VA, USA
e-mail: hlp5d@uvahealth.org

G. Smith
St. Mary's Hospital Rehabilitation Unit, Mayo Clinic, Rochester, MN, USA

Neurological Rehabilitation Division, Department of Physical Medicine and Rehabilitation, Mayo Clinic, Rochester, MN, USA
e-mail: smith.geoffrey@mayo.edu

A. K. Wagner, J. Weppner (eds.), *Acute Care Neuroconsultation and Neurorehabilitation Management*, https://doi.org/10.1007/978-3-031-42830-2_10

Introduction

Autonomic dysreflexia (AD) is a potentially life-threatening complication of spinal cord injury (SCI) commonly affecting individuals with complete injuries at or above thoracic level six (T6). AD is defined by episodic hypertension with or without concomitant heart rate abnormalities initiated by unmodulated sympathetic reflexes, usually in response to a noxious stimulus [1, 2]. Symptoms of AD classically include anxiety, flushing, and sweating above the level of injury; however, many patients report atypical symptoms or may be asymptomatic [3]. Untreated AD may lead to serious complications including intracranial hemorrhage, retinal detachment, seizures, and death [2, 4]. Accordingly, the prevention, immediate recognition, and management of AD in order to mitigate its clinical complications are crucial SCI rehabilitation management principles to consider for individuals with SCI in the acute care setting. This chapter will focus on the pathophysiology, risk factors, clinical characteristics, and impact of AD in adult and pediatric patients with SCI.

Pathophysiology

The hallmark of AD is episodic hypertension generated by unmodulated sympathetic reflexes [2]. Within the literature, the precise criteria for the magnitude of hypertension required to define an episode of AD is unclear. The Consortium for Spinal Cord Medicine guidelines recommend that AD be considered for an abrupt elevation in systolic blood pressure (SBP) of 20–40 mmHg above baseline in adults, 15–20 mmHg above baseline in adolescents, and 15 mmHg above baseline in children [1]. Practitioners should bear in mind that blood pressure readings representing AD in SCI patients may be considered normal or high-normal in age-matched peers without SCI [1, 2, 5]. In extreme cases, blood pressure values in excess of 300 mmHg have been documented [2, 6, 7].

Cardiovascular dysfunction following SCI in both the acute and chronic phases poses numerous challenges for management. In the acute phase following high thoracic or cervical SCI, patients are at risk for neurogenic shock defined by hypotension and bradycardia due to dysregulation of vasomotor activity below the level of injury. The severity of neurogenic hypotension is often proportionate to the level and severity of the SCI and may persist for up to 5 weeks after injury [8, 9]. Over time, patients with an SCI level T6 or above will display systolic blood pressure on average 15–20 mmHg lower than uninjured subjects and may suffer symptomatic orthostatic hypotension [6]. Orthostatic blood pressure drops may compromise cerebral perfusion, exacerbate fatigue, and hinder the ability of spinal cord injured patients to tolerate upright positioning and transfers required to participate in rehabilitation programs. Even moderate resting hypotension (SBP below 110 mmHg) has been linked to diminished cognitive performance [6]. As spinal circuitry is reorganized to create a hyper-excitable sympathetic reflex state in the setting of interrupted descending inhibitory pathways, patients can become predisposed to AD, with the highest incidence of onset between the second and fifth months postinjury [2, 9, 10].

Typically, AD is activated by a noxious visceral or somatic stimulus below the level of injury. In the intact central nervous system, vasomotor control is modulated by supraspinal vasomotor neurons that send projections to the sympathetic preganglionic neurons residing in the intermediolateral cell column extending throughout the T1-L2 spinal cord segments. These sympathetic preganglionic neurons in turn control blood vessel diameter directly via the sympathetic chain ganglia and indirectly via endocrine function of the adrenal medulla [2]. Acutely following a high SCI, sympathetic preganglionic neurons are denervated. Eventually, a hyperexcitable state of the spinal sympathetic preganglionic neurons is created, accounting for the aberrant reflex activation featured in AD. In addition to the spinal mechanisms described, there is evidence from human and animal studies that adrenergic hypersensitivity in the peripheral vasculature caudal to the lesion contributes to the exaggerated pressor response observed in AD [2].

Clinical Features

In addition to the cardinal objective sign of elevated blood pressure, the presenting symptoms reported by SCI patients are diverse. Symptoms may range from minimal to severe, and many patients may be asymptomatic. Classic AD symptoms include pounding headache, sweating, and flushing above the level of injury, with pale, cool skin below this level [5]. A severe occipital, bifrontal, or bitemporal headache has been noted in over half the patients reporting AD [11]. Patients may also experience piloerection, shivering, blurry vision, paresthesia, nasal stuffiness, increased spasticity, malaise, anxiety, nausea, or chest pressure. Most symptoms are explained by reflex vasodilatation occurring above the level of injury mediated by intact baroreceptor function in an attempt to counteract systemic hypertension resulting from loss of central inhibition in the disordered spinal cord [11]. Though bradycardia (defined as heart rate <60 in adults), or a relative decrease in heart rate from baseline, is generally considered a regular feature of AD, reports of bradycardia have been variable and numerous studies have reported tachycardia and/or tachy-arrhythmias with AD [4, 12].

Risk Factors

The T6 neurologic level is an anatomical landmark for AD risk because the splanchnic vascular bed, which can receive approximately 25% of total cardiac output, is innervated by splanchnic nerves arising from spinal segments T5-T12 [2]. Damage to the spinal cord above these levels results in the loss of inhibitory vasomotor inputs, placing the splanchnic vessels under the control of only the interspinal neurons. While AD has been reported in patients with a SCI neurological level below T6, these cases are rare and are generally characterized by milder changes in heart rate and blood pressure [2, 5]. AD is reported among individuals with SCI at or above T6 range at a prevalence of 48–91%, with differences attributed to such factors as completeness of injury, variability of criteria utilized to define AD, and time since injury [2]. While the majority of cases present in the chronic stage of SCI (3–6 months postinjury), the development of AD has been reported within the first 7 days after SCI [13]. Early presentation of AD, while uncommon, poses unique considerations for management as episodic hypertension may be compounded by pressor support agents, which are often required in acute high-level SCI [14, 15]. Another potential cause of hypertension related to autonomic dysregulation in a trauma patient, which is distinct from AD, is paroxysmal sympathetic hyperactivity (PSH). PSH may be associated with traumatic brain injury (TBI), which has a reported co-occurrence rate of 16–59% with SCI. PSH should be ruled out when a diagnosis of early AD is being considered in the intensive care setting [16]. In the absence of sepsis, PSH can usually be distinguished from AD based on the elevated heart rates and hyperthermia associated with the former.

Injury severity is related to AD risk and is highest among individuals with complete injuries (American Spinal Injury Association [ASIA] impairment scale [AIS] A), attributable to a more pronounced loss of descending vasomotor control. A retrospective study evaluating the incidence of AD requiring intervention during acute admission was 23% in patients with AIS A injuries compared to 13% of patients with AIS B SCI, and only 4% in patients with AIS C and D SCI (motor incomplete) [10]. Another study evaluating patients with chronic SCI (at least 4 months postinjury) reported a prevalence of AD in 43.5% in AIS A SCI compared to 10% in patients with AIS D SCI [17]. Because the average acute hospital length of stay (LOS) following initial injury has declined in recent years, it is important to note that incidence rates of AD in the acute setting are relatively low because hospital discharge (average LOS 16.8 days) will often precede the mean onset of AD postinjury (3–6 months) [2, 10]. Increase in recognition, prevention, and management of SCI may also contribute to decreased AD prevalence in recent years [10].

A variety of different mechanisms and stimuli have been identified as precipitating factors for AD. The most common and well-known trigger is bladder distention, accounting for 75–85% of all cases [18]. This occurs most frequently from bladder distension in acute care patients without an indwelling bladder catheter, but it may occur as a result of indwelling catheter dysfunction or blockage, or defects in catheter tubing or drainage bags. Patients with cervical SCI have poor gastric motility manifested by delayed gastric and colonic emptying as well as dissociation of antral and duodenal motility. Exacerbation of gastroparesis following abdominal surgery in patients with cervical SCI has been reported to trigger AD [19]. In patients with SCI who have required gastrostomy tube placement for feeding, manual venting or closed enteral decompression systems may be utilized to decrease discomfort from gastric distention. Other causes of AD include fecal impaction, infection or pathology of the rectum or bladder, fractures, lacerations, ingrown toenails, labor and delivery, soft tissue pressure injuries, restrictive clothing, and a variety of other conditions.

Pediatric AD

AD in children with SCI is defined by a sudden increase in blood pressure of 15 mmHg above baseline with a reported prevalence of 51% in children with injuries at or above level T6 [20]. As discussed in the adult SCI demographic, typical symptoms such as headache, facial flushing, and diaphoresis have been reported in pediatric SCI. However, depending on age and developmental level, children may not be able to effectively communicate symptoms and may present with crying, irritability, or lethargy. To promptly recognize AD, it is important to be familiar with normative blood pressure values in the pediatric population. With age, blood pressure increases and heart rate decreases in a stepwise fashion in pediatric patients with SCI. This physiologic progression is similar to that observed in typically developing children. There is additional variation in blood pressure and heart rate depending on level and completeness of injury as well as diurnal variation. A retrospective study by Hwang et al. evaluating SCI patients aged newborn to 18 years found that mean SBP was lower in youths with high cervical injuries (C1–C4) and those with complete injuries. Blood pressure and heart rates were highest in the late afternoon compared to values obtained in the morning; however, diurnal variation was not observed in those with cervical injuries [21]. A survey of caregivers and patients with SCI aged 1 to 21 years by Schottler et al. noted a higher prevalence of AD in traumatic injuries (44%) versus non-traumatic injuries (24%), as well as higher prevalence in ages 6–13 at injury group (45%) versus in ages 0–5 at injury group (19%) [22].

Clinical Complications

Complications from AD should be considered as a precipitating factor for acute care admission in any patient living with SCI. Consultants should be aware of and assist acute care providers in monitoring closely for these complications when managing patients at risk for AD during hospitalization. Although several studies have identified respiratory etiology as the most common cause of death in the chronic SCI population, cardiovascular diseases have gained recognition as a significant cause of mortality [23]. A large, retrospective study evaluating SCI patients in Taiwan over a 4-year period found an increased cumulative incidence rate of stroke in SCI (2.4% vs. 0.8% in the comparison group) [24]. SCI patients had greater rates of both hemorrhagic and ischemic stroke, with a more pronounced risk of ischemic stroke. Hypertension, the most important modifiable risk factor for stroke, is not thought to be more prevalent in SCI given lower average pressures at rest. However, the majority of reported cases of fatal complications of AD are due to central nervous system events, particularly intracranial hemorrhage and ischemic strokes [24, 25]. A literature review describing life-threatening cases of AD also reported seizures, myocardial ischemia, arrhythmia, and pulmonary edema [25]. Sympathetic hyperactivity has also been linked to diminished lymphocyte activity and immunosuppression contributing to the increased susceptibility of SCI patients to infections [2, 26]. A study evaluating hospitalizations in 226 veterans with SCI/spinal cord disorder reported at least one hospital-acquired infection occurring in 33.2% of the 549 hospitalizations studied. Hospital-acquired infections were most commonly of urinary tract source and occurred at a rate of 35 cases per 1000 patient days in this study population of predominately chronic SCI, which is significantly higher than that reported in other populations (range of 2.2–15.0 cases per 1000 patient days). Greater LOS was associated with increased risk of hospital-acquired infection [27].

Prevention and Management

The mainstay of AD management is identification and elimination of the inciting stimulus, ideally before pharmacologic measures are instituted. An essential role of the rehabilitation provider is to inform patients, caregivers, and medical staff involved in the care of individuals with SCI of the signs and symptoms of AD to enable prompt recognition. For immediate AD management, we recommend the algorithm outlined in Fig. 10.1, which was developed utilizing the Consortium for Spinal Cord Medicine Clinical Practice Guidelines [1]. Once symptoms are identified, resting blood pressure should be assessed. If determined to be representative of AD based on the patient's known baseline, the patient should be positioned upright with legs in the dependent position. Pulse and blood pressure should be monitored every 3–5 min during examination and treatment. Tight clothing and compression garments, to include stockings and abdominal binders, should be loosened or removed. Because AD is most often triggered by bladder distention, voiding routines should be evaluated to include bladder irrigation if an indwelling catheter is in place or draining the bladder with clean intermittent catheterization employing topical anesthetic. Indwelling catheters should be flushed with no more than 15 mL of fluid and should be removed and replaced if there is continued malfunction despite irrigation.

Fecal impaction should be considered if bladder drainage fails to resolve AD. If blood pressure is persistently above 150 mmHg systolic, pharmacologic management should be considered prior to assessment of the rectal vault. The recommended agent for acute AD is 2% nitroglycerin paste, 0.5–1 in. applied above the level of SCI due to its rapid onset and short duration [1, 2, 28]. Nitroglycerin paste should be wiped off once the therapeutic effect has been achieved. If impaction is noted, the rectum should be gently disimpacted following the application of topical anesthetic (lidocaine or dibucaine) to avoid introducing additional noxious stimulus. If blood pressure remains persistently above 150 mmHg systolic, additional doses of nitroglycerin paste may be considered with caution not to induce hypotension while less common triggers of AD are pursued.

There is a paucity of research regarding the management of AD in pediatric SCI. McGinnis et al. of Shriners Hospitals for Children have proposed adding the measurement of body temperature to initial vital signs given the potential for

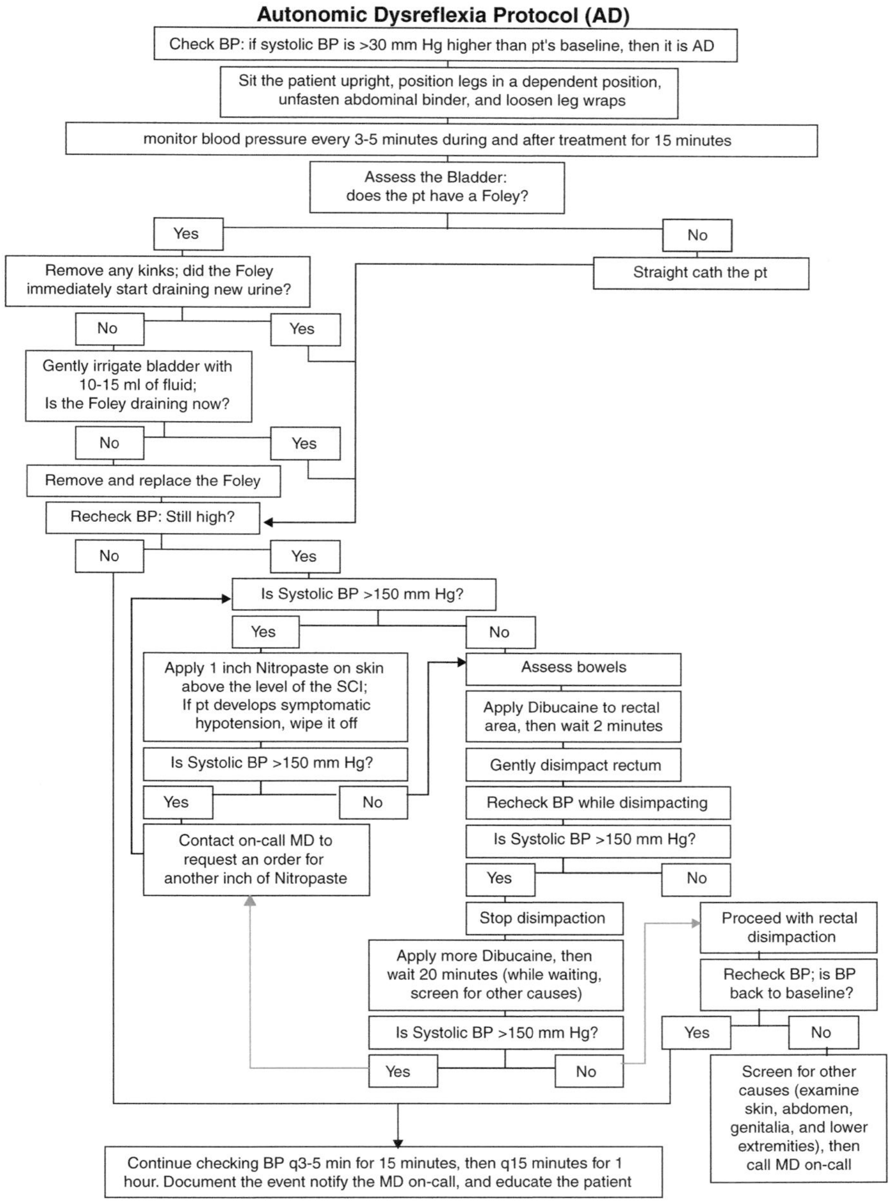

Fig. 10.1 University of Virginia autonomic dysreflexia protocol for adult in patient rehabilitation

environmentally responsive thermoregulatory dysfunction in children with SCI as a precipitating factor for AD. This reference also suggests age group-based thresholds for consideration of antihypertensives [29]. The consortium guidelines recommend bladder irrigation for indwelling catheters be limited to 5–10 mL for children under 2 years of age and 10–15 mL in older children and adolescents to avoid overdistension of the bladder [1].

While acute episodes of AD are often quickly reversible with usual remedies, many cases are protracted and/or recurrent and have no readily identifiable cause. The most effective strategy for AD prevention is education regarding its causes, establishment of appropriate bowel and bladder programs, and vigilant skin protection as reviewed in Chap. 12 [28]. The rehabilitation practitioner should work to identify and eliminate specific triggers unique to each individual living with SCI. Captopril and nifedipine have been utilized in acute AD; however, concerns have been raised regarding the risk of hypoperfusion with nifedipine. In severe refractory cases, intravenous sodium nitroprusside may resolve hypertension [2]. As this medication is delivered via intravenous drip, administration should occur in a closely monitored setting in consultation with the patient's intensivist. Epidural anesthesia is recommended to prevent AD in labor and delivery.

Case Illustration

Michael is a 7-year-old boy with a history of complete tetraplegia due to a C4 AIS A SCI sustained in a motor vehicle accident. He is admitted to the Pediatric Intensive Care Unit for management of ventilator-associated pneumonia. His past medical history is remarkable for recurrent episodes of AD associated with bradycardia requiring implantation of a pacemaker and tracheostomy placement. A gastrostomy tube is utilized for supplemental nutrition and he has experienced frequent abdominal distention due to bowel gas. One morning Michael's nurse contacts his physician after she records a blood pressure of 130/90, which she notes to be significantly higher than his baseline blood pressure of 95/65. Michael's nurse contacts his physician after having already positioned him upright and performed catheterization for bladder drainage. His temperature is 37.1 °C. The physician arrives to find Michael sitting upright in bed in no obvious distress and reporting no symptoms. He is wearing no compression garments or restrictive clothing. A repeat blood pressure measurement taken after 5 min is 122/87 with a normal-range pulse and oxygen saturation. Suspecting gastric distention, the physician requests ventilation of Michael's gastrostomy tube and after 3 min his blood pressure improves to 108/76. His blood pressure is monitored at 5-min intervals and gradually normalizes after 20 min.

Summary and Key Points

Autonomic dysreflexia is a clinical emergency in patients living with SCI, which is often underrecognized outside of rehabilitation settings. Episodes of sympathetically mediated hypertension caused by disruption of descending central inhibitory pathways may be drastic and rapid in onset. AD symptoms are variable in character and range from non-existent to unbearable. Adults and children at highest risk for AD are those with higher thoracic (T6) and cervical lesions as well as those with more complete lesions who are in the chronic phase of SCI. The optimization of daily routine cares for patients with SCI should be reinforced as an essential prevention strategy. Education and empowerment of patients and their care teams to quickly recognize AD, identify and eliminate its triggers, and control hypertension is critical to mitigating AD's potentially grave ramifications for multiple organ systems.

References[1]

1. Consortium for Spinal Cord Medicine. Acute management of autonomic dysreflexia: individuals with spinal cord injury presenting to health-care facilities. J Spinal Cord Med. 2002;25(Suppl 1):S67–88.
2. Eldahan KC, Rabchevsky AG. Autonomic dysreflexia after spinal cord injury: systemic pathophysiology and methods of management. Auton Neurosci. 2018;209:59–70. https://doi.org/10.1016/j.autneu.2017.05.002.
3. Linsenmeyer TA, Campagnolo DI, Chou IH. Silent autonomic dysreflexia during voiding in men with spinal cord injuries. J Urol. 1996;155(2):519–22.
4. Krassioukov AV, Furlan JC, Fehlings MG. Autonomic dysreflexia in acute spinal cord injury: an under-recognized clinical entity. J Neurotrauma. 2003;20(8):707–16. https://doi.org/10.1089/089771503767869944.
5. Blackmer J. Rehabilitation medicine: 1. Autonomic dysreflexia. CMAJ. 2003;169(9):931–5.
6. Claydon VE, Steeves JD, Krassioukov A. Orthostatic hypotension following spinal cord injury: understanding clinical pathophysiology. Spinal Cord. 2006;44(6):341–51. https://doi.org/10.1038/sj.sc.3101855.
7. Krassioukov A, Warburton DE, Teasell R, Eng JJ. A systematic review of the management of autonomic dysreflexia after spinal cord injury. Arch Phys Med Rehabil. 2009;90(4):682–95. https://doi.org/10.1016/j.apmr.2008.10.017.
8. Guly HR, Bouamra O, Lecky FE. The incidence of neurogenic shock in patients with isolated spinal cord injury in the emergency department. Resuscitation. 2008;76(1):57–62. https://doi.org/10.1016/j.resuscitation.2007.06.008.
9. Krassioukov A, Claydon VE. The clinical problems in cardiovascular control following spinal cord injury: an overview. Prog Brain Res. 2006;152:223–9. https://doi.org/10.1016/s0079-6123(05)52014-4.
10. Helkowski WM, Ditunno JF Jr, Boninger M. Autonomic dysreflexia: incidence in persons with neurologically complete and incomplete tetraplegia. J Spinal Cord Med. 2003;26(3):244–7. https://doi.org/10.1080/10790268.2003.11753691.
11. Karlsson AK. Autonomic dysreflexia. Spinal Cord. 1999;37(6):383–91. https://doi.org/10.1038/sj.sc.3100867.
12. Collins HL, Rodenbaugh DW, DiCarlo SE. Spinal cord injury alters cardiac electrophysiology and increases the susceptibility to ventricular arrhythmias. Prog Brain Res. 2006;152:275–88. https://doi.org/10.1016/s0079-6123(05)52018-1.
13. Weaver LC. What causes autonomic dysreflexia after spinal cord injury? Clin Auton Res. 2002;12(6):424–6. https://doi.org/10.1007/s10286-002-0076-0.

[1] Key References [1, 2, 7, 15, 24].

14. Inoue T, Manley GT, Patel N, Whetstone WD. Medical and surgical management after spinal cord injury: vasopressor usage, early surgerys, and complications. J Neurotrauma. 2014;31(3):284–91. https://doi.org/10.1089/neu.2013.3061.
15. Ploumis A, Yadlapalli N, Fehlings MG, Kwon BK, Vaccaro AR. A systematic review of the evidence supporting a role for vasopressor support in acute SCI. Spinal Cord. 2010;48(5):356–62. https://doi.org/10.1038/sc.2009.150.
16. Nott M, Baguley I, Heriseanu R, et al. Effects of concomitant spinal cord injury and brain injury on medical and functional outcomes and community participation. Top Spinal Cord Inj Rehabil. 2014;20(3):225–35.
17. Furusawa K, Tokuhiro A, Sugiyama H, et al. Incidence of symptomatic autonomic dysreflexia varies according to the bowel and bladder management techniques in patients with spinal cord injury. Spinal Cord. 2011;49(1):49–54. https://doi.org/10.1038/sc.2010.94.
18. Shergill I, Arya M, Hamid R, Khastgir J, Patel H, Shah P. The importance of autonomic dysreflexia to the urologist. BJU Int. 2004;93:923–6.
19. Pacheco M, Garstang S. Gastric dysmotility after abdominal surgery in persons with cervical spinal cord injury: a case series. J Spinal Cord Med. 2007;30(4):378–84.
20. Hickey KJ, Vogel LC, Willis KM, Anderson CJ. Prevalence and etiology of autonomic dysreflexia in children with spinal cord injuries. J Spinal Cord Med. 2004;27(Suppl 1):S54–60. https://doi.org/10.1080/10790268.2004.11753786.
21. Hwang M, Zebracki K, Betz R, Mulcahey M, Vogel L. Normative blood pressure and heart rate in pediatric spinal cord injury. Top Spinal Cord Inj Rehabil. 2013;19(2):87–95.
22. Schottler J, Vogel L, Chafetz R, Mulcahey MJ. Patient and caregiver knowledge of autonomic dysreflexia among youth with spinal cord injury. Spinal Cord. 2009;47(9):681–6. https://doi.org/10.1038/sc.2009.12.
23. Garshick E, Kelley A, Cohen SA, et al. A prospective assessment of mortality in chronic spinal cord injury. Spinal Cord. 2005;43(7):408–16. https://doi.org/10.1038/sj.sc.3101729.
24. Wu JC, Chen YC, Liu L, et al. Increased risk of stroke after spinal cord injury: a nationwide 4-year follow-up cohort study. Neurology. 2012;78(14):1051–7. https://doi.org/10.1212/WNL.0b013e31824e8eaa.
25. Wan D, Krassioukov AV. Life-threatening outcomes associated with autonomic dysreflexia: a clinical review. J Spinal Cord Med. 2014;37(1):2–10. https://doi.org/10.1179/2045772313y.0000000098.
26. Brommer B, Kopp M, Laginha I, JM S. Secondary immunodeficiancy (immune paralysis) following spinal cord injury. e-Neuroforum. 2010;1:43–51.
27. Evans C, LeVela S, Weaver F, et al. Epidemiology of hospital-acquired infections in verterans with spinal cord injury and disorder. Infect Control Hosp Epidemiol. 2008;29(3):234–42.
28. Krassioukov A, Eng JJ, Claxton G, Sakakibara BM, Shum S. Neurogenic bowel management after spinal cord injury: a systematic review of the evidence. Spinal Cord. 2010;48(10):718–33. https://doi.org/10.1038/sc.2010.14.
29. McGinnis KB, Vogel LC, McDonald CM, et al. Recognition and management of autonomic dysreflexia in pediatric spinal cord injury. J Spinal Cord Med. 2004;27(Suppl 1):S61–74. https://doi.org/10.1080/10790268.2004.11753787.

Chapter 11
Geriatric Considerations: Age-Related Functional Changes in Acquired Neurologic Injury

Shanti M. Pinto

Chapter Objectives

1. Discuss the physiologic changes that occur with aging and how these changes impact long-term function and development of the rehabilitation program.
2. Summarize the epidemiology and outcomes of traumatic brain and spinal cord injuries in older adults.
3. Understand how the aging process impacts those with disabilities.

Introduction

With the aging of the general population, there is great need for physicians to understand management of geriatric patients. Increasing age is a known risk factor for multiple medical complications that can lead to functional impairments, such as stroke, malignancy, and anoxic brain injury resulting from cardiac arrest. Additionally, older individuals are at increased risk of traumatic injury, particularly because of fall. This acute care rehabilitation consultant resource has two chapters that focus on the aging population. This chapter will summarize age-related functional changes and how they are associated with acquired neurologic injury. Chapter 17 discusses medical considerations for the geriatric population with acquired neurological injuries.

S. M. Pinto (✉)
Department of Physical Medicine and Rehabilitation, University of Texas - Southwestern, Dallas, TX, USA
e-mail: shanti.pinto@utsouthwestern.edu

A. K. Wagner, J. Weppner (eds.), *Acute Care Neuroconsultation and Neurorehabilitation Management*, https://doi.org/10.1007/978-3-031-42830-2_11

Literature-Based Assessment of Key Concepts

Age-Related Physiologic Changes and Association with Injury

Multiple physiologic changes occur during the normal aging process, and these changes have a profound impact on function. Overall, there is a decrease in muscle mass and cross-sectional area, which is associated with a decrease in muscle strength and aerobic capacity [1–3]. There is selective loss of the glycolytic type II fibers with little impact on the oxidative and fatigue-resistant type I fibers due to selective denervation and decline in satellite cell number [4–6]. These changes are associated with decreased muscle strength and an age-related decline in aerobic capacity. Patients with lower peak aerobic capacity experience greater levels of exertion during basic tasks such as ambulation and compensate by decreasing habitual gait speed [7].

Older patients are at increased risk for deconditioning because of immobility. A 10-day period of bed rest has been associated with significant decline in total body and lower extremity lean muscle mass, lower extremity strength, and peak aerobic capacity in healthy older adults [8]. Bed rest is associated with decrease in functional skills [8], and the impact of immobility is particularly noted during hospitalization. In one study of older adults admitted to a general medical service, those who were placed on bed rest or had mobility limited to being out of bed to a chair had high rate of a decline in self-care abilities and discharge to skilled nursing facility [9]. Functional decline is more pronounced in those who have restricted oral intake during hospitalization [3].

The brain also undergoes crucial changes during normal aging. White matter volume increases during the first 40 years of life and begins to rapidly decline after 60. These changes are associated with depression, cognitive decline, and increased risk for cerebrovascular disease [3, 10]. Hypertension, atherosclerosis, and diabetes (known cerebrovascular risk factors) are more highly prevelant in the aging population, further increasing the risk of cerebrovascular disease, which affects over 9% of patients aged 70 and older [1, 10].

Epidemiology of Traumatic Injury in the Aging Population

Over one-third of older adults experience falls annually, leading to significant morbidity and mortality. Older adults are at increased risk for falls due to the age-related declines in lower extremity strength and gait speed. Visual impairments from changes within the lens and retina of the eye, sensory and proprioceptive deficits due to peripheral neuropathy, orthostatic hypotension, cardiac arrhythmias, and medication side effects are other risk factors for falls [3, 11]. Significant injury can occur even after ground level falls, and falls are the most common cause of injury for both traumatic brain injury (TBI) and spinal cord injury (SCI) in the geriatric population [12–20]. In fact, hospitalization after TBI is highest in those over the age of 65 [13, 14, 16, 18, 21]. Overall, TBI and SCI most frequently affect men, but this disparity with incidence diminishes with increasing age [12, 15, 17, 19, 22]. Older individuals are more likely to suffer cervical level and incomplete injuries than younger patients [15, 18, 23]. Central cord syndrome commonly occurs due to cervical hyperextension during fall, and these individuals present with motor and sensory impairments that affect the arms more than legs.

Prognosis and Outcomes

Overall prognosis and outcomes are worse with increasing age. This is due in large part to higher rate of co-morbid medical conditions and decreased neural plasticity. Additionally, older individuals with traumatic injury are more susceptible to higher degree of injury with seemingly minor insult. Older adults have a higher rate of mortality after TBI and SCI than younger adults [14, 16, 18, 20, 22, 24–29]. Increased mortality rates are noted not only during acute hospitalization but also in the first year following discharge from inpatient rehabilitation (IPR) [17, 30]. The increase in TBI mortality with each year of advancing age at time of injury begins in the fourth decade of life, with the sharpest increase in mortality beginning in the eighth decade [25, 31]. Individuals with TBI and traumatic SCI have greater degree of disability and lower rate of functional independence at IPR discharge despite suffering less severe neurologic injuries than younger individuals [23, 27, 32–34]. When comparing age-related differences in a group of individuals with paraplegia that were matched based on level of injury, those 60 or older demonstrated less functional improvements during inpatient rehabilitation stay despite longer IPR length of stay (LOS) [35]. Likewise, older individuals have greater functional deficits, lower functional recovery, and greater disability following stroke rehabilitation program [36–38].

Considerations for Rehabilitation Referrals in the Geriatric Population

At present, there are no guidelines regarding the specific therapeutic interventions for geriatric patients after acquired neurologic injury. Older adults do make progress with intensive rehabilitation programs, and many individuals can be successfully discharged back to the community; however, the gains are typically slower for older individuals following TBI, traumatic SCI, or stroke [12, 17, 32, 34–36, 39]. There is no consensus on how IPR LOS varies based on age with some studies showing that older individuals having longer IPR LOS [32, 35, 39], others showing no difference [12, 34], and finally shorter IPR LOS for older individuals [36]. In general, there is no difference in daily rehabilitation costs based on age; however, rehabilitation costs to achieve the same functional improvements are greater for older compared with younger individuals following TBI [32, 39]. Though older individuals can be successfully discharged to the community, older age patients are more likely to be discharged to a skilled nursing facility following IPR after stroke, TBI, or SCI [12, 16, 17, 23, 32, 34, 40].

Older individuals who experience a later onset of an SCI tend to require more daily nursing hours and may have a higher number of co-morbidities and secondary complications [15, 41–43]. They may also experience a decline in self-sufficiency and are more likely to require institutional care post-discharge [44]. Personalized acute inpatient rehabilitation plans can significantly improve patient autonomy and reduce the rate of institutionalization, which can lessen the long-term burden on healthcare systems [43, 45]. Therefore, when consulting with a geriatric patient for inpatient rehabilitation, a physiatrist should approach them with a comprehensive and individualized plan that focuses on the potential for secondary complications and community discharge planning. This approach, tailored to the patient's unique needs, can help maximize their autonomy and potential for rehabilitation while minimizing the likelihood of institutionalization.

Older adults are less likely to have access to inpatient rehabilitation services. A retrospective study using the National Trauma Data Bank found that older individuals were more likely to be discharged to skilled nursing facilities rather than IPR from the acute hospital following TBI [14]. Older individuals are also less likely to receive the same level of rehabilitation services during IPR. Dijkers et al. [17] compared the therapeutic interventions for adults admitted to IPR after TBI based on age at time of admission. They found that older patients have shorter IPR LOS and receive less overall therapy services during IPR admission; furthermore, therapy sessions for older adults were more frequently focused on basic gait training rather than advanced mobility and self-care skills provided to younger patients. They also found that older patients were less likely to receive psychology services and to participate in community reintegration activities than younger patients following TBI [17].

The rehabilitation program should be tailored to meet the specific needs of the older individual following acquired neurologic conditions to best maximize function and overall health. Aerobic conditioning can enhance mitochondrial functioning, leading to improved aerobic capacity and gait speed. Aerobic training has additionally been shown to improve function and decrease symptoms related to arthritis, chronic obstructive pulmonary disease, cardiovascular disease, and diabetes mellitus [1, 46]. Progressive resistance training programs lead to muscle fiber hypertrophy and can reverse some of the age-related loss of muscle strength, particularly in the lower extremities. This can lead to improvements in functional mobility and balance, leading to decreased fall risk [4, 5, 11]. Additionally, the rehabilitation program should be tailored to the individual patient's associated medical co-morbidities as severity of associated medical co-morbidities is often predictive of overall functional change during the rehabilitation program [47]. Arthritis and chronic musculoskeletal conditions are common in older adults, which can lead to decreased range of motion and cause pain with use of the joint. Any therapy program, including neurorehabilitation programs in the acute care and IPR settings, should incorporate exercises and modalities to decrease pain and improve range of motion of the affected joints. Older individuals may have poor endurance during therapy sessions due to underlying cardiac and pulmonary disease. These individuals would benefit from incorporated rest breaks between exercises to help achieve functional goals. Use of a perceived exertion scale may help guide the intensity of therapeutic activities. Ambulation goals may be limited to only short household distances with use of an assistive device, such as an attendant-propelled manual wheelchair, for long community distances. Patients should be educated on energy conservation techniques.

Aging with Disability

Due to advances in health care, individuals with disabilities are living longer, with life expectancies near that of able-bodied individuals. In 2015, approximately 12–15 million older adults were living in the USA with a disability that began in childhood through young adulthood. This represents nearly 15% of older adults [48] and is an important but often overlooked population. These patients frequently experience new or worsening functional limitations during normal aging and can experience further functional decline during hospitalization due to the acute medical illness and relative immobility.

One study of adults at least 20 years post-SCI found age-related decline in muscle strength and energy level was associated with decreased participation in active recreation activities due to need to conserve energy to maintain independence with activities of daily living [49]. Assistive devices utilized for mobility and self-care may need to be reassessed during the aging process. For example, a paraplegic patient previously independent with mobility in a manual wheelchair may benefit from addition of power features for energy conservation. Patients may develop orthopedic injuries of the impaired limbs due to overuse, and this may cause further loss of functional independence and need for reassessment of adaptive equipment and strategies for mobility and completing ADLs. Patients frequently experience changes in caregiver support with increased time since disability. This typically occurs due to loss of a caregiver or changes in the health of an aging caregiver.

Understanding the impact of age on the prolonged outcomes of TBI necessitates a focus on both the persistent and developing effects of TBI, as well as alterations in health and functionality associated with aging. Increased age and prolonged duration of TBI are associated with worse functional outcomes [50–52]. The enduring and escalating functional challenges in individuals a decade after experiencing TBI indicate a need for reconsidering the delivery methods of rehabilitation services. Although the advantages of brain injury rehabilitation are well-recognized, these services are generally concentrated at the early stages, overlooking the later development and handling of chronic health issues and affected neurocognitive aging [31, 52–55]. There is a need for (1) specific management for elderly individuals who have suffered a moderate-severe TBI, and (2) continuous monitoring of persons who experience a moderate-severe TBI at any stage of life [52, 56]. The increased risk of co-morbid health conditions could potentially negatively impact the function in those growing older with TBI, and these chronic conditions (i.e., arthritis, sleep disorders, neurosensory impairments, stroke) could be detected and mitigated through appropriate physiatry intervention [56, 57]. A more comprehensive, long-term approach to TBI rehabilitation, which includes early detection and intervention for co-morbid conditions, could significantly improve the quality of life for individuals as they age post-TBI.

Case Illustrations

The two cases below help illustrate important rehabilitation concepts for geriatric patients. The first case discusses a previously independent elderly patient who suffers an acute neurologic injury. The second case discusses a patient who suffered

SCI while young and has experienced additional complications due to aging. This chapter focuses on functional rehabilitation aspects of these patients, and the cases will be revisited in Chap. 17 with focus on medical considerations.

TBI in Geriatric Patient

A 95-year-old, previously independent male with history of mild cognitive impairment suffered a complex mild TBI due to a ground level fall. He was walking outside and tripped over a curb. There was no loss of consciousness. His initial GCS was 14 due to confusion, which was worse than baseline. CT of the head showed a small intracranial hemorrhage as well as a left zygomaxillary fracture. Both injuries were non-operatively managed, and he was not prescribed anti-epileptic medication for seizure prophylaxis due to small size of the hemorrhage. Prior to admission, he lived alone and was independent for mobility and basic self-care without assistive device. His daughter and son-in-law lived nearby and assisted with driving, groceries, and household chores. He walked to the assistive living facility across the street to spend time with a friend daily. During his acute care hospitalization, he was noted to be confused and impulsive, requiring the use of an enclosure bed for safety. The early rehabilitation program focused on strategies to improve his orientation to the situation and decrease risk of delirium. Staff implemented scheduled time out of bed to the wheelchair, using a rear-fastening seatbelt for safety. Attempts were made to ensure regular sleep hours with limited overnight interruptions. Signs with large print were placed in his room to reorient him to the date, location, and reason for admission. The acute hospital therapists noted chronic right knee pain. On the rehabilitation consultant's examination, he demonstrated bilateral genu varum upon standing. X-rays of the knees showed evidence of bilateral knee osteoarthritis, right more severe than the left. The rehabilitation consultant recommended use of a neoprene sleeve for the right knee to provide proprioceptive support and a short course of NSAIDs to help with the arthritis pain to facilitate participation in the therapy program. Once admitted to IPR, his therapy program included exercises for stretching and strengthening of the knees. Ambulation was limited to only short distances to simulate a home environment, and he was educated on wheelchair skills for longer distances.

He was admitted to IPR 7 days after injury. At the time of admission, he required minimal to maximum assistance for all self-care, minimal to moderate assistance for all transfers, and moderate assistance with stand by assistance of a second person due to safety concerns during ambulation. He was discharged to home with daughter and son-in-law after 22 days in IPR, at which time, he required minimal assistance to supervision for mobility and basic self-care activities. He had moderate to severe cognitive deficits and required initial constant supervision. He was provided a transport chair at discharge due to decreased endurance with mobility. At an outpatient follow-up appointment 6 weeks later, his daughter reported that he was back to his baseline prior to the injury. He was independent for all mobility and basic self-care activities. His cognition had improved back to his baseline, and he was being transitioned back to his home to live independently.

Aging with SCI

A 68-year-old, right-hand dominant male who suffered C6 ASIA A SCI due to motor vehicle accident 50 years ago was hospitalized due to atrial fibrillation with rapid ventricular rate. He was seen by a physiatrist during this admission. The patient currently lives in an accessible home with his wife, his primary caretaker. He completed college and law school after his injury and worked for nearly 30 years as a district attorney. He utilized a manual wheelchair for the first 25 years after his injury but switched to a power wheelchair with static seating system in his mid-40s due to bilateral shoulder pain. He performs pressure relief by hooking his arm behind his chair and leaning forward. He drives a wheelchair accessible van using hand controls. His wife assists him with all transfers and self-care tasks, and he notes that he has required more assistance with these tasks as he has aged due to the shoulder pain. He reports an increase in his right shoulder pain over the past 6 months, which began acutely while he was performing a pressure relief maneuver. He recently had an ultrasound of the shoulder that showed subacute total thickness tear of the subscapularis tendon with bursitis as well as chronic tear of the supraspinatus tendon, acromioclavicular joint arthritis, and glenohumeral joint arthritis. The tear of the subscapularis tendon was estimated to have occurred 6 months ago when he noted the acute pain onset; the other findings were attributed to overuse of the shoulder.

He is evaluated by physical and occupational therapy during his hospitalization and is at his baseline status for transfers and self-care tasks. His wife demonstrates that she is able to perform the skills needed at home. To address his shoulder pain, he is recommended to modify his weight shifts to preferentially activate the latissimus dorsi to compensate for the subscapularis tendon rupture. He is given exercises to strengthen the latissimus dorsi muscle. He is recommended to switch to a wheelchair with power seating options to better perform pressure relief maneuvers; however, he is reluctant to make this change as he feels that it would represent a loss of independence.

Summary/Key Points

Aging is associated with a number of physiologic changes that lead to important changes in function. Older adults are at increased risk for falls, which can lead to severe injuries. Older adults with traumatic and non-traumatic neurologic injuries to the brain have higher number of medical co-morbidities and usually suffer worse outcomes than younger individuals. Despite these challenges, older individuals can achieve good functional gains during IPR, and many can be successfully discharged to the community. Rehabilitation programs should be tailored to account for these medical co-morbidities. Additionally, longer IPR LOS may be needed as these gains occur more slowly over time. Patients aging with pre-morbid disability note increased functional changes that lead to a loss of independence, requiring reassessment of durable medical equipment and techniques used for mobility and self-care. It is important for the acute care consultant to be aware of the challenges faced by older individuals following acquired neurologic injury to tailor the goals of the rehabilitation program appropriately.

References[1]

1. Bean JF, Vora A, Frontera WR. Benefits of exercise for community-dwelling older adults. Arch Phys Med Rehabil. 2004;85(7 Suppl 3):S31–42; quiz S43–44.
2. Fleg JL, Morrell CH, Bos AG, et al. Accelerated longitudinal decline of aerobic capacity in healthy older adults. Circulation. 2005;112(5):674–82. https://doi.org/10.1161/CIRCULATIONAHA.105.545459.
3. Rosenthal RA, Kavic SM. Assessment and management of the geriatric patient. Crit Care Med. 2004;32(4 Suppl):S92–105.
4. Kirkendall DT, Garrett WE. The effects of aging and training on skeletal muscle. Am J Sports Med. 1998;26(4):598–602. https://doi.org/10.1177/03635465980260042401.
5. Nilwik R, Snijders T, Leenders M, et al. The decline in skeletal muscle mass with aging is mainly attributed to a reduction in type II muscle fiber size. Exp Gerontol. 2013;48(5):492–8. https://doi.org/10.1016/j.exger.2013.02.012.
6. Verdijk LB, Koopman R, Schaart G, Meijer K, Savelberg HHCM, van Loon LJC. Satellite cell content is specifically reduced in type II skeletal muscle fibers in the elderly. Am J Physiol Endocrinol Metab. 2007;292(1):E151–7. https://doi.org/10.1152/ajpendo.00278.2006.
7. Fiser WM, Hays NP, Rogers SC, et al. Energetics of walking in elderly people: factors related to gait speed. J Gerontol A Biol Sci Med Sci. 2010;65(12):1332–7. https://doi.org/10.1093/gerona/glq137.
8. Coker RH, Hays NP, Williams RH, Wolfe RR, Evans WJ. Bed rest promotes reductions in walking speed, functional parameters, and aerobic fitness in older, healthy adults. J Gerontol A Biol Sci Med Sci. 2015;70(1):91–6. https://doi.org/10.1093/gerona/glu123.
9. Brown CJ, Friedkin RJ, Inouye SK. Prevalence and outcomes of low mobility in hospitalized older patients. J Am Geriatr Soc. 2004;52(8):1263–70. https://doi.org/10.1111/j.1532-5415.2004.52354.x.
10. Liu H, Yang Y, Xia Y, et al. Aging of cerebral white matter. Ageing Res Rev. 2017;34:64–76. https://doi.org/10.1016/j.arr.2016.11.006.
11. Enderlin C, Rooker J, Ball S, et al. Summary of factors contributing to falls in older adults and nursing implications. Geriatr Nurs. 2015;36(5):397–406. https://doi.org/10.1016/j.gerinurse.2015.08.006.
12. Cifu DX, Huang ME, Kolakowsky-Hayner SA, Seel RT. Age, outcome, and rehabilitation costs after paraplegia caused by traumatic injury of the thoracic spinal cord, conus medullaris, and cauda equina. J Neurotrauma. 1999;16(9):805–15. https://doi.org/10.1089/neu.1999.16.805.
13. Coronado VG, Thomas KE, Sattin RW, Johnson RL. The CDC traumatic brain injury surveillance system: characteristics of persons aged 65 years and older hospitalized with a TBI. J Head Trauma Rehabil. 2005;20(3):215–28.
14. Dams-O'Connor K, Cuthbert JP, Whyte J, Corrigan JD, Faul M, Harrison-Felix C. Traumatic brain injury among older adults at level I and II trauma centers. J Neurotrauma. 2013;30(24):2001–13. https://doi.org/10.1089/neu.2013.3047.
15. DeVivo MJ, Kartus PL, Rutt RD, Stover SL, Fine PR. The influence of age at time of spinal cord injury on rehabilitation outcome. Arch Neurol. 1990;47(6):687–91. https://doi.org/10.1001/archneur.1990.00530060101026.
16. Devivo MJ. Epidemiology of traumatic spinal cord injury: trends and future implications. Spinal Cord. 2012;50(5):365–72. https://doi.org/10.1038/sc.2011.178.
17. Dijkers M, Brandstater M, Horn S, Ryser D, Barrett R. Inpatient rehabilitation for traumatic brain injury: the influence of age on treatments and outcomes. NeuroRehabilitation. 2013;32(2):233–52. https://doi.org/10.3233/NRE-130841.
18. Fassett DR, Harrop JS, Maltenfort M, et al. Mortality rates in geriatric patients with spinal cord injuries. J Neurosurg Spine. 2007;7(3):277–81. https://doi.org/10.3171/SPI-07/09/277.
19. Harvey LA, Close JCT. Traumatic brain injury in older adults: characteristics, causes and consequences. Injury. 2012;43(11):1821–6. https://doi.org/10.1016/j.injury.2012.07.188.

[1] Key References [1, 3, 39].

20. Jabbour P, Fehlings M, Vaccaro AR, Harrop JS. Traumatic spine injuries in the geriatric population. Neurosurg Focus. 2008;25(5):E16. https://doi.org/10.3171/FOC.2008.25.11.E16.
21. DeVivo MJ, Chen Y. Trends in new injuries, prevalent cases, and aging with spinal cord injury. Arch Phys Med Rehabil. 2011;92(3):332–8. https://doi.org/10.1016/j.apmr.2010.08.031.
22. Susman M, DiRusso SM, Sullivan T, et al. Traumatic brain injury in the elderly: increased mortality and worse functional outcome at discharge despite lower injury severity. J Trauma. 2002;53(2):219–23; discussion 223–24.
23. DeVivo MJ, Shewchuk RM, Stover SL, Black KJ, Go BK. A cross-sectional study of the relationship between age and current health status for persons with spinal cord injuries. Paraplegia. 1992;30(12):820–7. https://doi.org/10.1038/sc.1992.158.
24. Daneshvar P, Roffey DM, Brikeet YA, Tsai EC, Bailey CS, Wai EK. Spinal cord injuries related to cervical spine fractures in elderly patients: factors affecting mortality. Spine J. 2013;13(8):862–6. https://doi.org/10.1016/j.spinee.2013.01.045.
25. Hukkelhoven CWPM, Steyerberg EW, Rampen AJJ, et al. Patient age and outcome following severe traumatic brain injury: an analysis of 5600 patients. J Neurosurg. 2003;99(4):666–73. https://doi.org/10.3171/jns.2003.99.4.0666.
26. McIntyre A, Mehta S, Aubut J, Dijkers M, Teasell RW. Mortality among older adults after a traumatic brain injury: a meta-analysis. Brain Inj. 2013;27(1):31–40. https://doi.org/10.3109/02699052.2012.700086.
27. Pennings JL, Bachulis BL, Simons CT, Slazinski T. Survival after severe brain injury in the aged. Arch Surg Chic Ill 1960. 1993;128(7):787–93; discussion 793–94.
28. Spaniolas K, Cheng JD, Gestring ML, Sangosanya A, Stassen NA, Bankey PE. Ground level falls are associated with significant mortality in elderly patients. J Trauma. 2010;69(4):821–5. https://doi.org/10.1097/TA.0b013e3181efc6c6.
29. Thompson HJ, Dikmen S, Temkin N. Prevalence of comorbidity and its association with traumatic brain injury and outcomes in older adults. Res Gerontol Nurs. 2012;5(1):17–24. https://doi.org/10.3928/19404921-20111206-02.
30. Harrison-Felix C, Whiteneck G, DeVivo M, Hammond FM, Jha A. Mortality following rehabilitation in the traumatic brain injury model Systems of Care. NeuroRehabilitation. 2004;19(1):45–54.
31. Thompson HJ, McCormick WC, Kagan SH. Traumatic brain injury in older adults: epidemiology, outcomes, and future implications. J Am Geriatr Soc. 2006;54(10):1590–5. https://doi.org/10.1111/j.1532-5415.2006.00894.x.
32. Frankel JE, Marwitz JH, Cifu DX, Kreutzer JS, Englander J, Rosenthal M. A follow-up study of older adults with traumatic brain injury: taking into account decreasing length of stay. Arch Phys Med Rehabil. 2006;87(1):57–62. https://doi.org/10.1016/j.apmr.2005.07.309.
33. McKinley W, Cifu D, Seel R, et al. Age-related outcomes in persons with spinal cord injury: a summary paper. NeuroRehabilitation. 2003;18(1):83–90.
34. New PW, Epi MC. Influence of age and gender on rehabilitation outcomes in nontraumatic spinal cord injury. J Spinal Cord Med. 2007;30(3):225–37.
35. Seel RT, Huang ME, Cifu DX, Kolakowsky-Hayner SA, McKinley WO. Age-related differences in length of stays, hospitalization costs, and outcomes for an injury-matched sample of adults with paraplegia. J Spinal Cord Med. 2001;24(4):241–50. https://doi.org/10.1080/10790268.2001.11753581.
36. Ergeletzis D, Kevorkian CG, Rintala D. Rehabilitation of the older stroke patient: functional outcome and comparison with younger patients. Am J Phys Med Rehabil. 2002;81(12):881–9. https://doi.org/10.1097/01.PHM.0000034952.83652.95.
37. Saposnik G, Kapral MK, Cote R, et al. Is pre-existing dementia an independent predictor of outcome after stroke? A propensity score-matched analysis. J Neurol. 2012;259(11):2366–75. https://doi.org/10.1007/s00415-012-6508-4.
38. Veerbeek JM, Kwakkel G, van Wegen EEH, Ket JCF, Heymans MW. Early prediction of outcome of activities of daily living after stroke: a systematic review. Stroke. 2011;42(5):1482–8. https://doi.org/10.1161/STROKEAHA.110.604090.
39. Cifu DX, Kreutzer JS, Marwitz JH, Rosenthal M, Englander J, High W. Functional outcomes of older adults with traumatic brain injury: a prospective, multicenter analysis. Arch Phys Med Rehabil. 1996;77(9):883–8. https://doi.org/10.1016/s0003-9993(96)90274-9.

40. Nguyen VQC, PrvuBettger J, Guerrier T, et al. Factors associated with discharge to home versus discharge to institutional care after inpatient stroke rehabilitation. Arch Phys Med Rehabil. 2015;96(7):1297–303. https://doi.org/10.1016/j.apmr.2015.03.007.
41. Krassioukov AV, Furlan JC, Fehlings MG. Medical co-morbidities, secondary complications, and mortality in elderly with acute spinal cord injury. J Neurotrauma. 2003;20:391–9. https://doi.org/10.1089/089771503765172345.
42. Roth EJ, Lovell L, Heinemann AW, Lee MY, Yarkony GM. The older adult with a spinal cord injury. Paraplegia. 1992;30:520–6. https://doi.org/10.1038/sc.1992.109.
43. Keusen P, Vuilliomenet T, Friedli M, Widmer M. Age at onset of spinal cord injury is associated with increased inpatient care needs, reduced independence at discharge and a higher risk of institutionalization after primary inpatient rehabilitation. J Rehabil Med. 2023;55:jrm00353. https://doi.org/10.2340/jrm.v54.4468. PMID: 36306176; PMCID: PMC9855980.
44. Jensen MP, Truitt AR, Schomer KG, Yorkston KM, Baylor C, Molton IR. Frequency and age effects of secondary health conditions in individuals with spinal cord injury: a scoping review. Spinal Cord. 2013;51:882–92. https://doi.org/10.1038/sc.2013.112.
45. Anzai K, Young J, McCallum J, Miller B, Jongbloed L. Factors influencing discharge location following high lesion spinal cord injury rehabilitation in British Columbia, Canada. Spinal Cord. 2006;44:11–8. https://doi.org/10.1038/sj.sc.3101778.
46. Roig RL, Worsowicz GM, Stewart DG, Cifu DX. Geriatric rehabilitation. 3. Physical medicine and rehabilitation interventions for common disabling disorders. Arch Phys Med Rehabil. 2004;85(7 Suppl 3):S12–7; quiz S27–30.
47. Patrick L, Knoefel F, Gaskowski P, Rexroth D. Medical comorbidity and rehabilitation efficiency in geriatric inpatients. J Am Geriatr Soc. 2001;49(11):1471–7.
48. LaPlante MP. Key goals and indicators for successful aging of adults with early-onset disability. Disabil Health J. 2014;7(1 Suppl):S44–50. https://doi.org/10.1016/j.dhjo.2013.08.005.
49. Lundström U, Wahman K, Seiger Å, Gray DB, Isaksson G, Lilja M. Participation in activities and secondary health complications among persons aging with traumatic spinal cord injury. Spinal Cord. 2017;55(4):367–72. https://doi.org/10.1038/sc.2016.153.
50. Bogner JA, Whiteneck GG, MacDonald J, Juengst SB, Brown AW, Philippus AM, Marwitz JH, Lengenfelder J, Mellick D, Arenth P, Corrigan JD. Test-retest reliability of traumatic brain injury outcome measures: a traumatic brain injury model systems study. J Head Trauma Rehabil. 2017;32:E1–16.
51. Howrey BT, Graham JE, Pappadis MR, Granger CV, Ottenbacher KJ. Trajectories of functional change following inpatient rehabilitation for traumatic brain injury. Arch Phys Med Rehabil. 2017;98:1606–13.
52. Rabinowitz AR, Kumar RG, Sima A, Venkatesan UM, Juengst SB, O'Neil-Pirozzi TM, Watanabe TK, Goldin Y, Hammond FM, Dreer LE. Aging with traumatic brain injury: deleterious effects of injury chronicity are most pronounced in later life. J Neurotrauma. 2021;38(19):2706–13. https://doi.org/10.1089/neu.2021.0038. Epub 2021 Jul 20. PMID: 34082606; PMCID: PMC8822416.
53. Corrigan JD, Hammond FM. Traumatic brain injury as a chronic health condition. Arch Phys Med Rehabil. 2013;94:1199–201.
54. Forslund MV, Perrin PB, Røe C, Sigurdardottir S, Hellstrøm T, Berntsen SA, Lu J, Arango-Lasprilla JC, Andelic N. Global outcome trajectories up to 10 years after moderate to severe traumatic brain injury. Front Neurol. 2019;10:219.
55. Cheng C, Chi NC, Williams E, Thompson HJ. Examining age-related differences in functional domain impairment following traumatic brain injury. Int J Older People Nurs. 2018;13:e12208.
56. Colantonio A, Ratcliff G, Chase S, Vernich L. Aging with traumatic brain injury: long-term health conditions. Int J Rehabil Res. 2004;27:209–14.
57. Chen YH, Kang JH, Lin HC. Patients with traumatic brain injury: population-based study suggests increased risk of stroke. Stroke. 2011;42:2733–9.

Chapter 12
Bowel, Bladder, and Skin Management

Aileen Giordano, William Ide, Geoffrey Smith, and Heather Asthagiri

Chapter Objectives

1. Review normal physiology of bladder, bowel, and skin
2. Consider characteristic pathophysiology of bladder, bowel, and skin after SCI
3. Discuss management of SCI-associated neurogenic bladder and bowel
4. Summarize the etiology, prevention, and treatment of pressure injuries

A. Giordano (✉)
Parham Doctors Hospital, Richmond, VA, USA
e-mail: alg8e@virginia.edu

W. Ide
Department of Physical Medicine and Rehabilitation, University of Virginia, Charlottesville, VA, USA

Kennedy Krieger Institute, Baltimore, MD, USA

Department of Physical Medicine and Rehabilitation, Johns Hopkins University School of Medicine, University of Virginia, Baltimore, MD, USA
e-mail: ide@kennedykrieger.org

G. Smith
St. Mary's Hospital Rehabilitation Unit, Mayo Clinic, Rochester, MN, USA

Neurological Rehabilitation Division, Department of Physical Medicine and Rehabilitation, Mayo Clinic, Rochester, MN, USA
e-mail: smith.geoffrey@mayo.edu

H. Asthagiri
Department of Physical Medicine and Rehabilitation, University of Virginia, Charlottesville, VA, USA
e-mail: hlp5d@uvahealth.org

A. K. Wagner, J. Weppner (eds.), *Acute Care Neuroconsultation and Neurorehabilitation Management*, https://doi.org/10.1007/978-3-031-42830-2_12

Introduction

In order to optimize each patient's function and quality of life (QOL), providers who treat patients with spinal cord injuries (SCIs) must understand both the physiology of normal bladder, bowel, and skin and these systems' characteristic pathophysiologies following SCI. Appropriate bladder and bowel management acutely after SCI is vital to protect kidney function, prevent severe constipation and discomfort, and allow ongoing nutrition. Skin protection following SCI is of the utmost importance, with advanced pressure injuries carrying significant morbidity, mortality, and health care costs.

Of note, for patients who have sustained an acute SCI and are admitted to a unit or hospital environment unfamiliar with SCI management, transfer to a unit (often a neurological unit) or hospital with appropriate expertise is recommended. Often, the physiatrist is integral to implementing safe and appropriate protocols for management of SCI bowel, bladder, and skin and to ensuring unit staff are educated in SCI care.

Bladder

Anatomy and Physiology of Normal Voiding Function

The urinary tract is divided into the upper tract (kidneys and ureters) and lower tract (bladder and urethra). The urethra has both an internal sphincter, which is under autonomic control, and an external sphincter, which is under volitional, somatic control [1].

Normal urine storage and elimination are dependent on coordination of multiple neuronal circuits. Anatomically, there are three primary locations along the neuroaxis that control voiding: the sacral micturition center (SMC), pontine micturition center (PMC), and cerebral cortex.

Starting caudally, the SMC (S2–S4) mediates the parasympathetic, non-volitional, sacral micturition reflex and is involved with input coordination from the higher micturition centers. Moving cranially, the PMC coordinates bladder contraction and internal urethral sphincter relaxation. Most superiorly, the cerebral cortex is overall inhibitory to the SMC and allows for volitional suppression of reflex voiding [1, 2].

Peripherally, control of urine storage and elimination involves both the autonomic and somatic nervous systems. Broadly speaking, the parasympathetic division of the autonomic nervous system promotes voiding. Efferent parasympathetic output travels via the pelvic nerve from the SMC to the bladder. Parasympathetic output stimulates bladder contraction via acetylcholine binding to muscarinic receptors in the bladder wall. Conversely, the sympathetic division of the autonomic nervous system promotes urine storage. Sympathetic efferents originate from the thoracolumbar spinal cord (T11-L2) and travel via the hypogastric nerve to both the bladder wall and internal urethral sphincter. Sympathetic output is mediated via the release of norepinephrine, which binds to beta-receptors in the bladder wall (promoting relaxation) and alpha-receptors in the urethra (promoting contraction). Finally, the external urethral sphincter is under volitional, somatic control mediated by the pudendal nerve, which originates from the S2–S4 segments of the spinal cord [1–3].

Pathophysiology of Voiding Dysfunction

Voiding dysfunction affects approximately 80% of individuals following SCI [2]. Hansen et al. surveyed 236 patients with chronic SCI and found that 43% reported ongoing urinary incontinence [4].

Spinal shock occurs acutely after SCI with an average duration of 4–12 weeks [5]. During full spinal shock, the bladder is atonic and areflexic, putting patients at high risk of urinary retention and bladder overdistention [6]. Following resolution of spinal shock, heralded by the return of reflexes, voiding dysfunction can be divided along anatomical lines into suprasacral (above the S2 neurologic level) and sacral (lower conus medullaris and cauda equina) injuries.

Individuals with suprasacral SCIs lack input from the cortex but have an intact SMC, which results in an upper motor neuron (UMN) pattern of dysfunction. UMN dysfunction is typified by uncoordinated reflex detrusor contractions and reflex sphincter contractions. Of note, because the PMC's input is interrupted, detrusor-sphincter dyssynergia (DSD) can develop, meaning both the bladder wall and sphincter contract at the same time, which causes high bladder pressures, incomplete voiding, vesicoureteral reflux, and potential long-term damage to the upper tract. Thus, in general, injuries above the sacral nerve root origins in the conus medullaris result in spastic, overactive bladders that have impaired storage capabilities as well as spastic sphincters that inhibit outflow [1, 2].

Following injury to the conus medullaris or cauda equina, voiding control from all three central micturition centers is interrupted, which results in lower motor neuron (LMN) bladder dysfunction. Complete LMN bladder dysfunction is characterized by acontractile, highly compliant bladders and flaccid sphincters. Thus, sacral SCIs can result in large, areflexic bladders that have impaired emptying capabilities as well as flaccid sphincters that increase the risk of overflow incontinence [1, 2].

Complications of Neurogenic Bladder

Urinary tract infections (UTIs) are a common complication after SCI [7]. When treating patients with SCIs, it is important to distinguish between bacteriuria, which is simply the presence of bacteria in the urine, and symptomatic UTI. Per the

NIDRR consensus statement, three criteria must be met to diagnose UTI: significant bacteriuria, pyuria, and symptoms [8].

Additional infectious complications of neurogenic bladder include urethritis, prostatitis, and epididymitis. Bladder stones, which occur in the setting of infection by urea-splitting bacteria, can cause significant irritative voiding symptoms and hematuria. Similarly, renal stones are a potential consequence of UTI [2].

Autonomic dysreflexia, which is often secondary to bladder distention, is an acute, dangerous complication of bladder dysfunction in SCI (Chap. 10).

Chronic complications from neurogenic bladder include both renal insufficiency secondary to longstanding vesicoureteral reflux and bladder cancer [2].

Management of Neurogenic Bladder

The goals for bladder management following SCI include maximizing continence and facilitating safe, low-pressure storage and elimination of urine to prevent upper and lower tract injuries.

Acute SCI Bladder Management

Neurogenic bladder is typically managed acutely after SCI with an indwelling Foley catheter, which is favored in patients undergoing fluid resuscitation, diuresis, multiple surgeries, treatment with multiple IV antibiotics, or with any other large volume influx and expected large volume output. Unless other injuries exist that would necessitate an indwelling Foley catheter, once the daily urinary output has stabilized below approximately 2.5 liters (L), the Foley catheter can be removed and an alternate neurogenic bladder program started. In general, after severe SCI (such as ASIA Impairment Scale [AIS] A or B), it is ideal to start a clean intermittent catheterization (CIC) program when urine output is low enough to allow for safe bladder volumes with every 4 h in-and-out catheterizations (I/O caths), such as when 24-h urine output is less than 2.5 L. For patients with less severe SCI (AIS C or D), a scheduled voiding trial with timed voids every 4–6 h and post-void bladder scans (and bladder scans if the patient is unable to void at scheduled time) can be tried, with instructions to perform I/O caths if scanned bladder volumes are elevated. The voiding trial should be converted to a scheduled CIC program if the patient is not voiding; conversely, the trial can be discontinued if the patient is consistently able to empty the bladder. If elevated urine output continues despite medical stability, a 2–2.5 L fluid restriction can be instituted if not otherwise contraindicated. To summarize:

- For AIS A or B SCI: when daily UOP is <2.5 L, the indwelling Foley catheter can be removed and a CIC program can be initiated.
  - Start a scheduled q4h CIC program and measure all catheterization volumes.

- The frequency of CIC should be adjusted to ensure I/O cath volumes are <500 mL.

- For AIS C or D SCI: when daily UOP is <2.5 L, the indwelling Foley catheter can be removed and a scheduled q4–6h voiding trial with post-void bladder scans can be initiated.
  - If the patient is unable to void at scheduled time, then perform a bladder scan.
  - If bladder scan volume is elevated (>300 mL is used as at our institution), then perform I/O cath.
  - If the bladder scan volume is 200–300 mL, then wait 2 h, re-attempt voiding, and repeat the bladder scan.
  - All scanned, voided, and I/O cath volumes should be recorded.
  - The voiding trial can be discontinued if post-void residuals (PVRs) are consistently low (<200 mL for three consecutive PVRs at our institution).

Long-term SCI Bladder Management

For persons with chronic SCI who are admitted to the hospital and can direct their care, it is optimal to allow these patients to give input on the preferred bladder program as long as it is safe and effective. Below are examples of long-term neurogenic bladder programs and their benefits and drawbacks.

For those with ongoing urinary retention at time of discharge from rehabilitation, CIC is the most commonly employed method of neurogenic bladder management [9]. Typical protocols involve catheterization every 4–6 h with goal catheterization volumes of less than 500 ml. Benefits of this method include low-pressure emptying, allowance of catheter-free periods, and lower infection risk than indwelling catheter. Drawbacks include risks of incontinence between catheterizations, bladder overdistention between catheterizations, and urethral trauma. Additionally, some individuals may lack the hand dexterity required to perform CIC [1, 2].

Alternatively, some patients choose long-term bladder management with indwelling catheters for continuous urine drainage. Indwelling catheters are classified as transurethral catheters or suprapubic catheters (SPCs). Benefits of indwelling catheters include continuous low-pressure emptying, ease of use, and minimization of incontinence. Drawbacks of transurethral catheters specifically include higher risk of UTIs, prostatitis, bladder and kidney stones, bladder cancer, and urethral erosions [1, 2]. Conversely, SPCs do not risk urethral injury and have a less negative impact on quality of life [10].

Reflex voiding is a method in which urine is eliminated using an intact parasympathetic reflex arc and collected in a condom catheter bag. Despite relative ease of employment, there are several important risks associated with this method including skin breakdown, incomplete bladder emptying, and upper tract damage due to vesicoureteral reflux [1]. This method should not be used unless proven safe on urodynamic testing.

For some, a safe, effective bladder management program may not be feasible without a procedure, as performed by urology. Surgical options include urethral stents, sphincterotomy, bladder augmentation with creation of a continent abdominal stoma, and continent urinary diversions [1, 2].

Additionally, medications can be useful adjuncts in managing neurogenic bladder. Anticholinergic agents promote urine storage by inhibiting parasympathetic input to the bladder and reduce bladder contractions that may result in incontinence—helpful for patients with bladder spasms or "kick-offs" between CIC [2]. Conversely, alpha-blockers promote urethral relaxation and urine elimination by inhibiting sympathetic input to the urethra [1].

Please note that many commonly used medications can interfere with bladder function, with a number of agents causing urinary retention, such as those with anticholinergic activity (e.g., antipsychotics, antidepressants, antihistamines, and anticholinergic respiratory agents), opioids and anesthetics, alpha-adrenoceptor agonists, benzodiazepines, NSAIDs, detrusor relaxants, and calcium channel antagonists [11]. It is particularly important to try to minimize these medications for patients on voiding trials or with incomplete bladder emptying. Also, constipation may to contribute to urinary retention and incontinence in non-SCI populations and should be avoided [12].

Bowel

Anatomy and Physiology of Normal Bowel Function

The hindgut consists of the colon and rectum. The distal aspect of the hindgut includes an internal anal sphincter (IAS), under autonomic control, and an external anal sphincter (EAS), under somatic, volitional control [13, 14].

Normal bowel function involves input from the autonomic and somatic nervous systems. Broadly, parasympathetic input stimulates peristalsis and bowel evacuation while sympathetic input stimulates sphincter closure. Parasympathetic input is delivered by the vagus nerve proximally and the pelvic nerve (S2–S4) distally. Sympathetic innervation is delivered via the superior and inferior mesenteric (T9–T12) and the hypogastric (T12-L3) nerves. The EAS receives somatic innervation via the pudendal nerve (S2–S4) [13, 15].

The role of the hindgut is to propel, store, and eliminate waste while allowing for continence. Waste propulsion is locally controlled by the enteric nervous system in the colon wall; however, peristalsis is augmented by spinal cord-mediated, parasympathetic reflex arcs. Specifically, chemical or mechanical stimulation of the rectum triggers the rectocolic reflex. This reflex is mediated at the sacral spinal cord and results in delivery of increased parasympathetic, propulsive output to the colon. When stool is delivered to the rectal vault, rectal stretch is detected, triggering the urge to defecate. Defecation occurs with voluntary relaxation of the EAS. Defecation can be delayed by voluntary contraction of the EAS. At rest, continence is primarily achieved through maintenance of IAS tone. IAS tone is inhibited with rectal distention as occurs with stool burden (known as the rectoanal inhibitory reflex) [13, 15].

Pathophysiology of Bowel Dysfunction

Bowel dysfunction is estimated to affect half of individuals after SCI and is associated with significant morbidity [16, 17] and poorer health related quality of life [15, 17].

Finding an effective bowel program acutely after severe SCI is often very difficult, and it is not uncommon for patients with AIS A or B injuries to go several days without a bowel movement, with imaging often consistent with ileus. Some reasons for ileus include surgeries and use of anesthesia, opioids, anticholinergic agents or medications with anticholinergic side effects, immobility, and the lack of GI reflexes (including the rectocolic reflex) during spinal shock, rendering suppositories and digital stimulation ineffective. Despite this, enteral feeding in acute SCI is typically safe and is most frequently interrupted for large gastric aspirates [18]. It is helpful to reduce constipating medications, start an SCI bowel program as outlined below, ensure adequate hydration, and mobilize the patient as able. Avoidance of enemas is recommended, as overuse of enemas, particularly sodium phosphate containing ones, can cause volume shifts and electrolyte abnormalities [19].

Following resolution of spinal shock, SCI-associated bowel dysfunction is categorized as either a UMN- or LMN-pattern injury.

Lesions above the S2 sacral anterior horn cells located in the conus medullaris are UMN injuries and result in hyperreflexic bowel. Because the sacral-gut connection is uninterrupted, the parasympathetic-mediated rectocolic reflex remains intact, which allows for reflex-assisted bowel evacuation. However, volitional control over the EAS is lost and the EAS exhibits high (spastic) tone, which causes fecal retention [13, 15, 20].

Conversely, lesions involving the S2-4 neurologic levels of the conus medullaris or cauda equina can result in LMN bowel dysfunction, characterized by decreased distal bowel reflexes. The sacral-mediated rectocolic reflex is interrupted (as evidenced on exam by absence of a bulbocavernosus reflex), which precludes reflex-assisted defecation. Again, volitional control over the EAS is lost, but, in LMN injuries, the EAS exhibits low tone, which contributes to fecal incontinence [13, 14, 20].

Complications of Neurogenic Bowel

Complications of neurogenic bowel include peri-anal problems (hemorrhoids, fissures, rectal prolapse) [21], evacuation problems (constipation, impaction, ileus, incontinence, diarrhea), autonomic dysreflexia (Chap. 10), and diverticulosis [13].

Management of Neurogenic Bowel

Neurogenic bowel dysfunction is typically managed via an individualized bowel program. The goals of a bowel program are to evacuate stool at a predicable time, to prevent incontinence, to minimize gastrointestinal symptoms and complications, and to maximize efficiency. Bowel programs involve prescription of the timing and type of bowel care (the process for assisted defecation) as well as management of fluid intake, diet, activity, assistive equipment, and medications [13].

The typical UMN bowel care routine involves placement of a stimulant against the rectal mucosa, followed by cycles of rectal stimulation that are repeated until successful evacuation occurs and subsequent stimulations do not produce stool. Initially, UMN bowel care is performed daily [13, 15] (Fig. 12.1).

The typical LMN bowel care routine—absent the rectocolic reflex needed for suppository efficacy or digital stimulation—involves manual disimpaction of stool. A gloved, lubricated finger is introduced into the rectal vault, and stool is digitally evacuated. LMN bowel care is performed several times per day to avoid incontinence [13, 15].

The optimal stool consistency for the UMN bowel program is soft and loosely-formed, while, for LMN bowel program, stool should be firm and well-formed. Stool consistency can be adjusted by titration of medications, fiber intake, and fluid intake [13].

Medications are used as adjuncts to bowel programs and, broadly, include bulk forming agents, stool softeners, laxatives, and prokinetic agents [13, 20]. One important practical note is the relative efficacy in terms of decreased time to defecation of polyethylene glycol-based bisacodyl suppositories and docusate mini-enemas compared to standard vegetable oil-based bisacodyl suppositories [22]. A common, standard UMN bowel management program includes the following medications, with suppository administration in the evening to allow for other activities during the day and followed by digital stimulation as per Fig. 12.1:

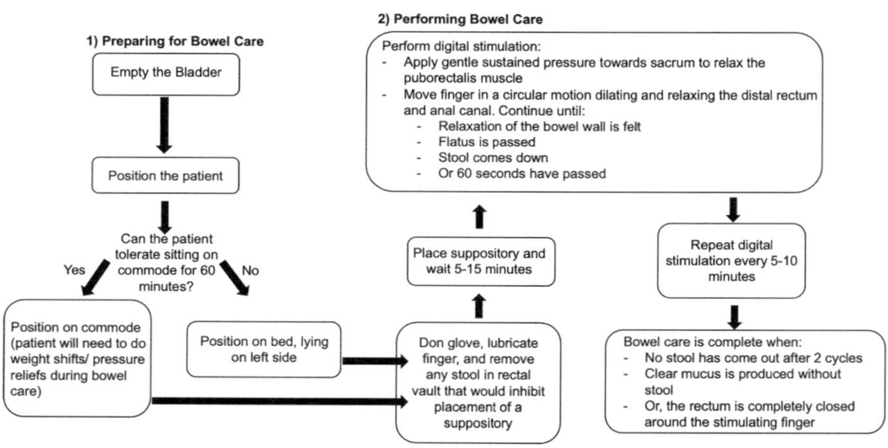

Fig. 12.1 Standard workflow for upper motor neuron pattern of dysfunction bowel care

- Docusate sodium 100 mg BID to TID, senna 17.2 mg at 2 pm, polyethylene glycol-based (Magic Bullet) bisacodyl suppository (or mini-enema) PR qPM. Dibucaine ointment may be used prior to suppository administration if the bowel program is painful or causes autonomic dysreflexia.

Of note, for persons with remote SCI who can direct their care, it is ideal to allow them to guide the preferred bowel management program if safe and effective. Many persons with UMN SCI wean off oral and rectal agents over time if digital stimulation alone produces desired results, and may perform a bowel program less frequently—often only three times per week. However, if admitted with large stool burden, new constipating medications, or with less effective digital stimulation, it may be necessary to restart suppositories/mini-enemas or oral medications as recommended above.

Surgical management of SCI-associated neurogenic bowel is typically reserved for extreme constipation, for individuals with significant sacral pressure injuries, and for individuals whose bowel care takes an inordinate amount of time. Surgical options include ileostomy and colostomy [13, 14]. Of note, if an ostomy is created as a result of other injuries sustained along with the acute SCI, the patient should be educated regarding neurogenic bowel potential should ostomy reversal be considered in the future.

Clostridium difficile colitis and other diarrhea-causing conditions may present a unique challenge for some patients with neurogenic bowel. For those with UMN bowel, the spastic EAS is helpful in sequestering the stool, and continuing an UMN bowel program at least daily to promote timed, scheduled bowel movements is recommended. For LMN bowel, frequent manual bowel disimpaction and diligent cleaning to avoid skin maceration and breakdown is key. Of note, rectal tubes should be used with extreme caution and vigilance in the SCI population, given the risk for skin breakdown, mucosal injury, rectal hemorrhage, and possibly fissures or sphincter damage [23, 24].

Skin

Skin Changes Following SCI

Skin functions as a protective barrier between the body and the environment. Following SCI, skin undergoes several changes that impair this function, including collagen catabolism and loss of adrenergic receptor density [25].

Pressure Injuries: Etiology, Risk Factors, Staging

Pressure injuries are the most common medical complication among chronic SCI patients and their prevalence increases with years since injury [26]. Pressure injuries also affect patients early after SCI, with Brienza et al. observing a 38% rate of pressure injury development during initial hospitalization and inpatient rehabilitation [27]. Pressure injuries have a significant association with mortality after SCI, and Krause et al. identified chronic pressure injury as the risk factor associated with greatest loss of life expectancy in SCI patients [28].

Pressure injuries involve the skin and/or underlying soft tissues and result from application of pressure with or without associated shear. Pressure injuries typically occur over bony prominences. Pressure can injure tissues via two mechanisms: ischemia and direct tissue deformity. Factors that influence the severity of pressure injuries include the degree, duration, and type of force applied to the tissues as well as the microclimate (the temperature and moisture at the tissue-support surface interface) [29].

Risk factors for the development of pressure injuries include immobility, impaired tissue perfusion, poor nutritional status, skin moisture (frequently related to incontinence), and impaired sensation [29]. Given the breadth of factors associated with pressure injury, multiple risk stratification tools have been proposed. Flett et al. found that lower admission Functional Independence Measure score (particularly a lower bed/chair transfer score) was most predictive of pressure injury development during acute rehabilitation [30].

Pressure injuries are graded based on degree of tissue loss:

1. Stage 1 injuries exhibit non-blanchable erythema with intact skin.
2. Stage 2 injuries are characterized by partial thickness dermis loss.
3. Stage 3 injuries exhibit full thickness dermis loss; while fat may be visible, bone, tendon, and muscle are not.
4. Stage 4 injuries demonstrate full thickness tissue loss with exposure of underlying tendon, muscle, or bone.

Full thickness skin ulcers whose bases are obscured by slough or eschar are termed unstageable. Finally, deep tissue injuries are areas of soft tissue injury with initially intact overlying skin; these injuries can evolve rapidly to deep, open ulcers [25, 29].

Pressure Injury Prevention

The primary tenants of pressure injury prevention are pressure redistribution and frequent skin inspection. Pressure redistribution includes frequent repositioning when lying down and pressure reliefs when seated. Pressure reliefs allow for reoxygenation of compressed tissues and include front leans, side leans, wheelchair pushups (discouraged due to risk of musculoskeletal injury), and tilting in a tilt-in-space wheelchair. Patients are typically instructed to perform pressure reliefs every 15–30 min [25]. Coggrave and Rose found that the mean duration of pressure relief required to raise tissue oxygenation levels back to their unloaded state was 2 min 51 s [31]; thus, patients should be encouraged to perform pressure reliefs of at least 3-min duration.

While hospitalized after initial injury, it is important to ensure that at least every 2 h turning from back to flank (at least 30° from the bed surface) to contralateral flank is being performed when the patient is in bed, and that every 20 min pressure reliefs are performed when the patients is in the bedside chair (ideally in a chair that converts to supine position for pressure relief and with a pressure relief cushion). For patients with AIS A SCIs, who are at markedly increased risk for pressure injury development during their acute care and acute inpatient rehabilitation stays [27], a progressive sitting protocol which allows for small increases in sitting duration every few days with post-sitting inspection of skin is ideal. For transfers in acute care from bed to stretcher or stretcher chair, an air-fluidized turn and positioning system (TAPS) can be utilized to reduce shear forces.

Comprehensive pressure injury prevention also involves nutritional optimization, exercise, appropriate equipment selection, and education [25]. Despite the emphasis on education and behavioral intervention historically espoused by the medical establishment, Cogan et al. found no evidence that these interventions prevent pressure injuries [32].

Pressure Injury Treatment

Once a pressure injury is identified, referrals should be placed to a wound care team and registered dietician if available. For acutely injured patients who develop pressure injuries, review of potential causes for breakdown such as lapses in turning while in bed or in sitting pressure reliefs, inappropriate contact surfaces, and skin maceration with ineffective bowel/bladder management should be identified and corrected. For patients with chronic SCI admitted with pressure injuries, it is important to investigate and address any preventable factors leading to the development of skin breakdown, such as changes in activity or spasticity/tone, ill-fitting or inappropriate equipment, poor nutrition, and adequacy of the bowel and bladder programs.

The goal of pressure injury treatment is to create a physiological wound environment to promote healing. The primary components of a pressure injury treatment plan include cleansing, debridement, dressing, positioning, and nutritional optimization. Cleansing removes devitalized tissue and bacteria to reduce risk of secondary infection. Debridement, which includes autolytic, enzymatic, mechanical, sharp, surgical, and maggot techniques, also removes devitalized tissue to promote healing. Dressings are used to control exudate, protect the wound, and eliminate dead space. Positioning is selected to avoid placing direct pressure on the injury, and pressure redistribution support surfaces are indicated if an individual has a pressure injury. Furthermore, individuals with sacral or ischial pressure injuries should consider eliminating sitting time to promote wound healing. If sitting is pursued, it should be minimized and done with a wheelchair cushion that provides low sitting pressures, ideally proven with pressure mapping [25, 29].

Additional therapeutic options used for stage III/IV injuries include electrical stimulation to promote wound closure and surgical intervention (typically a flap procedure) [25, 29].

Case Illustration

A 33-year-old, previously healthy man is admitted to the ICU following a motor vehicle accident; he undergoes emergent decompression and fusion for an unstable cervical spine. Despite successful surgical stabilization, the patient continues to exhibit paralysis of both legs, and, on hospital day 3, the ICU team consults a physiatrist for management of the patient's acute SCI. The physiatrist's initial exam is consistent with a C8 AIS A SCI. The physiatrist notes flaccid tone of the lower extremities and absence of reflexes below the level of injury (consistent with spinal shock). The physiatrist carefully inspects the patient's skin and finds there are no pressure injuries. Currently, a Foley catheter is in place (with 24-h urine output of 3.3 L), and the patient has not had a bowel movement since admission. An abdominal X-ray shows partial ileus. Initially, the physiatrist recommends continuation of the Foley catheter (with close monitoring of daily urine output). The physiatrist reviews the patient's medication list and recommends minimization of opiates and anticholinergics as much as possible. The physiatrist recommends initiation of a bowel regimen that includes docusate 100 mg BID, senna 17.2 mg at 2:00 pm, and nightly polyethylene glycol-based (Magic Bullet) bisacodyl suppository. The physiatrist counsels both the patient and the ICU team that, given the ongoing spinal shock, the suppository may be relatively ineffective until spinal shock resolves and manual disimpaction may be required nightly. The physiatrist begins education with the patient on the importance of skin inspection and pressure reliefs. The physiatrist recommends the ICU team perform at least q2 hour turning when the patient is in bed and q20 minute pressure reliefs when the patient is up in a chair and also recommends utilization of an air fluidized turning and positioning system (TAPS) for transfers. Two days later, 24-h urine output has decreased to 2 L, and the patient has had a large incontinent bowel movement. The physiatrist recommends initiation of q4 hour CIC (with monitoring to ensure I/O cath volumes remain <500 mL) and continuation of the current bowel program. The physiatrist again reinforces the importance of nightly suppository placement and digital stimulation with additional manual disimpaction as needed while sacral reflexes transition out of spinal shock. By hospital day 10, the patient is consistently having bowel movements during nightly bowel cares (although he continues to have bowel incontinence between bowel cares). On hospital day 11, he is transitioned to acute inpatient rehabilitation for ongoing SCI education and rehabilitation.

Summary

SCI is a chronic condition that causes predictable patterns of bladder, bowel, and skin dysfunction. SCI-associated neurogenic bladder and neurogenic bowel can be dichotomized as either UMN or LMN dysfunction. Management of bladder and bowel after SCI is predicated on correctly identifying the dysfunction pattern to select the intervention that will promote safe elimination/evacuation while maximizing continence and avoiding complications. Similarly, skin dysfunction following SCI is managed by interventions directed at protecting skin integrity and preventing breakdown. In summation, by understanding normal physiology, patterns of pathophysiology, and common complications, SCI-associated bladder, bowel, and skin dysfunction can be successfully managed to maximize each patient's function and quality of life.

References[1]

1. Consortium for Spinal Cord Medicine. Bladder management for adults with spinal cord injury: a clinical practice guideline for health-care providers. J Spinal Cord Med. 2006;29(5):527–73.
2. Taweel WA, Seyam R. Neurogenic bladder in spinal cord injury patients. Res Rep Urol. 2015;7:85–99. https://doi.org/10.2147/rru.s29644.
3. Weledji EP, Eyongeta D, Ngounou E. The anatomy of urination: what every physician should know. Clin Anat. 2019;32(1):60–7. https://doi.org/10.1002/ca.23296.
4. Hansen RB, Biering-Sorensen F, Kristensen JK. Urinary incontinence in spinal cord injured individuals 10-45 years after injury. Spinal Cord. 2010;48(1):27–33. https://doi.org/10.1038/sc.2009.46.
5. Ko H-Y. Revisit spinal shock: pattern of reflex evolution during spinal shock. Korean J Neurotrauma. 2018;14(2):47–54.
6. Rossier AB, Fam BA, Dibenedetto M, Sarkarati M. Urodynamics in spinal shock patients. J Urol. 1979;122(6):783–7. https://doi.org/10.1016/s0022-5347(17)56603-3.
7. Manack A, Motsko SP, Haag-Molkenteller C, et al. Epidemiology and healthcare utilization of neurogenic bladder patients in a US claims database. Neurourol Urodyn. 2011;30(3):395–401. https://doi.org/10.1002/nau.21003.
8. National Institute on Disability and Rehabilitation Research Consensus Statement. The prevention and management of urinary tract infections among people with spinal cord injuries. J Am Paraplegia Soc. 1992;15(3):194–204. https://doi.org/10.1080/01952307.1992.11735873.
9. Afsar SI, Yemisci OU, Cosar SN, Cetin N. Compliance with clean intermittent catheterization in spinal cord injury patients: a long-term follow-up study. Spinal Cord. 2013;51(8):645–9. https://doi.org/10.1038/sc.2013.46.
10. Adriaansen JJ, van Asbeck FW, Tepper M, et al. Bladder-emptying methods, neurogenic lower urinary tract dysfunction and impact on quality of life in people with long-term spinal cord injury. J Spinal Cord Med. 2017;40(1):43–53. https://doi.org/10.1179/2045772315y.0000000056.
11. Verhamme K, Sturkenboom M, Stricker B, Bosch R. Drug-induced urinary retention: incidence, management and prevention. Drug Saf. 2008;31(5):373–88.
12. Malik R, Cohn J, Bales G. Urinary retention in elderly women: diagnosis & management. Curr Urol Rep. 2014;15(1):454.

[1] Key References [1, 2, 25, 29].

13. Consortium for Spinal Cord Medicine. Clinical practice guidelines: neurogenic bowel management in adults with spinal cord injury. Spinal Cord Medicine Consortium. J Spinal Cord Med. 1998;21(3):248–93. https://doi.org/10.1080/10790268.1998.11719536.
14. Stiens SA, Bergman SB, Goetz LL. Neurogenic bowel dysfunction after spinal cord injury: clinical evaluation and rehabilitative management. Arch Phys Med Rehabil. 1997;78(3):86–102. https://doi.org/10.1016/s0003-9993(97)90416-0.
15. Han TR, Kim JH, Kwon BS. Chronic gastrointestinal problems and bowel dysfunction in patients with spinal cord injury. Spinal Cord. 1998;36(7):485–90. https://doi.org/10.1038/sj.sc.3100616.
16. Glickman S, Kamm MA. Bowel dysfunction in spinal-cord-injury patients. Lancet. 1996;347(9016):1651–3. https://doi.org/10.1016/s0140-6736(96)91487-7.
17. Liu CW, Huang CC, Yang YH, Chen SC, Weng MC, Huang MH. Relationship between neurogenic bowel dysfunction and health-related quality of life in persons with spinal cord injury. J Rehabil Med. 2009;41(1):35–40. https://doi.org/10.2340/16501977-0277.
18. Rowan C, Gillanders L, Paice R, Judson J. Is early enteral feeding safe in patients who have suffered spinal cord injury? Injury. 2004;35(3):238–42.
19. Ori Y, Rozen-Zvi B, Chagnac A, et al. Fatalities and severe metabolic disorders associated with the use of sodium phosphate enemas: a single center's experience. Arch Intern Med. 2012;172(3):263–5.
20. Krassioukov A, Eng JJ, Claxton G, Sakakibara BM, Shum S. Neurogenic bowel management after spinal cord injury: a systematic review of the evidence. Spinal Cord. 2010;48(10):718–33. https://doi.org/10.1038/sc.2010.14.
21. Adriaansen JJ, van Asbeck FW, van Kuppevelt D, Snoek GJ, Post MW. Outcomes of neurogenic bowel management in individuals living with a spinal cord injury for at least 10 years. Arch Phys Med Rehabil. 2015;96(5):905–12. https://doi.org/10.1016/j.apmr.2015.01.011.
22. House JG, Stiens SA. Pharmacologically initiated defecation for persons with spinal cord injury: effectiveness of three agents. Arch Phys Med Rehabil. 1997;78(10):1062–5. https://doi.org/10.1016/s0003-9993(97)90128-3.
23. Tiwari A, Sharma H, Qamar K, Alastal Y, Sodeman T, Nawras A. The traumatic tude: bleeding rectal ulcer caused by flexi-seal device. Case Rep Gastrointest Med. 2017;2017:5278971.
24. Ousey K. An easily forgotten tube. AORN J. 2015;101(6):718, 696. https://doi.org/10.1016/j.aorn.2015.03.006.
25. Consortium for Spinal Cord Medicine. Pressure ulcer prevention and treatment following spinal cord injury: a clinical practice guideline for health-care professionals. J Spinal Cord Med. 2001;24(1):40–101. https://doi.org/10.1080/10790268.2001.11753592.
26. McKinley WO, Jackson AB, Cardenas DD, DeVivo MJ. Long-term medical complications after traumatic spinal cord injury: a regional model systems analysis. Arch Phys Med Rehabil. 1999;80(11):1402–10. https://doi.org/10.1016/s0003-9993(99)90251-4.
27. Brienza D, Krishnan S, Karg P, Sowa G, Allegretti AL. Predictors of pressure ulcer incidence following traumatic spinal cord injury: a secondary analysis of a prospective longitudinal study. Spinal Cord. 2018;56(1):28–34. https://doi.org/10.1038/sc.2017.96.
28. Krause JS, Saunders LL. Health, secondary conditions, and life expectancy after spinal cord injury. Arch Phys Med Rehabil. 2011;92(11):1770–5. https://doi.org/10.1016/j.apmr.2011.05.024.
29. National Pressure Ulcer Advosiry Panel, European Pressure Ulcer Advisory Panel, Pan Pacific Pressure Injury Alliance. Prevention and Treatment of Pressure Ulcers. 2014.
30. Flett HM, Delparte JJ, Scovil CY, Higgins J, Laramee MT, Burns AS. Determining pressure injury risk on admission to inpatient spinal cord injury rehabilitation: a comparison of the FIM, spinal cord injury pressure ulcer scale, and braden scale. Arch Phys Med Rehabil. 2019;100(10):1881–7. https://doi.org/10.1016/j.apmr.2019.04.004.
31. Coggrave MJ, Rose LS. A specialist seating assessment clinic: changing pressure relief practice. Spinal Cord. 2003;41(12):692–5. https://doi.org/10.1038/sj.sc.3101527.
32. Cogan AM, Blanchard J, Garber SL, Vigen CL, Carlson M, Clark FA. Systematic review of behavioral and educational interventions to prevent pressure ulcers in adults with spinal cord injury. Clin Rehabil. 2017;31(7):871–80. https://doi.org/10.1177/0269215516660855.

Chapter 13
Pulmonary and Venous Thromboembolism Care

Shanti M. Pinto

Chapter Objectives

1. Understand the pulmonary complications that may arise in patients with acquired CNS injury.
2. Discuss the specifics of respiratory management in a patient with spinal cord injury (SCI).
3. Understand risk factors, prevention, and treatment of VTE.

Introduction

Pulmonary complications and venous thromboembolism (VTE) cause significant morbidity and mortality in patients with acquired injury to the central nervous system (CNS). This chapter summarizes these important medical conditions and appropriate management.

S. M. Pinto (✉)
Department of Physical Medicine and Rehabilitation, University of Texas - Southwestern, Dallas, TX, USA
e-mail: shanti.pinto@utsouthwestern.edu

A. K. Wagner, J. Weppner (eds.), *Acute Care Neuroconsultation and Neurorehabilitation Management*, https://doi.org/10.1007/978-3-031-42830-2_13

Pulmonary

Pulmonary Complications

Medical Complications

Medical complications involving the respiratory system are common in hospitalized patients. Hospital-acquired pneumonia is the second most common hospital-acquired infection, only behind urinary tract infections. Risk factors include more severe injury or illness at hospital admission, intubation, older age, and pre-morbid pulmonary disease. Dysphagia is an important risk factor as aspiration of oral secretions, gastric contents, or enteral intake can lead to pneumonitis and pneumonia [1]. Early swallowing evaluation by a speech-language pathologist (SLP) is essential to ensure appropriate diet and medications administration. Patients should be fed while in an upright position, and the head of bed should be elevated to 30–45° for patients on tube feeds, to decrease the risk of aspiration. Acute respiratory distress syndrome (ARDS) is a severe form of acute lung injury that occurs due to widespread inflammation and edema of the lungs. ARDS can occur as a result of traumatic injury (particularly to the head or chest), pneumonia, sepsis, or massive transfusion, among other causes. ARDS carries a high rate of mortality and requires aggressive respiratory management within the intensive care unit (ICU).

Trauma-Related Complications

Patients may also suffer trauma-related pulmonary complications. Rib fractures frequently occur as a result of thoracic blunt force trauma. Pain can cause impaired respiratory function and decreased respiratory capacity; therefore, aggressive pain management is required. Fracture of adjacent ribs in two or more locations may lead to independent movement of a segment of the chest wall, known as "flail chest." Surgical fixation may be required. Pneumothorax, collection of air in the pleural space, and hemothorax, collection of blood in the pleural space, can both occur following thoracic trauma. Placement of a chest tube allows for re-expansion of the lung.

Complication Management

Tracheostomy

Tracheostomy is frequently performed in patients with severe neurologic injury, typically due to prolonged mechanical ventilation and impaired secretion management. Other indications for tracheostomy include upper airway obstruction due to severe injury to the head and neck [2]. To date there is no consensus regarding appropriate timing of tracheostomy. Some studies report shorter time of mechanical ventilation and ICU length of stay when tracheostomy is placed within seven days of intubation. No difference in mortality or overall hospital length of stay has been found [2, 3]. Current evidence suggests that patients with severe acquired brain injury may benefit from an early tracheostomy due to improved clinical outcomes, including decreased mechanical ventilation duration and intensive care unit length of stay, compared to late tracheostomy. At this time, further multi-institutional studies are needed to develop evidence-based guidelines [4–7]. Either open or percutaneous techniques can be used for tracheostomy placement [3]. The percutaneous technique is preferred for patients with normal anatomy and no contraindications due to decreased rate of infection and improved closure after decannulation. Percutaneous tracheostomy can be performed bedside in the ICU, which is advantageous for patients that may be too unstable to transfer to the operating room [2, 3].

The inspired air through a tracheostomy should be heated and humidified as to improve consistency of secretions and improve mucociliary transport. This can be accomplished through the use of artificial exchangers in patients on mechanical ventilation or use of humidified tracheostomy mask for those off ventilation [2]. Tracheostomy tube exchange may begin as early as 7 days post-procedure, which allows for the formation of a tracheocutaneous tract. When neither mechanical ventilation nor a risk of gross aspiration is present, the tracheostomy tube cuff should be deflated. The tracheostomy tube can be changed to a cuffless device once cuff inflation is not needed for mechanical ventilation or airway protection in cases of gross aspiration. Oral vocalization can be attained through the use of a one-way valve, such as a Passy-Muir valve, which allows for inspiratory airflow through the tracheostomy tube but closes during expiration to force airflow through the larynx [2]. Use of a one-way valve should only be initiated in the presence of a trained professional, typically SLP, and patients should be monitored for desaturation or other signs of respiratory distress. Capping of the tracheostomy prevents airflow in and out of the tracheostomy tube, forcing the patient to breathe through the mouth or nose. This is typically trialed as a step toward decannulation, and supplemental oxygen can be provided through a nasal cannula. A clinically stable patient may be decannulated after 24–48 h of continuous capping [2].

SCI-Specific Pulmonary Management

Pulmonary complications are a leading cause of morbidity and mortality after SCI [8, 9]. Patients with tetraplegia due to cervical or upper thoracic SCI develop restrictive lung disease due to paralysis of the respiratory muscles (Table 13.1). Inspiration is primarily controlled by the diaphragm while intercostal, scalene, trapezius, and sternocleidomastoid muscles provide important support [9–11]. Expiration is typically a passive process; however, the rectus abdominis, transversus abdominis, and internal and external oblique muscles assist in expiration when minute ventilation is increased and during cough [9, 10]. Loss of abdominal muscle tone leads to changes in respiratory biomechanics, which presents most notably when the patient is seated.

Table 13.1 Muscles involved in respiration. (a) Muscles involved in inspiration. (b) Muscles involved in expiration

A. Inspiration		
Muscle	Spinal nerve roots	Function
Diaphragm	C3–C5	Provides 65% of tidal volume during inspiration
Sternocleidomastoid	C1–C4 (plus CN XI)	Elevates rib cage
Trapezius	C1–C4 (plus CN XI)	Elevates rib cage
Scalene muscles	C4–C8	Elevates rib cage
Intercostal muscles	T1–T11	Expands chest wall
B. Expiration		
Muscle	Spinal nerve roots	
Rectus abdominis	T7–T11	
Transversus abdominis	T7–T11	
External obliques	T7–T12	
Internal obliques	T6–L1	

Abdominal contents are pulled downward by gravity when the patient is in an upright position, leading to increased lung volume and decreased efficiency of diaphragm function resulting in lower forced vital capacity and forced expiratory volume in 1 s (FEV1). An abdominal binder can provide additional support to the abdominal muscles, elevating the diaphragm. This causes improved diaphragm muscle function, leading to decreased functional reserved capacity, improved peak expiratory flow and FEV1, greater tidal volume, and decreased perceived exertion during functional tasks [10, 12].

Mechanical ventilation is required for most patients with acute SCI, particularly those with upper cervical injuries. Tracheostomy placement has been associated with decreased mortality, lower pulmonary complication rates, and earlier ventilator independence in patients with cervical SCI [9]. Use of high tidal volumes at 15–20 mL/kg may assist with ventilator weaning by preventing atelectasis [9, 10]. Progressive ventilator-free breathing (PVFB) can decrease time to wean off the ventilator in patients with high cervical SCI. PFVB is a weaning strategy where the patient is taken off the ventilator for a period to allow for independent breathing. These sessions are initially short in duration and lengthened as the patient gains respiratory muscle strength. The sessions may be repeated multiple times per day, with sufficient rest breaks to allow the diaphragm to recover [9].

Secretion management is important to acute SCI management. Loss of sympathetic tone with cervical and upper thoracic SCI leads to unopposed parasympathetic activity, increased mucous production, and decreased mucociliary clearance. Additionally, expiratory muscle weakness decreases efficacy of secretion clearance from cough [9, 10]. Physical techniques, such as intrapulmonary percussive ventilation (IPV) and chest physiotherapy, help loosen secretions to aide in removal. In IPV, high frequency pulsations of pressurized air occur at 100–300 cycles/min with use of a one-way flutter valve [10]. Chest physiotherapy requires use of external force to aide in loosening of secretions through either percussion, which refers to manual rhythmic tapping force on the chest wall, or a device that provides vibration force to the chest wall [9]. Postural drainage refers to changes in body position, holding each for 5–10 min, to allow for mobilization of secretions into the main airways to help with clearance [9, 10]. Contraindications to chest physiotherapy are all relative and include bleeding diathesis, including therapeutic anticoagulation, discomfort due to physical positions or manipulations, elevated intracranial pressure, recent hemoptysis, rib fractures, and vertebral fractures or osteoporosis [13–15]. Techniques to enhance efficacy of cough include use of mechanical insufflation-exsufflation (MIE) device and quad cough. Cough Assist is a type of MIE that is frequently used in clinical practice that provides an initial positive pressure to the airway (insufflation) followed immediately by an immediate negative pressure force (exsufflation), typically with pressures of positive and negative 40 cm H_2O. This is done for a total of 6–8 cycles followed by rest [9, 10].

Unopposed vagal tone due to the loss of sympathetic innervation after cervical or upper thoracic SCI can lead to bronchospasm [9, 10]; thus, bronchodilators can be effective in respiratory management of patients with tetraplegia. Inhaled beta-agonists and anticholinergic medications may also improve spirometric test results in patients with tetraplegia without history of intrinsic lung disease [16, 17].

VTE Care

Epidemiology

Patients with acquired CNS injury are at increased risk for VTE development, either deep venous thrombosis (DVT) or pulmonary embolism (PE). Asymptomatic VTE rates may be as high as 39% in patients with acute SCI [18] and 25% in patients with isolated traumatic brain injury (TBI) [19] based on venous Doppler ultrasound. VTE is associated with important medical consequences. Though population specific investigations are needed for TBI, PE is the most common cause of death two to four weeks following acute CVA [20], and patients diagnosed with VTE have higher odds of in-hospital mortality after acute SCI [21]. Patients diagnosed with VTE prior to admission to inpatient rehabilitation were found to have increased inpatient rehabilitation length of stay and rate of acute hospital transfer, making acute care diagnosis and treatment of paramount importance for safe and uninterrupted transitions of care [22].

Multiple risk factors for VTE in hospitalized patients have been identified (Table 13.2). VTE risk increases with acute medical illness, surgery, or traumatic injury. Patients with TBI or SCI, and those with more severe injury, are at greatest risk [16–21]. Patients with paraplegia and motor complete injuries are more likely to develop VTE than those with tetraplegia and motor incomplete injury, respectively [21, 23, 24]. Older age is frequently cited as a known risk factor for VTE in adults [24–30].

Table 13.2 Identified risk factors for development of VTE

Demographics	Trauma-related factors	Hospital-related factors
Older age	TBI with AIS ≥3	Surgery performed
History of DVT or PE	SCI	Blood transfusions
History of cancer or active cancer	Lower extremity fracture with AIS ≥3	Prolonged immobility
Myeloproliferative or sickle cell disease	Higher injury severity score (ISS)	Longer ICU length of stay
Obesity	Presentation in shock	Spine fixation for instability
Hypercoagulable condition	Extrication from MVA at scene	Placement of femoral/central line
History of cardiac disease	Spine fracture	Longer time of mechanical ventilation
Varicose veins	Chest injury with AIS ≥3	Presence of ventriculostomy
Use of hormonal therapy	Abdominal injury	
Recent or current pregnancy		
History of inflammatory bowel disease		

Prevention

Pharmacologic prophylaxis is effective in decreasing the rate of VTE and should be instituted for all hospitalized patients with acute medical illness, trauma, or major surgery [31]. Mechanical means of prophylaxis, such as intermittent pneumatic compression, should be used with patients who are unable to receive pharmacologic chemoprophylaxis due to high bleeding risk until the bleeding risk resolves [31]. In patients with TBI, pharmacologic VTE prophylaxis can be safely initiated 48–72 h after injury with stable head CT [32–34]. Medications commonly used for pharmacologic VTE prophylaxis are summarized in Table 13.3a. Low molecular weight heparin (LMWH), such as enoxaparin, is preferred due to superiority over low dose unfractionated heparin (LDUH) [23, 31, 35]. Pharmacologic prophylaxis typically continues through inpatient rehabilitation (IPR) admission for those with impaired mobility [31] and at least 8 weeks following acute SCI [23]. Inferior vena cava (IVC) filters should not be used routinely for prophylaxis [23, 31]. No randomized trials have studied the prophylactic use of IVC filters in any patient population with neurologic injury. Furthermore, IVC filter use is associated with both short-term and long-term complications and may result in inappropriate delays in the use of effective thromboprophylaxis as well as increased risk of DVT at the vascular access site and in the IVC [36–40].

Individual hospitals typically utilize a formal VTE prevention strategy to ensure appropriate VTE initiation and maintenance prophylaxis [31]. Delayed initiation, and missed doses of pharmacologic prophylaxis, have been associated with increased VTE rates [23, 41, 42]. Education, alerts in the electronic medical record, and unit-based approaches to assess VTE risk are effective for increasing prescription of pharmacologic prophylaxis and decreasing VTE rates.

Table 13.3 Medication management for VTE prevention and treatment. (a) Prevention of VTE. (b) Treatment of VTE

A. Prevention of VTE		
Medication	Dose	Comments
Heparin	5000U Q8H or Q12H	No dose adjustment needed for renal impairment
Enoxaparin	CrCl >30 mL/kg: 40 mg Q24H or 30 mg Q12H CrCl <30 mL/kg: 30 mg Q24H	Should not be used in hemodialysis
Fondaparinux	CrCl >50 mL/kg: 2.5 mg daily CrCl 30–50 mL/kg: 1.25 mg daily	Safe to use in heparin-induced thrombocytopenia (HIT) Contraindicated if weight <50 kg or CrCl <30 mL/kg Caution for CrCl 30–50 mL/kg; heparin is preferred

B. Treatment of VTE			
Medication	Dose	Reversal/antidoate	Comments
Unfractionated heparin	Start at 12 U/kg/h with or without initial bolus of 60–70 U/kg (up to 5000 U) Adjust rate to achieve aPTT 50–75 s	Protamine sulfate	No dose adjustment needed for renal impairment
Enoxaparin	CrCl >30 mL/kg 1 mg/kg Q12H CrCl <30 mL/kg: 1 mg/kg Q24H	Protamine sulfate may help neutralize enoxaparin but is not as effective as with heparin	Should not be used in hemodialysis
Fondaparinux	Weight <50 kg: 5 mg daily Weight 50–100 kg: 7.5 mg daily Weight >100 kg: 10 mg daily	None	Safe to use in patients with history of HIT Caution for CrCl <50 mL/kg and contraindicated for CrCl <30 mL/kg
Argatroban	Start at 2 mcg/kg/min Adjust rate to achieve aPTT 1.5–3 times initial baseline value	None	Used for treatment of HIT Impacts INR value
Warfarin	Dose to achieve INR 2–3 Bridge with unfractionated or low molecular weight heparin	Vitamin K Unactivated prothrombin complex concentrate (PCC)	Geriatric patients usually require lower doses due to changes in metabolism
Rivaroxaban (Xarelto)	15 mg twice daily for 21 days then 20 mg daily	Coagulation factor Xa (recombinant), inactivated (Andexxa) can be used with life-threatening bleed	Take with food Avoid with CrCl <30 mL/kg

(continued)

Table 13.3 (continued)

A. Prevention of VTE			
Medication	Dose	Comments	
Apixaban (Eliquis)	10 mg twice daily for 7 days then 5 mg twice daily	Coagulation factor Xa (recombinant), inactivated (Andexxa) can be used with life-threatening bleed	Use caution with CrCl <25 mL/kg or moderate hepatic impairment due to lack of evidence in these patients
Dabigatran (Pradaxa)	150 mg twice daily Requires 5–10 days initial treatment with unfractionated or low molecular weight heparin	Idarucizumab (Praxbind) Hemodialysis Antifibrinolytic agent can be used with life-threatening bleed	Use caution with CrCl <30 mL/kg as not studied in these patients

Diagnosis

DVT should be suspected in the case of pain or swelling of the affected limb. The skin may be warm, erythematous, or have evidence of swollen veins. Limbs may be tender to the touch, and in the case of lower extremity DVT, passive dorsiflexion of the foot on the affected limb may elicit pain, known as a positive Homans sign. PE can present as sudden onset of chest pain, shortness of breath, or hypoxia. Tachycardia and tachypnea may be seen, and electrocardiogram (ECG) may show a new right bundle branch block, T wave inversions, right axis deviation, or the classic $S_1Q_3T_3$ pattern, which includes deep S wave in lead I, Q wave in lead III, and T wave inversion in lead III.

Early VTE detection and treatment are important to decrease complications. Venous Doppler ultrasound has a sensitivity of 96.5% and specificity of 94.2% for DVT diagnosis when compared with contrast venography, making it the preferred method for diagnosis [43]. Serum d-dimer testing is of limited utility as a screening tool because it is non-specific and is frequently elevated in the acutely ill and injured patient [43]. In fact, d-dimer can be elevated for at least eight weeks following TBI [44]. CT angiography (CTA) of the chest is the preferred diagnostic technique for PE. This technique requires contrast dye; therefore, it is contraindicated in patients with contrast allergies and patients with renal failure. Ventilation-perfusion (V/Q) scans can be used in those cases.

There is significant debate regarding the use of routine Doppler ultrasound to screen for lower extremity DVT in asymptomatic patients. Early detection and treatment of asymptomatic lower extremity DVT is associated with lower PE rates in patients admitted to the neurosurgical ICU [45] but not in patients with traumatic pelvic or acetabular fracture [30]. Routine use of Doppler ultrasound to diagnosis asymptomatic lower extremity DVT at admission to IPR has been found cost-effective per life-year saved in patients admitted with TBI or SCI but not stroke, presumably due to lower life expectancy after injury [44, 46, 47]. However, the most recent American College of Chest Physicians (ACCP) clinical practice guidelines recommend against use of venous Doppler ultrasound in asymptomatic patients unless they are high risk—SCI, major TBI, or lower extremity/pelvic fracture—and received suboptimal pharmacologic prophylaxis [31]. Also, SCI-specific guidelines published by the Paralyzed Veterans of America recommend against the use of Doppler ultrasound in asymptomatic patients regardless of the level of injury, patient acuity, and time post-injury [23].

VTE Treatment

Prompt VTE treatment is recommended to prevent further morbidity and mortality. Treatment duration should be three months for patients with a provoked DVT or PE due to hospitalization, medical illness, surgery, or trauma. Traditionally, either an unfractionated heparin drip or LMWH as bridge to warfarin has been recommended to treat non-cancer patients; however, the most recent ACCP guidelines recommend non-vitamin K oral anticoagulant (NOAC) over warfarin due to lower bleeding rates and greater convenience (Table 13.3b) [48]. No specific NOAC is more effective than another. Warfarin should still be considered for patients with impaired renal function or in patients where a reversal agent is desired, such as those with high fall risk. LMWH should be utilized in patients with cancer as it is reportedly superior to warfarin, and no comparative studies using NOACs have been completed [48]. IVC filters should be used in patients who are unable to be anticoagulated due to significant hemorrhage risk at time of VTE diagnosis. If required, retrievable filters should be used, and they should be removed once the patient is treated with anticoagulant medications. IVC filter placement in addition to full anticoagulation us is not recommended [48].

Case Illustration

A 19-year-old male who weighs 70 kg is involved in a helmeted motorcycle accident. He is intubated on hospital arrival due to respiratory failure and diagnosed with right pneumothorax, for which a chest tube is placed. CT scan shows multiple fractures in the cervical spine with evidence of instability, and he undergoes surgical fixation. Neurologic examination 72 h after injury is consistent with C5 ASIA A SCI. His chest tube is removed on hospital day 4, and he is started on prophylactic doses of enoxaparin to prevent VTE. He is diagnosed with pneumonia on hospital day 5 and is treated with antibiotics. He has difficulties weaning from the ventilator due to secretions and respiratory muscle paralysis. On hospital day 7, he undergoes percutaneous tracheostomy in the ICU. Post-operatively, he is started on nebulized treatments of ipratropium-albuterol to decrease bronchospasm. Mechanical ventilation tidal volume is set at 1200 mL (17.1 mL/kg) to decrease atelectasis. He begins PVFB on hospital day 8. Two weeks after injury he is off all mechanical ventilation but continues to have secretions that require suctioning through the tracheostomy tube. On hospital day 18, he has erythema and swelling of his right leg, and Doppler ultrasound confirms the diagnosis of DVT. He is started on treatment dose of enoxaparin 70 mg every 12 hours and is transitioned to NOAC for the duration of his 3-month treatment on hospital day 22. His tracheostomy tube is changed to a smaller uncuffed tube on hospital day 28, and he is transferred to IPR. Abdominal binder is used when out of bed to provide additional support of the paralyzed abdominal muscles for respiration. For secretion management, he is continued on nebulized ipratropium-albuterol, and the respiratory therapist uses MIE to enhance secretion clearance. His family begins training on quad cough techniques. SLP begins using a one-way speaking valve to allow for communication. He is capped and subsequently decannulated six weeks following injury. He is eventually discharged to home with his parents, who perform quad cough three times daily for secretion clearance.

Summary/Key Points

Pulmonary complications and VTE frequently occur in patients with acquired CNS injury. Traumatic pulmonary injuries can include rib fractures, pulmonary contusion, and hemothorax. SCI leads to both obstructive and restrictive lung pathology due to changes in autonomic function and respiratory muscle paralysis, respectively. Aggressive management for secretion clearance is needed. VTE commonly occurs after TBI, SCI, and stroke, and it can be a life-threatening condition. Appropriate use of pharmacologic prophylaxis has been shown to decreased rate of VTE. Systematic screening during acute care may be a low-cost way to reduce VTE and unplanned acute IPR discharges.

References[1]

1. American Thoracic Society, Infectious Diseases Society of America. Guidelines for the management of adults with hospital-acquired, ventilator-associated, and healthcare-associated pneumonia. Am J Respir Crit Care Med. 2005;171(4):388–416. https://doi.org/10.1164/rccm.200405-644ST.
2. De Leyn P, Bedert L, Delcroix M, et al. Tracheotomy: clinical review and guidelines. Eur J Cardiothorac Surg. 2007;32(3):412–21. https://doi.org/10.1016/j.ejcts.2007.05.018.
3. Cheung NH, Napolitano LM. Tracheostomy: epidemiology, indications, timing, technique, and outcomes. Respir Care. 2014;59(6):895–915; discussion 916-9. https://doi.org/10.4187/respcare.02971.
4. Robba C, Galimberti S, Graziano F, et al. Tracheostomy practice and timing in traumatic brain-injured patients: a CENTER-TBI study. Intensive Care Med. 2020;46(5):983–94. https://doi.org/10.1007/s00134-020-05935-5.
5. McShane EK, Sun BJ, Maggio PM, Spain DA, Forrester JD. Improving tracheostomy delivery for trauma and surgical critical care patients: timely trach initiative. BMJ Open Qual. 2022;11(2):1589. https://doi.org/10.1136/bmjoq-2021-001589.

[1] Key References [3, 9, 23, 31, 48].

6. Marra A, Vargas M, Buonanno P, Iacovazzo C, Coviello A, Servillo G. Early vs. late tracheostomy in patients with traumatic brain injury: systematic review and meta-analysis. J Clin Med. 2021;10(15):3319. https://doi.org/10.3390/jcm10153319.
7. de Sabrina Araujo F, Wagner MT, Wellingson SP, Manoel JT. Benefits of early tracheostomy in TBI patients. In: Zamzuri I, editor. Advancement and new understanding in brain injury. London: IntechOpen; 2020.
8. DeVivo MJ, Krause JS, Lammertse DP. Recent trends in mortality and causes of death among persons with spinal cord injury. Arch Phys Med Rehabil. 1999;80(11):1411–9. https://doi.org/10.1016/s0003-9993(99)90252-6.
9. Galeiras Vázquez R, Rascado Sedes P, Mourelo Fariña M, Montoto Marqués A, Ferreiro Velasco ME. Respiratory management in the patient with spinal cord injury. Biomed Res Int. 2013;2013:168757. https://doi.org/10.1155/2013/168757.
10. Berlly M, Shem K. Respiratory management during the first five days after spinal cord injury. J Spinal Cord Med. 2007;30(4):309–18. https://doi.org/10.1080/10790268.2007.11753946.
11. Zimmer MB, Nantwi K, Goshgarian HG. Effect of spinal cord injury on the neural regulation of respiratory function. Exp Neurol. 2008;209(2):399–406. https://doi.org/10.1016/j.expneurol.2007.05.015.
12. Schilero GJ, Spungen AM, Bauman WA, Radulovic M, Lesser M. Pulmonary function and spinal cord injury. Respir Physiol Neurobiol. 2009;166(3):129–41. https://doi.org/10.1016/j.resp.2009.04.002.
13. Demers B. Contraindications for chest physiotherapy. Chest. 1986;89(6):902–3. https://doi.org/10.1378/chest.89.6.902b.
14. Bott J, Blumenthal S, Buxton M, et al. Guidelines for the physiotherapy management of the adult, medical, spontaneously breathing patient. Thoras. 2009;64:1–52.
15. Spapen HD, De Regt J, Honore PM. Chest physiotherapy in mechanically ventilated patients without pneumonia-a narrative review. J Thorac Dis. 2017;9(1):E44–9. https://doi.org/10.21037/jtd.2017.01.32.
16. Almenoff PL, Alexander LR, Spungen AM, Lesser MD, Bauman WA. Bronchodilatory effects of ipratropium bromide in patients with tetraplegia. Paraplegia. 1995;33(5):274–7. https://doi.org/10.1038/sc.1995.62.
17. Grimm DR, Schilero GJ, Spungen AM, Bauman WA, Lesser M. Salmeterol improves pulmonary function in persons with tetraplegia. Lung. 2006;184(6):335–9. https://doi.org/10.1007/s00408-006-0011-6.
18. Furlan JC, Fehlings MG. Role of screening tests for deep venous thrombosis in asymptomatic adults with acute spinal cord injury: an evidence-based analysis. Spine. 2007;32(17):1908–16. https://doi.org/10.1097/BRS.0b013e31811ec26a.
19. Denson K, Morgan D, Cunningham R, et al. Incidence of venous thromboembolism in patients with traumatic brain injury. Am J Surg. 2007;193(3):380–3; discussion 383-4. https://doi.org/10.1016/j.amjsurg.2006.12.004.
20. Viitanen M, Winblad B, Asplund K. Autopsy-verified causes of death after stroke. Acta Med Scand. 1987;222(5):401–8. https://doi.org/10.1111/j.0954-6820.1987.tb10956.x.
21. Selassie AW, Varma A, Saunders LL. Current trends in venous thromboembolism among persons hospitalized with acute traumatic spinal cord injury: does early access to rehabilitation matter? Arch Phys Med Rehabil. 2011;92(10):1534–41. https://doi.org/10.1016/j.apmr.2011.04.018.
22. Pinto SM, Galang G. Venous thromboembolism as predictor of acute care hospital transfer and inpatient rehabilitation length of stay. Am J Phys Med Rehabil. 2017;96(6):376–3.
23. Consortium for Spinal Cord Medicine. Prevention of venous thromboembolism in individuals with spinal cord injury. 3rd ed. Paralyzed veterans of America; 2016. https://pva.org/wp-content/uploads/2021/09/cpg_thrombo_fnl.pdf.
24. Giorgi Pierfranceschi M, Donadini MP, Dentali F, et al. The short- and long-term risk of venous thromboembolism in patients with acute spinal cord injury: a prospective cohort study. Thromb Haemost. 2013;109(1):34–8. https://doi.org/10.1160/th12-06-0390.

25. Azarbal A, Rowell S, Lewis J, et al. Duplex ultrasound screening detects high rates of deep vein thromboses in critically ill trauma patients. J Vasc Surg. 2011;54(3):743–7; discussion 747-8. https://doi.org/10.1016/j.jvs.2011.02.058.
26. Cipolle MD, Wojcik R, Seislove E, Wasser TE, Pasquale MD. The role of surveillance duplex scanning in preventing venous thromboembolism in trauma patients. J Trauma. 2002;52(3):453–62. https://doi.org/10.1097/00005373-200203000-00007.
27. Schwarcz TH, Quick RC, Minion DJ, Kearney PA, Kwolek CJ, Endean ED. Enoxaparin treatment in high-risk trauma patients limits the utility of surveillance venous duplex scanning. J Vasc Surg. 2001;34(3):447–52. https://doi.org/10.1067/mva.2001.117146.
28. Bajenaru O, Antochi F, Balasa R, et al. Assessment of venous thromboembolism prophylaxis in neurological patients with restricted mobility - VTE-NEURO study. Maedica. 2014;9(1):6–14.
29. Beckman MG, Hooper WC, Critchley SE, Ortel TL. Venous thromboembolism: a public health concern. Am J Prev Med. 2010;38(4):495–501. https://doi.org/10.1016/j.amepre.2009.12.017.
30. Moed BR, Miller JR, Tabaie SA. Sequential duplex ultrasound screening for proximal deep venous thrombosis in asymptomatic patients with acetabular and pelvic fractures treated operatively. J Trauma Acute Care Surg. 2012;72(2):443–7. https://doi.org/10.1097/TA.0b013e318241090d.
31. Geerts WH, Bergqvist D, Pineo GF, et al. Prevention of venous thromboembolism: American College of Chest Physicians evidence-based clinical practice guidelines (8th edition). Chest. 2008;133(6):381–453. https://doi.org/10.1378/chest.08-0656.
32. Abdel-Aziz H, Dunham CM, Malik RJ, Hileman BM. Timing for deep vein thrombosis chemoprophylaxis in traumatic brain injury: an evidence-based review. Crit Care. 2015;19(1):96. https://doi.org/10.1186/s13054-015-0814-z.
33. Saadeh Y, Gohil K, Bill C, et al. Chemical venous thromboembolic prophylaxis is safe and effective for patients with traumatic brain injury when started 24 hours after the absence of hemorrhage progression on head CT. J Trauma Acute Care Surg. 2012;73(2):426–30. https://doi.org/10.1097/TA.0b013e31825a758b.
34. Scudday T, Brasel K, Webb T, et al. Safety and efficacy of prophylactic anticoagulation in patients with traumatic brain injury. J Am Coll Surg. 2011;213(1):148–53; discussion 153-4. https://doi.org/10.1016/j.jamcollsurg.2011.02.027.
35. Chen HL, Wang XD. Heparin for venous thromboembolism prophylaxis in patients with acute spinal cord injury: a systematic review and meta-analysis. Spinal Cord. 2013;51(8):596–602. https://doi.org/10.1038/sc.2013.48.
36. McMurty AL, Owings JT, Anderson JT, al. e. Increased use of prophylactic vena cava filters in trauma patients failed to decrease overall incidence of pulmonary embolism. J Am Coll Surg. 1999;189:314–20.
37. Patton JH, Fabian TC, Croce MA, et al. Prophylactic greenfield filters: acute complications and long-term follow-up. J Trauma. 1996;41:231–6.
38. Decousus H, Leizorovicz A, Parent F, et al. A clinical trial of vena caval filters in the prevention of pulmonary embolism in patients with proximal deep-vein thrombosis. N Engl J Med. 1998;338:409–15.
39. Blebea J, Wilson R, Waybill P, et al. Deep venous thrombosis after percutaneous insertion of vena caval filters. J Vasc Surg. 1999;30:821–8.
40. Karmy-Jones R, Jurkovich GJ, Velmahos GC, et al. Practice patterns and outcomes of retrievable vena cava filters in trauma patients: an AAST multicenter study. J Trauma. 2007;62:17–25.
41. Louis SG, Sato M, Geraci T, et al. Correlation of missed doses of enoxaparin with increased incidence of deep vein thrombosis in trauma and general surgery patients. JAMA Surg. 2014;149(4):365–70. https://doi.org/10.1001/jamasurg.2013.3963.
42. Salottolo K, Offner P, Levy AS, Mains CW, Slone DS, Bar-Or D. Interrupted pharmocologic thromboprophylaxis increases venous thromboembolism in traumatic brain injury. J Trauma. 2011;70(1):19–24; discussion 25-6. https://doi.org/10.1097/TA.0b013e318207c54d.

43. Bates SM, Jaeschke R, Stevens SM, et al. Diagnosis of DVT: antithrombotic therapy and prevention of thrombosis, 9th ed: American College of Chest Physicians evidence-based clinical practice guidelines. Chest. 2012;141(2 Suppl):e351S–418S. https://doi.org/10.1378/chest.11-2299.
44. Meythaler JM, DeVivo MJ, Hayne JB. Cost-effectiveness of routine screening for proximal deep venous thrombosis in acquired brain injury patients admitted to rehabilitation. Arch Phys Med Rehabil. 1996;77(1):1–5. https://doi.org/10.1016/s0003-9993(96)90210-5.
45. Misra M, Roitberg B, Ebersole K, Charbel FT. Prevention of pulmonary embolism by combined modalities of thromboprophylaxis and intensive surveillance protocol. Neurosurgery. 2004;54(5):1099–102; discussion 1102-3. https://doi.org/10.1227/01.neu.0000119352.71531.29.
46. Kadyan V, Clinchot DM, Colachis SC. Cost-effectiveness of duplex ultrasound surveillance in spinal cord injury. Am J Phys Med Rehabil. 2004;83(3):191–7. https://doi.org/10.1097/01.phm.0000113401.47681.a6.
47. Wilson RD, Murray PK. Cost-effectiveness of screening for deep vein thrombosis by ultrasound at admission to stroke rehabilitation. Arch Phys Med Rehabil. 2005;86(10):1941–8. https://doi.org/10.1016/j.apmr.2005.05.009.
48. Kearon C, Akl EA, Ornelas J, et al. Antithrombotic therapy for VTE disease: CHEST guideline and expert panel report. Chest. 2016;149(2):315–52. https://doi.org/10.1016/j.chest.2015.11.026.

Chapter 14
Heterotopic Ossification

Justin Weppner and Amy K. Wagner

Chapter Objectives
1. Review the clinical presentation and diagnosis of neurogenic HO.
2. Summarize the levels of evidence for the prevention and treatment of neurogenic HO.
3. Describe early interventions for the prevention and treatment of neurogenic HO.

Introduction

Heterotopic ossification (HO) is defined as the formation of extra-skeletal bone in muscle and soft tissues. HO may develop around joints after central neurologic injury, including traumatic brain injury (TBI) and spinal cord injury (SCI). The reported incidence for HO associated with TBI ranges from 11% to 73%, with clinically significant HO ranging from 10% to 20% [1, 2]. The reported incidence of HO varies greatly in the SCI population, ranging from 10% to 78% [3, 4]. Patients with severe spasticity, impaired cognition, tracheostomy, pneumonia, and/or urinary tract infections are at a higher risk [5]. Generally, HO following SCI is formed caudal to the level of injury, whereas HO following closed TBI may occur around any large joint, including the hip, knee, elbow, and shoulder [6]. Development of neurogenic

J. Weppner (✉)
Virginia Tech Carilion School of Medicine, Edward Via College of Osteopathic Medicine, Roanoke, VA, USA
e-mail: jlweppner@carilionclinic.org

A. K. Wagner
Department of Physical Medicine and Rehabilitation, University of Pittsburgh School of Medicine, Pittsburgh, PA, USA
e-mail: wagnerak@upmc.edu

A. K. Wagner, J. Weppner (eds.), *Acute Care Neuroconsultation and Neurorehabilitation Management*, https://doi.org/10.1007/978-3-031-42830-2_14

HO generally occurs within 4–12 weeks after injury to the central nervous system (CNS) and progresses over the years. Although it is still unclear how CNS insults initiate a sequence of events that lead to juxta-articular HO, it is known that central and peripheral neurotransmitters may affect osteoblast formation and osteogenic activity [5, 7, 8].

Clinical Presentation

Individuals who develop HO experience pain, which is the most common symptom; other symptoms include loss of range of motion (ROM), swelling, redness, warmth, and low-grade fever [9]. The three stages of HO are early/inflammatory, intermediate, and mature [10]. In the early/inflammatory stage of HO development, immature heterotopic bone is made up of well-ordered collagen fibers with occasional fibroblasts and small islands of calcification. In this early/inflammatory stage, HO presents with localized pain, tenderness, and swelling that may mimic other pathologies such as cellulitis, thrombophlebitis, osteomyelitis, or tumor [9, 11]. In the intermediate stage of development, an intense inflammatory process follows initial calcification, with invasion by vascular channels and eventual bone formation. In this phase, both bone scan and radiographic changes are discernible. Radiographs at this stage show immature periarticular bone formation with a poorly defined cortex. In the mature stage of development, mature bone has formed and radiographs show mature bone formation with a well-delineated cortex.

Individuals who sustain an SCI with abnormal sensation below the level of the injury may not report pain in the affected area while individuals with severe TBI may not report pain due to the inability to communicate. In SCI, HO may manifest as autonomic dysreflexia while HO may present as dysautonomia, or paroxysmal sympathetic hyperactivity, in the TBI population (Chap. 10). In TBI and SCI populations, neurogenic HO usually develops in the impaired limbs, occurs more often in the spastic than in flaccid limbs, and forms in the muscle planes surrounding the joints rather than within the muscles or joints themselves. In the SCI population, the hip is more commonly involved, followed by the knee, elbow, and shoulder. In the TBI population as well, the hip joint is most often affected, followed by the elbow, shoulder, and knee. Small peripheral joints such as the wrists, ankles, hands, and feet are almost never involved in both populations [12]. The mean time of presentation is approximately 2 months post neurologic injury, but it can range from 2 weeks to 1 year post injury [10]. Thus, the early recognition of symptoms and physical findings associated with HO, as well as preventive measures in the acute care setting for those at high risk for HO after injury, is an important part of the neurorehabilitation consultation evaluation.

There are no established screening guidelines or algorithms for neurologic HO, and early diagnosis is often based on clinical signs and symptoms. Applying literature-based guidance from non-neurologic and neurologic patient populations combined with traditional physiatric principles can inform the acute care consultant in addressing screening prevention and early phase HO treatment. In addition, physiatry consultation prior to and following surgical treatment for chronic HO can support ongoing rehabilitation for this patient population.

HO Pathophysiology

HO pathophysiology after TBI and SCI is poorly understood. Although CNS influences on heterotopic bone formation likely occur, the peripheral effects of TBI- and SCI-associated polytrauma (including surgical intervention) [13–17] and burns [18] likely have a significant influence on HO incidence, pathophysiology, and associated functional limitations. However, evidence suggests that CNS processes facilitate HO bone formation in what may either be a temporally distinct or temporally coordinated mechanistic process.

For example, preclinical models suggest that osteoblast exposure to sera collected 48 h after experimental closed head injury leads to increased ALP activity by 11 days and mineralization 21 days after application [19]. Interestingly, this same study showed that sera collected 24 h after injury, and applied to osteoblasts, induced mitogenic (proliferative) effects [19]. Clinical work parallels these findings by suggesting patients with long bone fractures in addition to TBI have two-fold faster union rates and up to 50% more callus formation [20]. Serum taken from patients with TBI contains circulating factors that stimulate the preferential differentiation of mesenchymal cells into osteoblast [21].

Bone remodeling is also subject to central control through the sympathetic nervous system, which is partially regulated by the endocannabinoid system. After experimental TBI, cannabinoid-mediated down-regulation of norepinephrine at osteoblasts contributes to increased bone formation [8]. Other research suggests that humeral factors in human CSF after TBI are osteoinductive. However, specific factors have not been identified [22]. Leptin, a metabolic protein, is also a potential mediator of HO through both central and peripheral mechanisms [23]. Further a recent review suggests that after SCI and TBI, growth factors, inflammatory markers, substance P, and neurotransmitters like glutamate can influence heterotopic bone production by supporting neurological mechanisms that drive HO [5].

Diagnosis of HO

The early diagnosis of HO is primarily based on clinical signs and symptoms such as severe joint pain, swelling, erythema, warmth, or loss of joint ROM. Consideration should be made for other conditions that have similar clinical manifestations, such as joint infection, deep venous thrombosis (DVT), cellulitis, or osteomyelitis. Radiography is often the first imaging modality used to detect HO; however, in the early stages of HO, radiography may show normal findings, with standard radiographs becoming positive at 4–6 weeks following evidence of HO on three-phase bone scan [24–26]. Initial radiographic findings associated with HO often include a soft tissue mass, and usual radiographic appearance of HO is a circumferential ossification with a lucent center.

Three-phase bone scan is the most sensitive imaging modality for early HO detection, as early as two and a half weeks after injury, and may be utilized to assess the maturity of HO [27–30]. Technetium-99m-labeled diphosphonate used in bone scanning has an affinity for newly developing bone. The three phases include dynamic blood flow phase obtained 60 s after injection, static blood pooled phase obtained 5 min after injection, and the delayed phase obtained 2–4 h later. In the early stage of lesions, only blood flow or blood pooled images may be positive, reflecting the hypervascularity of early HO. Soft tissue uptake in the delayed phase subsequently develops within 1 week of the appearance of blood flow or pool abnormalities. Activity on delayed bone scans usually peaks a few months after injury, after which the intensity of activity on these scans progressively lessens. Most bone scan findings return to baseline within 12 months. However, during the pathophysiological course of the HO, the delayed phase may show increased activity even after the blood flow and blood pool images have returned to normal and the underlying HO has become mature [27–29, 31, 32].

In the SCI population, ultrasonography has been used for diagnosis of HO around the hip. In the early pre-radiographic phase, a chaotic disruption of the normal structure of the lamella of the skeletal muscle will be evident on ultrasound images. This disruption progresses to a mass-like, peripherally echogenic, and centrally hypoechoic pattern. Once early mineralization becomes radiographically visible, sheets or irregular clumps of echogenic material with acoustic shadowing will be evident on ultrasound images. Mature lesions show echogenicity and dense shadowing of the cortical bone [33]. However, ultrasonography is an operator-dependent examination, and no data are available on the value of ultrasonography in the diagnosis of HO in other joints.

For early diagnosis of HO, serum alkaline phosphatase (ALP) is a sensitive but nonspecific indicator whose level increases with worsening of clinical signs and symptoms such as stiffness, loss of ROM, swelling, erythema, and pain. Moreover, serum ALP levels become abnormal at around 2 weeks following the onset of symptoms and peak at 3.5 times of the normal levels at approximately 10 weeks [25].

HO Prevention

The prevention of HO requires a multipronged approach combining pharmacologic intervention with ROM exercises focusing on three basic principles: (1) disrupting the inductive signaling pathways, (2) altering the osteoprogenitor cells, and (3) modifying the environment. Since the development of neurogenic HO can occur within weeks of the initial injury, the prophylaxis should begin relatively early. Although there is no consensus on which medication should be used and when prophylaxis should begin, several drugs have successfully been used. Nonsteroidal anti-inflammatory medications (NSAIDs) inhibit prostaglandin-mediated bone remodeling and inhibit the differentiation of osteoprogenitor cells while bisphosphonates can affect bone formation at the stage of mineralization, preventing the conversion of amorphous calcium phosphate to hydroxyapatite [11, 34]. In the acute hospital setting a high index of suspicion for and surveillance of HO should be combined with preventative measures.

ROM

In the literature, although ROM exercises have not been shown to inhibit HO, physical therapy may be an adjunct in HO prevention. Gentle ROM may help maintain joint mobility and prevent secondary soft tissue contractures. Active ROM may be limited in patients with intact sensation, because of the associated discomfort. In addition, mobilization of joints may be limited by spasticity, which can be treated with phenol, botulinum toxin, or oral medications such as baclofen, dantrolene, or tizanidine [10, 35]. Multimodal treatment of spasticity in the acute setting should be utilized to reduce tone and assist with maintaining joint ROM.

Nonsteroidal Anti-inflammatory Medications (NSAIDs)

NSAIDs have successfully reduced the incidence of HO in the orthopedic population although gastrointestinal and bleeding complication has been associated with the use of nonselective NSAIDs [36, 37]. In the neurotrauma population, this may increase the risk of treatment discontinuation and could interfere with thromboprophylaxis after major trauma. In a study comparing celecoxib versus indomethacin for the prevention of HO following total hip arthroplasty, a significantly greater number of patients in the indomethacin group had to discontinue treatment as a result of excessive bleeding and gastrointestinal side effects compared to celecoxib [38]. At the same time, COX-2 inhibitors have been related to increased cardiovascular risk [39, 40] although a large randomized double-blind trial with celecoxib demonstrated no difference in cardiovascular risk compared with nonselective NSAIDs [37]. In the orthopedic population, subjects administered celecoxib directly following total hip arthroplasty did not have any adverse bleeding complications or delayed healing requiring revision demonstrating the safety of selective NSAIDs [41]. Following spine surgery, the use of NSAIDs around the time of spinal fusion is controversial with the inability to make clinical recommendations on the appropriate use of NSAIDs in this context. Considering the current literature available, a perioperative exposure to NSAIDs most likely does not cause an adverse effect [42]. Considering the orthopedic literature, in the SCI population, early administration of NSAIDs within close proximity to injury may not delay healing nor increase bleeding risk after orthopedic surgery. The safety of NSAIDs in the severe TBI population has not been well studied, and the safety of NSAID administration following severe TBI has not been established.

Two randomized controlled clinical trial studies have examined the use of NSAIDs for the prophylaxis of HO in the SCI population, within 3 weeks of injury, and found significant reductions in the development of HO [3, 43]. Thirty-three SCI patients were randomized to treatment or placebo groups, with the treatment group receiving 3 weeks of slow-release indomethacin at 75 mg daily for HO prophylaxis. Patients were followed longitudinally to determine those who developed HO based on clinical presentation, nuclear bone scans, or radiographs. As a result, a significantly lower incidence of HO was found in the treatment group (25.0%) than in the placebo group (64.7%) ($p < 0.001$). Treated patients also experienced HO symptoms later than those in the placebo group (31.7 vs. 19.2 days; $p < 0.048$). Upper abdominal discomfort was the most common symptom in both groups; however, this symptom did not result in medication discontinuation [3].

In a second study, 76 persons with early SCI were randomized into two groups: the treatment group prophylactically received 25 mg of rofecoxib daily for 4 weeks, a medication subsequently withdrawn voluntarily from the market for reported increased risk of cardiovascular side effects. HO was diagnosed based on clinical presentation and nuclear bone scans, and a significantly lower incidence of HO was found in the rofecoxib group (13.4%) than in the placebo group (33.3%: $p < 0.05$). Moreover, treated patients had 2.5 times lower relative risk of HO development than patients in the placebo group (95% confidence interval, 2.3–6) [43]. This Level 1 evidence supports that NSAIDs, rofecoxib and indomethacin, reduced the incidence of HO when administered early in the first 3 weeks after SCI [3, 43].

Bisphosphonates

In the acquired brain injury (ABI) population, one small study has investigated etidronate administration to prevent HO [44]. In this cohort study, patients ($n = 10$) were administered etidronate prophylactically within a week of injury for 6 months. Those receiving etidronate were compared to a retrospective untreated control group ($n = 10$). Radiographic and clinical evidence revealed that those receiving etidronate had a significantly ($p < 0.025$) lower incidence of HO than those without treatment. This study provides Level 2 evidence that etidronate reduces the development of HO in severe ABI patients [44].

HO Acute and Chronic Treatments in the Acute Care Setting

Treatment of HO includes maintenance of functional ROM through stretching and exercises. Early initiation of treatment with bisphosphonates such as etidronate may lead to decreased disease severity. Although some of the newer bisphosphonates such as alendronate may have a more favorable side effect profile and are more effective for treating disorders of bone such as osteoporosis, the use of alendronate has not been evaluated for the treatment of heterotopic ossification. Radiation therapy may also be considered in the SCI population to halt the progression of HO and if severe ankylosis or functional limitations occur, surgical wedge resection may be considered.

Bisphosphonates

Etidronate for the management of HO was investigated prospectively in 46 SCI patients. The diagnosis of HO was made based on bone scan and radiographic evaluation. Patients were divided into two groups: Group 1 comprised 33 patients with positive bone scan and negative evidence of HO and Group 2 included 13 patients with positive bone scintigraphy and positive radiographic evidence of HO. Etidronate was started intravenously (300 mg/day) for 3 days followed by oral therapy for 6 months (20 mg/kg/day). In Group 1, etidronate therapy prevented HO in 79% of patients; in the remaining 21% of patients, a low degree of tissue ossification was found, which was not clinically significant. In Group 2, an inhibitory effect of etidronate on the progression of soft tissue ossification was noted in six patients. The remaining seven patients did not respond to therapy and showed HO progression. The authors concluded that etidronate may prevent HO in most of the patients when administered at an early stage of HO development prior to positive radiographic findings and in higher doses than are routinely recommended [45].

Another study investigated 27 consecutive patients with a diagnosis acute onset of HO based on bone scan following SCI [46]. Etidronate 300 mg was administered intravenously daily for 3–5 days. After intravenous etidronate, 20 of 27 patients (74.1%) showed a rapid decrease of soft tissue swelling over 1–2 days ($p < 0.01$), and no side effects were associated with the intravenous administration. Also, these patients were compared with 11 patients treated with oral etidronate alone for a period of 6 months. No significant difference was noted with HO development between those who received etidronate both intravenously and orally and those who only received etidronate orally [46].

There is Level 2 evidence that etidronate can halt post-SCI HO progression if initiated early before radiographic evidence of HO is present.

ROM

A retrospective chart study reviewed clinical data of 16 patients with TBI and radiograph positive HO, an average of 3.6 months after head injury, who participated in forceful ROM therapy. Indications for forceful ROM therapy were uncontrolled spasticity, voluntary muscle guarding, or early bony ankylosis. Initial improvement in ROM was reported for 82% of the patients with 64% showing ROM maintenance or further ROM gain through rehabilitation. This study presented Level 4 evidence that forceful joint manipulation improves ROM among patients with TBI [47].

Radiation

Radiation treatment may prevent HO development by disrupting the differentiation process of mesenchymal cells into osteoblasts. In one study, 49 SCI patients were treated with low-field radiation during the inflammatory phase of early HO formation. Of the 49 patients (70 joints, 65 hips, three knees, one shoulder, one elbow), 71% of the joints did not show progression of HO over a median follow-up period of 11 months. However, there are theoretical concerns that patients subjected to radiation treatment would be at risk for radiation-induced sarcoma; despite its rarity, this is a serious complication [48]. In another study, 36 patients underwent radiotherapy early in the course of the disease, with 30 irradiated patients showing no progression of HO. In three patients, recurrent ossification after therapy caused a moderate decrease in joint mobility. No relevant adverse effects were observed [49]. Results from these two case studies provide Level 4 evidence that radiotherapy halts the progression of HO post-SCI [48, 49].

Surgical Resection

Surgical indications for HO removal include improvement of function and standing posture, sitting or ambulation, and independent dressing, feeding, and hygiene. Excision should also be considered for patients in whom an underlying bone mass contributes to repeated pressure injuries [50]. The timing of surgery has been controversial with some studies reporting that HO must reach maturity before surgery, while others have reported that surgery can be safely carried out prior to HO maturity to reduce stiffness postoperatively [5, 51–54]. Waiting for HO maturity to avoid recurrence exposes the patient to prolonged pain and loss of joint motion, which may reduce functional ability and probably neurological recovery and increase the risk of postoperative complications such as hematoma or fracture [30]. Reported rates of radiographic recurrence of HO ranged from 0% to 92% [53, 55, 56]. Although the timing of surgery and follow-up varies among studies, the incidence of radiographic recurrence in asymptomatic patients who underwent surgery is more frequent than that of symptomatic clinical recurrence, and it is not clear if the timing of surgery influences clinical recurrence. Early consultation with an orthopedic surgeon should be considered in patients with HO resulting in severe loss of motion or decreased function. The consulting physiatrist, in coordination with the inpatient multidisciplinary therapy team, may provide useful information to orthopedics by clearly determining the functional impact of HO in the setting of a neurologic disorder. In addition to the importance of ongoing orthopedic engagement, the consulting physiatrist should optimize the patient by managing risk factors that might influence HO recurrence such as treating spasticity, early identification and treatment of urinary tract infections, preventing pressure injury, and maximizing function prior to excision.

Case Illustration

A 19-year-old male patient was admitted to an acute hospital following severe TBI secondary to a motor vehicle accident. His 41-day acute hospital course was complicated by prolonged coma, respiratory failure requiring tracheostomy placement, pneumonia, sepsis, dysphagia with percutaneous endoscopic gastrostomy placement, spastic left hemiplegia, and bilateral lower extremity DVT. A physical medicine and rehabilitation (PM&R) consultation requested post-acute care recommendations. On examination, passive ROM of the left hip was limited and painful. HO was clinically suspected by the consultation team, and a pelvic X-ray was ordered and unremarkable. Given the high clinical suspicion for HO, a three-phase bone scan was performed and revealed positive findings for early HO of the left hip. Serum ALP level was elevated at 267 U/L (reference, 44–147 U/L). The consultation service formulated a treatment plan that included ROM exercises and dantrolene to reduce spasticity. He was subsequently admitted for inpatient rehabilitation and continued to experience impairments in mobility, transfers, and activities of daily living despite medical management. Subsequently, he underwent surgical resection of HO. Following surgery, PM&R was consulted and on examination the patient showed immediate improvement in left hip passive ROM. A physical therapy prescription was ordered by the PM&R consultant at discharge, which included passive ROM, active ROM, and a strengthening program. The patient made gradual improvements in active ROM and function over an 8-week course of physical therapy.

Summary and Key Points

HO is the abnormal formation of mature lamellar bone within extra-skeletal soft tissues where bone does not exist. A three-phase bone scan is the most sensitive imaging modality for early detection and assessment of HO maturity. Prevention strategies include ROM, NSAIDs, and bisphosphonates. Nonsurgical treatment with bisphosphonates and radiation therapy is appropriate for early treatment of

HO. Although bisphosphonates are effective prophylaxis if initiated shortly after the trauma, mineralization of the bone matrix resumes after drug discontinuation. During the acute inflammatory stage, the patient should rest the affected joint in a functional position; once acute inflammatory signs subside, passive ROM exercises and continued mobilization are indicated. Surgical indications for excision of HO include improvement of function and standing posture, sitting or ambulation, independent dressing, feeding and hygiene, and repeated pressure injuries from underlying bone mass. The optimal timing of surgery is currently not established with new evidence suggesting that it is not necessary to wait for the maturation of HO prior to surgical excision. The consulting physiatrist, in coordination with the inpatient multidisciplinary therapy team, may provide useful information to orthopedics by clearly determining the functional impact of HO in the setting of a neurologic disorder. In addition to the importance of ongoing orthopedic engagement, the consulting physiatrist should optimize the patient by managing risk factors that might influence HO recurrence such as treating spasticity, early identification and treatment of urinary tract infections, preventing pressure injury, and maximizing function prior to excision.

References [1]

1. Cullen N, Bayley M, Bayona N, Hilditch M, Aubut J, Group E. Management of heterotopic ossification and venous thromboembolism following acquired brain injury. Brain Inj. 2007;21(2):215–30. https://doi.org/10.1080/02699050701202027.
2. Simonsen LL, Sonne-Holm S, Krasheninnikoff M, Engberg AW. Symptomatic heterotopic ossification after very severe traumatic brain injury in 114 patients: incidence and risk factors. Injury. 2007;38(10):1146–50. https://doi.org/10.1016/j.injury.2007.03.019.
3. Banovac K, Williams JM, Patrick LD, Haniff YM. Prevention of heterotopic ossification after spinal cord injury with indomethacin. Spinal Cord. 2001;39(7):370–4. https://doi.org/10.1038/sj.sc.3101166.
4. van Kuijk AA, Geurts AC, van Kuppevelt HJ. Neurogenic heterotopic ossification in spinal cord injury. Spinal Cord. 2002;40(7):313–26. https://doi.org/10.1038/sj.sc.3101309.
5. Sullivan MP, Torres SJ, Mehta S, Ahn J. Heterotopic ossification after central nervous system trauma: a current review. Bone Jt Res. 2013;2(3):51–7. https://doi.org/10.1302/2046-3758.23.2000152.
6. Ranganathan K, Loder S, Agarwal S, et al. Heterotopic ossification: basic-science principles and clinical correlates. J Bone Joint Surg. 2015;97(13):1101–11. https://doi.org/10.2106/JBJS.N.01056.
7. Reichel LM, Salisbury E, Moustoukas MJ, Davis AR, Olmsted-Davis E. Molecular mechanisms of heterotopic ossification. J Hand Surg Am. 2014;39(3):563–6. https://doi.org/10.1016/j.jhsa.2013.09.029.
8. Tam J, Trembovler V, Di M, et al. The cannabinoid CB1 receptor regulates bone formation by modulating adrenergic signaling. FASEB J. 2008;22(1):285–94.
9. Jensen LL, Halar E, Little JW, Brooke MM. Neurogenic heterotopic ossification. Am J Phys Med. 1987;66(6):351–63.

[1] Key References [2, 5, 10].

10. Cipriano CA, Pill SG, Keenan MA. Heterotopic ossification following traumatic brain injury and spinal cord injury. J Am Acad Orthop Surg. 2009;17(11):689–97.
11. Vanden Bossche L, Vanderstraeten G. Heterotopic ossification: a review. J Rehabil Med. 2005;37(3):129–36. https://doi.org/10.1080/16501970510027628.
12. Garland D. Heterotopic ossification. In: Orthopaedic rehabilitation. London: Churchill Livingstone; 1992.
13. Vermesan D, Prejbeanu R, Haragus H, et al. Clinical relevance of altered bone immunopathology pathways around the elbow. Eur Rev Med Pharmacol Sci. 2014;18(19):2846–50.
14. Kent WT, Shelton TJ, Eastman J. Heterotopic ossification around the knee after tibial nailing and ipsilateral antegrade and retrograde femoral nailing in the treatment of floating knee injuries. Int Orthop. 2018;42(6):1379–85. https://doi.org/10.1007/s00264-018-3845-7.
15. Kaempffe FA, Bone LB, Border JR. Open reduction and internal fixation of acetabular fractures: heterotopic ossification and other complications of treatment. J Orthop Trauma. 1991;5(4):439–45. https://doi.org/10.1097/00005131-199112000-00009.
16. Keret D, Harcke HT, Mendez AA, Bowen JR. Heterotopic ossification in central nervous system-injured patients following closed nailing of femoral fractures. Clin Orthop Relat Res. 1990;256:254–9.
17. Horne LT, Blue BA. Intraarticular heterotopic ossification in the knee following intramedullary nailing of the fractured femur using a retrograde method. J Orthop Trauma. 1999;13(5):385–8. https://doi.org/10.1097/00005131-199906000-00013.
18. Kornhaber R, Foster N, Edgar D, et al. The development and impact of heterotopic ossification in burns: a review of four decades of research. Scars Burn Heal. 2017;3:2059513117695659. https://doi.org/10.1177/2059513117695659.
19. Klein BY, Shohami E, Reikhinshtein Y, Ben-Bassat H, Liebergall M. Serum-mediated osteogenic effects of head injury on cultured rat marrow stromal cells. Calcif Tissue Int. 1999;65(3):217–22. https://doi.org/10.1007/s002239900686.
20. Cadosch D, Gautschi OP, Thyer M, et al. Humoral factors enhance fracture-healing and callus formation in patients with traumatic brain injury. J Bone Joint Surg. 2009;91(2):282–8. https://doi.org/10.2106/JBJS.G.01613.
21. Cadosch D, Toffoli AM, Gautschi OP, et al. Serum after traumatic brain injury increases proliferation and supports expression of osteoblast markers in muscle cells. J Bone Joint Surg. 2010;92(3):645–53. https://doi.org/10.2106/JBJS.I.00097.
22. Gautschi OP, Toffoli AM, Joesbury KA, Skirving AP, Filgueira L, Zellweger R. Osteoinductive effect of cerebrospinal fluid from brain-injured patients. J Neurotrauma. 2007;24(1):154–62.
23. Chauveau C, Devedjian JC, Delecourt C, Jeanfils J, Hardouin P, Broux O. Leptin receptors and beta2-adrenergic receptor mRNA expression in brain injury-related heterotopic ossification. J Recept Signal Transduct Res. 2008;28(4):347–59.
24. Kransdorf MJ, Meis JM. From the archives of the AFIP. Extraskeletal osseous and cartilaginous tumors of the extremities. Radiographics. 1993;13(4):853–84. https://doi.org/10.1148/radiographics.13.4.8356273.
25. Orzel JA, Rudd TG. Heterotopic bone formation: clinical, laboratory, and imaging correlation. J Nucl Med. 1985;26(2):125–32.
26. Mysiw WJ, Tan J, Jackson RD. Heterotopic ossification. The utility of osteocalcin in diagnosis and management. Am J Phys Med Rehabil. 1993;72(4):184–7.
27. Drane WE. Myositis ossificans and the three-phase bone scan. AJR Am J Roentgenol. 1984;142(1):179–80. https://doi.org/10.2214/ajr.142.1.179.
28. Freed JH, Hahn H, Menter R, Dillon T. The use of the three-phase bone scan in the early diagnosis of heterotopic ossification (HO) and in the evaluation of Didronel therapy. Paraplegia. 1982;20(4):208–16. https://doi.org/10.1038/sc.1982.39.
29. Banovac K. The effect of etidronate on late development of heterotopic ossification after spinal cord injury. J Spinal Cord Med. 2000;23(1):40–4. https://doi.org/10.1080/10790268.2000.11753507.
30. Shehab D, Elgazzar AH, Collier BD. Heterotopic ossification. J Nucl Med. 2002;43(3):346–53.

31. Muheim G, Donath A, Rossier AB. Serial scintigrams in the course of ectopic bone formation in paraplegic patients. Am J Roentgenol Radium Therapy, Nucl Med. 1973;118(4):865–9.
32. Tanaka T, Rossier AB, Hussey RW, Ahnberg DS, Treves S. Quantitative assessment of para-osteo-arthropathy and its maturation on serial radionuclide bone images. Radiology. 1977;123(1):217–21. https://doi.org/10.1148/123.1.217.
33. Bodley R, Jamous A, Short D. Ultrasound in the early diagnosis of heterotopic ossification in patients with spinal injuries. Paraplegia. 1993;31(8):500–6. https://doi.org/10.1038/sc.1993.81.
34. Francis MD, Russell RG, Fleisch H. Diphosphonates inhibit formation of calcium phosphate crystals in vitro and pathological calcification in vivo. Science. 1969;165(3899):1264–6. https://doi.org/10.1126/science.165.3899.1264.
35. Garland DE, Lilling M, Keenan MA. Percutaneous phenol blocks to motor points of spastic forearm muscles in head-injured adults. Arch Phys Med Rehabil. 1984;65(5):243–5.
36. Leese PT, Hubbard RC, Karim A, Isakson PC, Yu SS, Geis GS. Effects of celecoxib, a novel cyclooxygenase-2 inhibitor, on platelet function in healthy adults: a randomized, controlled trial. J Clin Pharmacol. 2000;40(2):124–32. https://doi.org/10.1177/00912700022008766.
37. Silverstein FE, Faich G, Goldstein JL, et al. Gastrointestinal toxicity with celecoxib vs nonsteroidal anti-inflammatory drugs for osteoarthritis and rheumatoid arthritis: the CLASS study: a randomized controlled trial. Celecoxib long-term Arthritis Safety Study. JAMA. 2000;284(10):1247–55. https://doi.org/10.1001/jama.284.10.1247.
38. Romanò CL, Duci D, Romanò D, Mazza M, Meani E. Celecoxib versus indomethacin in the prevention of heterotopic ossification after total hip arthroplasty. J Arthroplast. 2004;19(1):14–8. https://doi.org/10.1016/s0883-5403(03)00279-1.
39. Bresalier RS, Sandler RS, Quan H, et al. Cardiovascular events associated with rofecoxib in a colorectal adenoma chemoprevention trial. N Engl J Med. 2005;352(11):1092–102. https://doi.org/10.1056/NEJMoa050493.
40. Graham DJ, Campen D, Hui R, et al. Risk of acute myocardial infarction and sudden cardiac death in patients treated with cyclo-oxygenase 2 selective and non-selective non-steroidal anti-inflammatory drugs: nested case-control study. Lancet. 2005;365(9458):475–81. https://doi.org/10.1016/S0140-6736(05)17864-7.
41. Lavernia CJ, Contreras JS, Villa JM, Rossi MD. Celecoxib and heterotopic bone formation after total hip arthroplasty. J Arthroplast. 2014;29(2):390–2. https://doi.org/10.1016/j.arth.2013.06.039.
42. Borgeat A, Ofner C, Saporito A, Farshad M, Aguirre J. The effect of nonsteroidal anti-inflammatory drugs on bone healing in humans: a qualitative, systematic review. J Clin Anesth. 2018;49:92–100. https://doi.org/10.1016/j.jclinane.2018.06.020.
43. Banovac K, Williams JM, Patrick LD, Levi A. Prevention of heterotopic ossification after spinal cord injury with COX-2 selective inhibitor (rofecoxib). Spinal Cord. 2004;42(12):707–10. https://doi.org/10.1038/sj.sc.3101628.
44. Spielman G, Gennarelli TA, Rogers CR. Disodium etidronate: its role in preventing heterotopic ossification in severe head injury. Arch Phys Med Rehabil. 1983;64(11):539–42.
45. Banovac K, Gonzalez F, Renfree KJ. Treatment of heterotopic ossification after spinal cord injury. J Spinal Cord Med. 1997;20(1):60–5. https://doi.org/10.1080/10790268.1997.11719457.
46. Banovac K, Gonzalez F, Wade N, Bowker JJ. Intravenous disodium etidronate therapy in spinal cord injury patients with heterotopic ossification. Paraplegia. 1993;31(10):660–6. https://doi.org/10.1038/sc.1993.106.
47. Garland DE, Razza BE, Waters RL. Forceful joint manipulation in head-injured adults with heterotopic ossification. Clin Orthop Relat Res. 1982;169:133–8.
48. Sautter-Bihl ML, Hültenschmidt B, Liebermeister E, Nanassy A. Fractionated and single-dose radiotherapy for heterotopic bone formation in patients with spinal cord injury. A phase-I/II study. Strahlenther Onkol. 2001;177(4):200–5.

49. Sautter-Bihl ML, Liebermeister E, Nanassy A. Radiotherapy as a local treatment option for heterotopic ossifications in patients with spinal cord injury. Spinal Cord. 2000;38(1):33–6.
50. Subbarao JV, Garrison SJ. Heterotopic ossification: diagnosis and management, current concepts and controversies. J Spinal Cord Med. 1999;22(4):273–83. https://doi.org/10.1080/10790268.1999.11719580.
51. Baird EO, Kang QK. Prophylaxis of heterotopic ossification - an updated review. J Orthop Surg Res. 2009;4:12. https://doi.org/10.1186/1749-799X-4-12.
52. Baldwin K, Hosalkar HS, Donegan DJ, Rendon N, Ramsey M, Keenan MA. Surgical resection of heterotopic bone about the elbow: an institutional experience with traumatic and neurologic etiologies. J Hand Surg Am. 2011;36(5):798–803. https://doi.org/10.1016/j.jhsa.2011.01.015.
53. Melamed E, Robinson D, Halperin N, Wallach N, Keren O, Groswasser Z. Brain injury-related heterotopic bone formation: treatment strategy and results. Am J Phys Med Rehabil. 2002;81(9):670–4. https://doi.org/10.1097/01.PHM.0000023268.24759.36.
54. Chalidis B, Stengel D, Giannoudis PV. Early excision and late excision of heterotopic ossification after traumatic brain injury are equivalent: a systematic review of the literature. J Neurotrauma. 2007;24(11):1675–86. https://doi.org/10.1089/neu.2007.0342.
55. Carlier RY, Safa DM, Parva P, et al. Ankylosing neurogenic myositis ossificans of the hip. An enhanced volumetric CT study. J Bone Joint Surg. 2005;87(3):301–5.
56. Sorriaux G, Denormandie P, Martin JN, Kiefer C, Judet T. Excision of heterotopic new bone around the elbow in patients with head injury: 51 cases. Rev Chir Orthop Reparatrice Appar Mot. 2005;91(5):415–22.

Chapter 15
Principles of Enteral Feeding and Nutrition

Julie Lanphere

Chapter Objectives

1. Understand the in-hospital complications associated with malnutrition in general and with the traumatic brain injury (TBI) and spinal cord injury (SCI) populations during acute care.
2. Understand the benefits of enteral feeding and the physiologic processes associated with its use.
3. Understand the benefits of early enteral nutrition for TBI and SCI patients.
4. Understand the evidence supporting the use of early enteral nutrition and its benefits for the TBI and SCI populations.
5. Understand percutaneous endoscopic gastrostomy tube insertion risks and benefits.
6. Understand microbiome and nutritional benefits in recovery associated with critical illness, TBI and SCI survivors, and their role in recovery.

Introduction

Malnutrition is both a debilitating and highly prevalent condition in the acute hospital setting. Hospitalization with the diagnosis of malnutrition has been associated with longer lengths of stay (LOS), higher healthcare costs, immune system depression, impaired wound healing, muscle wasting, and up to five times the risk of mortality compared to other hospitalized adults. Early nutritional intervention may reduce complication rates, morbidity, mortality, and hospital resource utilization [1, 2]. The Academy of Nutrition and Dietetics and the American Society for Parenteral

J. Lanphere (✉)
Intermountain Medical Center, Murray, UT, USA
e-mail: julie.lanphere@imail.org

A. K. Wagner, J. Weppner (eds.), *Acute Care Neuroconsultation and Neurorehabilitation Management*, https://doi.org/10.1007/978-3-031-42830-2_15

and Enteral Nutrition-Society of Critical Care Medicine (ASPEN-SCCM) recommend that a standardized set of diagnostic characteristics be used to identify and document adult malnutrition in routine acute care practice [3, 4]. ASPEN-SCCM evidence-based guidelines recommend using immune-modulated enteral formulations supplemented for appropriate populations, including trauma. Ketogenic diets and micronutrients (i.e., minerals, vitamins, and trace elements) are unresolved approaches and need future research [4, 5]. Level IIA evidence suggests that feeding patients to attain basal caloric replacement at least by the fifth day and at most by the seventh day post-injury will decrease mortality [6].

Malnutrition in critically ill patients promotes endocrine dysfunction, multiorgan failure, impaired immunity, and increased mortality. Nutritional therapy aims to prevent malnutrition and its complications. There are shifts in metabolism and gastrointestinal dysfunction that contribute to the nutritional deficits associated with TBI and other neuroinflammatory conditions such as polytrauma, sepsis, stroke, and coronavirus disease 2019 (COVID-19) [7]. Nutritional and metabolic needs after neurotrauma are not well understood, and the literature surrounding these populations focuses on nutrition and supplementation optimization to improve outcomes. Optimal energy and protein targets vary due to the extent of hypermetabolism and catabolism that are dependent on ventilation status, sedation, and injury severity. It is a notable challenge to accurately estimate energy expenditure and protein needs for any individual patient, and no consensus exists in the literature [8]. There are also varying practices and resources available for unit nutritionists, and monitoring parameters also vary across systems that manage these patients. Generalized predictive equations can be somewhat inaccurate in determining nutritional needs when compared to more direct, yet invasive, methodologies such as indirect calorimetry and nitrogen balance studies [8, 9].

Indirect calorimetry is the gold standard for assessing kcal needs. Dieticians use a machine to measure indirect calorimetry, with most only using it for intubated intensive care unit (ICU) patients. For critically ill patients, dieticians follow an early feeding protocol in which patients are assessed within 25–48 h of hospital admission, and high-risk patients are reassessed every 3–5 days. In patients where indirect calorimetry is possible, the ASPEN Guidelines recommend a weight-based calculation. Given the lack of support for weight-based calculations and inaccuracy of formulas, dieticians use more than one calculation and take into account weight, height, age, and follow ASPEN standards of care for the diagnosis [4, 10]. The practicality of what happens in hospitals is due to a limited ability to conduct indirect calorimetry studies. In addition, a complete physical focused exam is done to assess for muscle loss/muscle wasting, followed by closely monitoring weight changes and providing as needed adjustments during the patient's hospital stay.

Nutritional and Metabolic Needs After Traumatic Brain Injury

TBI injuries are classified as primary and secondary injuries. The primary injury involves mechanical damage to the central nervous system (CNS) with characteristic tissue disruption, axonal shearing, and blood-brain barrier (BBB) dysfunction.

The secondary injury occurs in response to the primary injury and typically includes cerebral edema, increased inflammatory cytokines, excitotoxicity, ischemia, reactive oxygen species, and immunosuppression. Together, these injuries affect cellular metabolism systemically by creating a hypermetabolic and hypercatabolic state that ultimately increases caloric expenditure [11]. Patients with severe TBI may lose 10–15% lean body mass in a week without adequate nutrition. Protein catabolism is a major contributor to this loss. Studies suggest that protein catabolism increases significantly in the acute phase of TBI, appears to peak at 8–14 days, and is related to TBI severity [12].

Energy expenditure also is highly variable among critically ill patients and among individual patients during various phases of illness. As a consequence, be aware that critically ill patients are at considerable risk of under- or overfeeding during ICU and post-ICU hospital stay [10].

Early initiation of nutritional support following TBI is crucial in off-setting the acute catabolic state observed with TBI. Early nutrition supports muscle mass preservation, decreases infection complications, promotes cerebral homeostasis, and improves functional outcomes. Ideally, nutritional support should be started within 24–48 h post-injury to provide 50% of resting energy expenditure (REE) within the first 2 weeks post-injury. Previous studies show that patients with TBI need about 100–150% of REE. The REE is ideally measured by indirect calorimetry (IC), which measures oxygen consumption (VO_2) and carbon dioxide production (VCO_2). If REE measurement is not possible by indirect calorimetry, administering 25 kcal/kg/day, or 70% of the estimated REE during the initial 7–10 days, is advised [8, 9]. Patients with TBI, similar to other trauma patients, are likely to require 2.0–2.5 g of protein/kg at a minimum, especially during the early period following injury [8]. There are some barriers with regard to nutrition for patients with TBI. They may have difficulty maintaining caloric intake due to pain, loss of appetite, feeding tube removal, and other co-injuries that include facial fracture, oral injuries, and cervical immobilization [9]. However, a review by Lee et al. suggests that failure to initiate nutritional support within 5–7 days post severe TBI was associated with increased mortality by two- to four-fold [5].

Individualized real-time nutrition therapy is the next step toward optimal patient care. IC is considered the gold standard to measure caloric needs in critically ill patients at bedside, and its use has been strongly recommended by the recent European Society for Clinical Nutrition and Metabolism (ESPEN) and American Society for Parenteral and Enteral Nutrition (ASPEN) guidelines [10]. IC is used to measure energy expenditure as a proxy for caloric requirement in ICU patients. However, the superiority of IC-guided nutritional therapy is not yet unequivocally proven in randomized clinical trials, and further research is urgently warranted. Nevertheless, IC has strong theoretical potential to improve nutritional status, and consequently, long-term outcomes for critically ill patients in various metabolic phases of critical illness. Increased knowledge of the practical use and theoretical benefits of IC among clinicians can contribute to more widespread and routine implementation, thereby promoting research opportunities and real-time targeted and personalized nutrition therapy [10]. It remains the gold standard compared to predictive equations. It can at times be difficult based on conditions; therefore, the resting metabolic rate is calculated using an equation. It must be used in nonobese patients who are critically ill, and the Penn

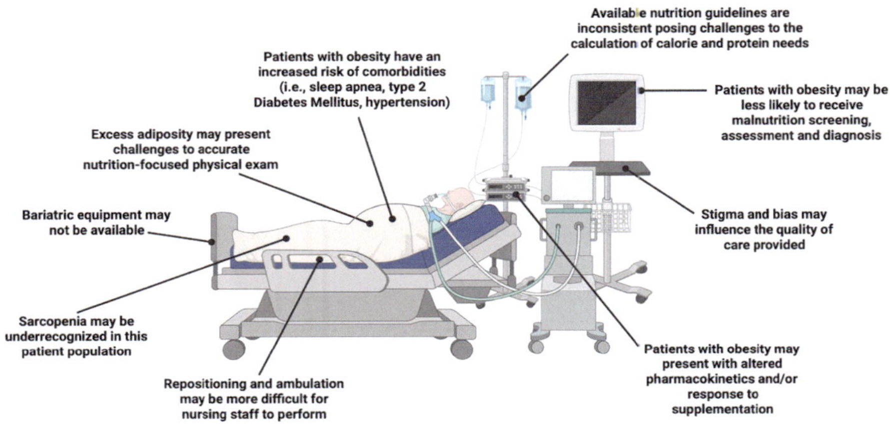

Fig. 15.1 This figure summarizes various factors that can complicate the care of critically ill patients with obesity. These factors are depicted visually to help better understand their interplay and potential impact on patient outcomes [17]. This is an open-access article distributed under the terms of the Creative Commons CC BY license, which permits unrestricted use, distribution, and reproduction in any medium, provided the original work is properly cited

State equation is considered to be the most accurate (REE = $(1.1 \times \text{value of HBE}) + (140 \times T_{max}) + (32 \times VE) - 5340$) [13].

The prevalence of obesity in patients admitted to the ICU has been reported to range between 28.2% and 36%, indicating an increasing trend in recent years [14–16]. Patients in the ICU that are overweight or obese require individualized nutrition plans due to underlying comorbidities, immunological factors such as inflammation, and changes in energy expenditure and metabolism. Despite ongoing research, knowledge gaps persist in recognizing and managing the complex nutritional needs of this population. Available malnutrition screening tools are limited in patients with obesity, and estimations of energy and protein demands are complex and may require the use of ideal, actual, or adjusted body weight [17]. The 2016 guidelines from ASPEN/SCCM recommend fewer calories and a high-protein diet for obese ICU patients [4]. A personalized approach to nutritional management that achieves higher protein intake without overfeeding energy is appropriate. While a high-protein regimen may be preferred, the duration and ideal protein delivery during hypocaloric feeding are debated. A target of 2–2.5 g/kg ideal body weight per day is considered reasonable for critically ill patients with obesity [11]. Monitoring patients for adequate protein is challenging, as proper interpretation of nitrogen balance results remains unclear (Fig. 15.1).

Nutritional and Metabolic Needs After Spinal Cord Injury

In contrast to other trauma patients, patients with SCI do not demonstrate hypermetabolism following injury. This patient population exhibits a negative nitrogen balance, and while this is typical, correcting this negative nitrogen balance by increasing caloric intake is problematic, as it can result in overfeeding. Overfeeding has its risks which include hypercapnia, hyperglycemia, uremia, and hypertriglyceridemia [18]. The time course over which overfeeding can cause these issues can vary depending on the individual and the amount of overfeeding. In general, hypercapnia and hyperglycemia may occur relatively quickly within a few hours or days of overfeeding. Uremia and hypertriglyceridemia may take longer to develop, potentially over several days or weeks of overfeeding. However, it is important to note that these risks can be mitigated by careful monitoring and individualized nutritional management in the ICU setting [18]. Due to the lack of rigorous SCI nutritional research, there are currently limited dietary recommendations that capture the unique nutrient needs for this population. A systematic review outlines recommended answers to three key clinical questions with regard to nutritional metabolic needs in patients with SCI. Multiple studies document metabolic abnormalities following SCI, including the obligatory negative nitrogen balance introduced above [19]. These patients have unique requirements mandating the development of specific treatment protocols. The recommendation was strong, and the data was moderate [18–20]. Equations overestimate and overfeed this population by as high as 70% [18, 20, 21]. With regard to methods applicable in evaluating metabolic demands among patients with SCI, the use of indirect calorimetry is most accurate. Indirect calorimetry measures oxygen consumption and carbon dioxide production to determine energy expenditure. It is performed by having the patient breathe into a mask or mouthpiece while measuring gas concentrations. However, the recommendation for indirect calorimetry is classified as weak due to limited data, despite the accuracy of the literature to date using this technique. Future multicenter clinical trials are needed to develop comprehensive, evidence-based dietary reference values specific for persons with SCI across the care continuum that rely on accurate, individualized energy needs assessments.

Given the state of the literature, it is difficult to provide recommendations around treatment protocols. Persons with SCI are instructed to adopt a healthy diet, the challenge is defining what a healthy diet for this population looks like. Evidence-based guidelines to ameliorate the risks of obesity and central metabolic syndrome did not exist for the SCI population until recently. The Paralyzed Veterans of America (PVA) guidelines are the first comprehensive publication to provide data-driven recommendations on healthy eating for individuals with SCI but do know that the quality of evidence is restrained by small sample sizes and known literature [20]. PVA guidelines recommend energetic assessment utilizing indirect calorimetry to determine energy expenditure and assess energy needs to implement a heart-healthy nutrition plan focusing on vegetables, fruits, poultry, fish, low-fat dairy products, whole grains, legumes, nuts, and non-tropical vegetable oils, while limiting sweets, sugar-sweetened beverages, and red meats [20].

Neurogenic Obesity

Although this chapter focuses on post-injury critical care, neurogenic obesity is important to consider in relation to this topic. Neurogenic obesity may result from changes in body composition, physical impairment, and endo metabolic physiology that occur when dietary intake exceeds energy expenditure. Given the post-injury reductions in lean body mass, sympathetic nervous system dysfunction, and anabolic deficiencies, energy balance is no longer in balance, and thereby an obesogenic environment can be easily created that facilitates cardiometabolic dysfunction. Accurate determination of metabolic rate can prevent excess caloric intake while promoting positive body habitus and mitigating obesity-related comorbidities [20].

Enteral Feeding

Enteral feeding is preferred to parenteral feeding. It is more physiologic and associated with fewer complications. It is highly supported that utilizing the gut with enteral nutrition helps to prevent gut atrophy, preserve normal gut flora, reduce endotoxin translocation, and maintain gut barrier function [22, 23]. Maintaining gut barrier function in TBI is important because studies have shown that the gut barrier can become compromised after TBI, leading to an increased risk of infections and sepsis. The gut barrier can be more permeable in patients with TBI than in trauma patients without TBI, and this increased permeability can contribute to the systemic inflammatory response commonly observed after TBI. Additionally, the disruption of the gut barrier in TBI shares similarities with blood-brain barrier (BBB) dysfunction after TBI, further emphasizing the importance of maintaining gut barrier function in these patients. Strategies for maintaining gut barrier function among patients with TBI may include early enteral feeding [24, 25]. Intestinal motility is affected by pathological processes such as fasting, mechanical ventilation while on paralytics, high-dose opioids, infection, sepsis, neurological compromise, and immobility [26].

Enteral nutrition is a routine aspect of in-hospital care that can have great benefit with regard to functional and clinical outcomes. Early enteral nutrition has been shown to significantly decrease mortality, the risk of metabolic derangements, pressure ulcer formation, and hepatobiliary dysfunction among patients with TBI. Enteral tube feeding is used to deliver nutrition and is most used during critical care—including in populations with dysphagia, altered mental state, intestinal and associated organ impairments, dysmotility, and other related diagnoses. If enteral feeds do not meet the metabolic demands within 5 days of injury, total parenteral nutrition should be started to ensure adequate caloric intake.

Several feeding strategies should be considered when initiating enteral nutrition. First, the patient's head needs to be elevated by 30–45° off the bed to decrease risk for reflux and aspiration. Second, graduated feeding may be attempted in patients initially intolerant to enteral nutrition. These patients can be started at 20 mL/h and advanced to their specific goal by 10–20 mL/h every 6–8 h. Further, continuous enteral nutrition is well tolerated compared to bolus enteral nutrition. However, bolus enteral feeds may have advantages once continuous enteral feeding goals are reached, mimicking gastric feeding and reducing the number of lines attached to restless and/or agitated patients.

Refeeding Syndrome

Refeeding syndrome can occur in patients with severe TBI and SCI during the initial phase of care. This condition is characterized by metabolic and electrolyte disturbances that can lead to serious complications, including cardiac failure, respiratory distress, seizures, and even death. Refeeding syndrome is caused by the rapid reintroduction of carbohydrates, fats, and proteins in malnourished individuals who have been fasting or receiving inadequate nutrition for an extended period. This sudden influx of nutrients can stimulate insulin secretion, leading to an increase in cellular uptake of potassium, phosphate, and magnesium. As a result, serum levels of these electrolytes may fall rapidly, leading to hypophosphatemia, hypokalemia, and hypomagnesemia. This condition can be prevented by early slow and cautious reintroduction of nutrition, close monitoring of serum electrolytes, and prompt correction of any imbalances. A multidisciplinary team including a physician and dietitian should work together to develop an individualized nutrition plan for each patient to minimize the risk of refeeding syndrome [4].

Percutaneous Endoscopic Gastrostomy (PEG) or Radiologically Inserted Gastrostomy (RIG) Tubes

When oral feeding is not possible, nasogastric, nasojejunal, and gastrostomy tube (in that order) may be necessary. Trans gastric-jejunal feeding is recommended to reduce the incidence of ventilator-associated pneumonia during critical illness. If the need for enteral nutrition exceeds 2–4 weeks, gastrostomy tube may be preferable. Evaluating timing of gastrostomy tube placement was studied in a large retrospective population study involving a TBI cohort; this study found that patients undergoing an early or late gastrostomy tube placement had a higher rate of in-hospital mortality, when compared with patients with a standard timing (7–14 days) of gastrostomy tube placement. Late placement was preferred in patients with higher Charleston index and trauma-related comorbidities, and these patients had a higher incidence of complications such as sepsis, urinary tract infection, acute respiratory distress syndrome/pneumonia, and deep vein thrombosis/pulmonary embolism [27]. It is important to note that a duotube/dobhoff can remain in place for an average of 29 days, with a variance of 5–151 days, based on a study for head and neck cancer patients who underwent radiation treatment. There were no serious medical complications associated with having the nasogastric tube in place [28].

Gastrostomy tube insertion is a common practice, whether in endoscopy suites or interventional radiology. Overall, procedure-related mortality is 1–2% [29]. However, there are associated risks, including failure of insertion, peristomal infection, leaking, and bleeding. Very low infection rates have been noted due to the use of prophylactic antibiotics [30]. Potentially serious complications include peritonitis, colonic perforation, and necrotizing fasciitis. Notably, a benign pneumoperitoneum is detectable on chest or abdominal radiography in 38% of patients after PEG insertion [31].

After gastrostomy placement, practitioners need to consider the appropriate time for removal. The patient must meet all caloric and hydration needs by mouth adequately and have minimal risk for aspiration to consider removal. Depending on body habitus, surgeon, and other complicating factors associated with the procedure or placement, a gastrostomy tube cannot be removed at the earliest, until 4–8 weeks post-procedure. Obese patients should wait for at least 6 weeks before gastrostomy tube removal.

Some patients experience diarrhea, reflux, aspiration, or low motility following injury. Caveats or considerations include tube feed formulations, medication options around PPI, H2 blockers, and probiotic use, need for a gastro-jejunal tube placement which bypasses the stomach, consistent bowel programs, and gut health evaluation. Medication options such as motility agents like Erythromycin or Reglan should be considered last given their side effect profiles. Erythromycin according to the National Institutes of Health is known to cause unpleasant side effects and is not approved by the FDA to treat gastroparesis. There have only been four studies demonstrating fair benefit with poor quality evidence. Side effects to note for erythromycin include stomach pain, nausea, vomiting, and diarrhea. Severe but rare side effects include hearing loss, allergic reactions, liver problems, heart arrhythmias, and bowel swelling [21]. Reglan should be used with caution in the TBI population, as it can impact recovery given this drug's dopamine D2 antagonist properties. Additionally, the FDA has a black box warning on Reglan due to its risk of tardive dyskinesia, citing up to 15% of patients who experience this complication. Reglan is most appropriate for short-term gastroparesis (approximately 3 weeks); any treatment beyond this timeframe has not been demonstrated to be effective and is associated with an increased risk for tardive dyskinesia. Additional side effects include acute dystonic reactions and akathisia. Risk-benefit needs to be evaluated prior to starting treatment in patients on antiseizure treatments, as well as patients with diabetes and liver disease [32].

Nutritional Supplements and the Gut Microbiome

A growing area of interest in understanding TBI and SCI pathophysiology is the role of nutritional support in mitigating injury sequelae. Nutritional support is essential given that the human brain consumes 20% of total resting energy. Nutritional deficits are often coupled with poor functional outcomes and optimization of nutritional care in critically ill patients is needed to improve short- and long-term recovery [7]. Timing and route of nutritional therapy are essential to treat TBI and SCI. Several new human and animal studies propose that probiotics contain large numbers of lactic acid-producing bacteria, which activate gut-associated immune cells that can inhibit inflammation. These immune cells (regulatory T cells) could prevent extra damage to the spinal cord after injury. Research into the role of the gut microbiota in modulating CNS function has been rapidly increasing in the past few decades, particularly in animal models. Growing preclinical and clinical evidence suggests that the gut microbiota is involved in the modulation of multiple cellular and molecular mechanisms fundamental to the progression of acute CNS injury-induced pathophysiological processes. The altered composition of gut microbiota after acute CNS injury damages the equilibrium of the bidirectional gut-brain axis, aggravating secondary brain injury, cognitive impairments, and motor dysfunctions, which leads to poor prognosis by triggering pro-inflammatory responses in both peripheral circulation and the CNS. Experimental models suggest a bidirectional communication between the gut and CNS in facilitating post-injury gut dysbiosis, intestinal lymphatic tissue-mediated neuroinflammation, and bacterial-metabolite-associated neurotransmission [33]. There are no formal management recommendations at this time with regard to pre- and probiotics, but it is a growing area of research.

In addition, there are several studies ongoing with regard to vitamins and minerals to improve outcomes. Support for using vitamins, minerals, and supplements in treating TBI has increased in recent years. These findings are concisely summarized in Tables 15.1 and 15.2 [7].

Table 15.1 Supplementation of vitamins and minerals in preclinical models of TBI [7]

Vitamins and minerals	Dosage used	Proposed/suggested mechanism	Findings
ATRA (vitamin A metabolite)	10 mg/kg	Anti-inflammatory and anti-apoptotic effects	Brain protective effects but no improvement in neurological and motor deficits in a mouse TBI model
Vitamin B2 (riboflavin) and magnesium	7.5 mg/kg (vitamin B2); 1 mmol/kg (magnesium)	Antioxidant effects	Reduced behavioral impairments, lesion size, edema formation, and expression of GFAP in a rat TBI model. Synergistic with magnesium
Magnesium sulfate and n-acetyl L tryptophan	30 mg/kg (magnesium); 2.5 mg/kg (n-acetyl L tryptophan)	Antioxidant effects	Reduced BBB permeability and improved functional outcomes in a rat TBI model
Vitamin B3 (nicotinamide)	50 mg/kg, 500 mg/kg, or continuous infusion of 12 mg/kg/h with LD of 75 mg/kg	Increased cellular energy as an NAD+ precursor	Neuroprotective effects and alleviation of behavioral deficits in a rat TBI model. Synergistic with progesterone
Vitamin B6 (pyridoxine)	300 mg/kg or 600 mg/kg	Increased oxygen delivery to damaged tissues	Alleviation of locomotor behavioral deficits in a rat TBI model. However, only the 600 mg/kg dose showed tissue sparing effect

(continued)

Table 15.1 (continued)

Vitamins and minerals	Dosage used	Proposed/suggested mechanism	Findings
Vitamin B9 (folic acid)	80 μg/kg or 800 μg/kg	Decreased homocysteine levels	(1) Early functional recovery in female TBI piglets treated with 80 μg/kg; (2) No improvement in behavioral outcomes in rats post-TBI treated with 80 μg/kg (low dose) or 800 μg/kg (high dose). Moreover, 800 μg/kg dose worsened neuronal loss
Vitamin B12 (cobalamin)	0.5 mg/kg or 1.5 mg/kg	Downregulation of the endoplasmic reticulum stress-related apoptosis	Improvement in neurological functional recovery in a mouse TBI model
Vitamin C (ascorbic acid) and vitamin E (α-tocopherol)	45 mg/kg or 60 mg/kg (vitamin C); 45 mg/kg or 60 mg/kg (vitamin E)	Improved SOD activity	Reduction of oxidative stress in a rat TBI model
Vitamin C (ascorbic acid) and simvastatin	20 mg/kg (ascorbic acid) and 15 mg/kg (simvastatin)	Diminished vascular inflammatory response	Combination treatment with ascorbic acid and simvastatin improved neurological recovery in a rat TBI model
Vitamin D and progesterone	1 μg/kg (vitamin D) and 16 mg/kg (progesterone)	Anti-inflammatory effects	Reduced markers of inflammation and neuronal cell death were observed in a rat TBI model Synergistic with progesterone
Vitamin E (α-tocopherol)	500 IU/kg	Involvement of BDNF and Sir2	Improved cognition scores in a mouse TBI model
Vitamin E (α-tocopherol)	2 IU/g chow diet	Reduction in lipid peroxidation	Decreased amyloidosis and improved memory impairment in Alzheimer's disease mouse post-TBI
Zinc	180 ppm	Attenuation of redox signaling	Reduced neuropsychiatric symptoms in a rat TBI model
Selenium	1.5 mg/kg	Antioxidant effect	Reduction in lipid peroxidation in a rat TBI model
Melatonin	5 mg/kg	Attenuation of oxidative stress	Reduction in lipid peroxidation in a rat TBI model

ATRA all-trans retinoic acid, *BBB* blood-brain barrier, *BNDF* brain-derived neurotrophic factor, *GFAP* glial fibrillary acidic protein, *NAD+*; *Sir2* silent information regulator 2, *SOD* superoxide dismutase, *TBI* traumatic brain injury

Table 15.2 Dietary supplement uses in clinical and preclinical models of TBI [7]

Dietary supplements	Dosage used	Proposed/suggested mechanism	Findings
Creatine	400 mg/kg	Increased phosphocreatine levels and ATP-buffering capability	Reduction of headache frequency, fatigue, and dizziness in a pilot study of 39 adolescents post-TBI. Up to 50% reduction of cortical damage in a rat TBI model
DHA	10 mg/kg/day or 40 mg/kg/day	Increase in antioxidant capacity molecules, including SOD and Sir2	Decreased axonal injury and apoptotic markers in a rat TBI model
Curcumin	500 ppm	Involvement of BDNF	Reduction in oxidative stress, conserved synaptic plasticity, and cognitive function in a rat TBI model
Resveratrol	100 mg/kg	(1) Action via heme oxygenase-1; (2) suppression of the NLRP3 inflammasome	Reduced neuroinflammation and secondary brain injury in a mice mTBI model
Enzogenol	1000 mg/day	Anti-inflammatory and antioxidant effects	Improved cognitive function in a phase II RCT in patients treated for mild TBI
Sulforaphane	5 mg/kg	Induction of Nrf2-driven genes	Reduced cerebral edema and BBB permeability in a rat TBI model. Working memory also improved
Ginseng	20–80 mg/kg	(1) Increased expression of NGF, GDNF, NCAM, and BrdU/nestin neural stem cells; (2) Decreased apoptotic cell death, downregulation of inflammatory cytokines, upregulation of anti-inflammatory interleukin-10, and increased SOD activity	Improved recovery of neurological function and reduced neuronal cell loss in a rat TBI model
Astaxanthin	25 mg/kg or 75 mg/kg	Increased BDNF, GAP-43, and SYP expression	Neuroprotection improved sensorimotor and enhanced cognitive function in a mouse TBI model
Melatonin	5 mg/kg	Attenuation of oxidative stress	Reduction in lipid peroxidation in a rat TBI model

(continued)

Table 15.2 (continued)

Dietary supplements	Dosage used	Proposed/suggested mechanism	Findings
N-Acetylcysteine	(1) 150 mg/kg (rat study); (2) 4 g loading dose followed by 4 g for 4 days and 3 g for 3 days (human study)	Attenuation of oxidative stress	(1) Reduction in lipid peroxidation in a rat TBI model; (2) Resolution of early sequelae of blast-induced mTBI
Pycnogenol	150 mg/kg	Attenuation of oxidative stress	Ameliorated oxidative stress, synaptic protein loss, and inflammatory cytokines in a rat TBI model

BBB blood-brain barrier, *BDNF* brain-derived neurotrophic factor, *BrdU* bromodeoxyuridine, *DHA* docosahexaenoic acid, *GDNF* glial cell line-derived neurotrophic factor, *NGF* nerve growth factor, *NCAM* neuronal cell adhesion molecule, *NSC* neural stem cell, *NLRP3* nucleotide-binding domain, leucine-rich-containing family, pyrin domain-containing-3, *Nrf2* nuclear factor erythroid 2-related factor 2, *RCT* randomized controlled trial, *Sir2* silent information regulator 2, *SOD* superoxide dismutase, *TBI* traumatic brain injury

Case Illustration

The PM&R consultation service is consulted on a 43-year-old male who suffered a severe traumatic brain injury (TBI) following a motor vehicle accident. He was admitted to the intensive care unit and required mechanical ventilation and sedation. His Glasgow Coma Scale (GCS) score was 5 on admission.

Feeding was started via an oro-gastric feeding tube using the standard ICU feeding protocol within 24–48 h of injury, with a polymeric 1.5 kcal/ml feed at 50 ml/h. Gastric residual volumes increased throughout the day up to 450 ml at every 4-h check. The unit feeding protocol stated that gastric aspirates should be replaced up to 250 ml and the remainder discarded. Due to the discarding of gastric aspirates and the inability to increase the feed rate because of poor enteral tolerance, the patient was unable to meet the target nutritional requirements. The PM&R consultation service recommended avoiding metoclopramide and starting erythromycin as a short-term prokinetic.

Due to ongoing high gastric residual volumes and failure to meet target enteral feed volumes, the dietitian recommended changing the patient to Peptamen® HN (1500 ml/day to provide 1995 kcal, 99 g protein). Gastric residual volumes reduced to between 0 and 160 ml at every 4-h check. Sedation and ventilation were being weaned, and the patient was beginning to awaken. Feeding was continued with Peptamen® HN but increased to 1750 ml/day due to a reassessment of nutritional requirements via the Harris-Benedict equation, physical examination, and daily weights. The new feed regimen provided 2188 kcal and 110 g of protein daily. Enteral absorption improved with this change, allowing the patient's total dietary needs to be met. The patient was extubated, and a duodenal tube was placed by nursing to allow for post-pyloric feeding as a precautionary measure.

As the patient's condition stabilized, he underwent early PEG tube placement as prolonged dysphagia was anticipated based on speech therapy assessment. The PEG tube was placed under endoscopic guidance, with a low-profile feeding device secured to the abdominal wall. Feeding was continued with Peptamen® HN via the PEG tube. In addition to the enteral formula, appropriate nutritional supplements were provided to the patient as recommended by the consult service. These included vitamin D and vitamin B12 supplements to prevent deficiencies that can occur with long-term enteral feeding. The patient also received fish oil supplements to support brain health and reduce inflammation. The patient was monitored for signs of refeeding syndrome, and electrolyte abnormalities were corrected as necessary. The patient's nutritional support was monitored and adjusted throughout his recovery, with regular reassessments of his dietary needs and tolerance by the treatment team and dietician.

Summary and Key Points

- Malnutrition is a highly prevalent complication in the acute hospital setting and requires immediate attention. It can have adverse outcomes on the TBI and SCI populations while critically ill.
- Early enteral nutrition has been demonstrated to improve functional and clinical outcomes in most clinical settings by reducing hospital LOS, cost, morbidity, and mortality.
- Early enteral nutrition is feasible and maintains intestinal physiologic preservation, and there are considerations around the gut microbiome and its connection to the CNS with growing animal and human trials looking at outcomes.
- PEG tube placement is a common practice that supports early enteral nutrition support with low risk; it is important to understand the timing for placement, removal, and situations that warrant gastro-jejunal tube use.

References[1]

1. Barker NN, Himchak MV. Environmental issues affecting elder abuse victims in their reception of community based services. J Gerontol Soc Work. 2006;48(1-2):233–55. https://doi.org/10.1300/J083v48n01_16.
2. Weiss AJ, Fingar KR, Barrett ML, et al. Statistical brief #210. Characteristics of hospital stays involving malnutrition, 2013. 2016.
3. White JV, Guenter P, Jensen G, et al. Consensus statement: Academy of Nutrition and Dietetics and American Society for Parenteral and Enteral Nutrition. J Parenter Enter Nutr. 2012;36(3):275–83. https://doi.org/10.1177/0148607112440285.
4. McClave SA, Taylor BE, Martindale RG, et al. Guidelines for the provision and assessment of nutrition support therapy in the adult critically ill patient: Society of Critical Care Medicine

[1] Key References [3–5, 12, 27].

(SCCM) and American Society for Parenteral and Enteral Nutrition (A.S.P.E.N.). JPEN J Parenter Enteral Nutr. 2016;40(2):159–211. https://doi.org/10.1177/0148607115621863.
5. Lee HY, Oh B-M. Nutrition management in patients with traumatic brain injury: a narrative review. Brain Neurorehabil. 2022;15(1):e4.
6. Dash HH, Chavali S. Management of traumatic brain injury patients. Korean J Anesthesiol. 2018;71(1):12–21. https://doi.org/10.4097/kjae.2018.71.1.12.
7. Nwafor D, Goeckeritz J, Hasanpour Z, Davidson C, Lucke-Wold B. Nutritional support following traumatic brain injury: a comprehensive review. Expl Res Hypothesis Med. 2022. https://doi.org/10.14218/ERHM.2022.00086.
8. Chapple LA, Chapman MJ, Lange K, Deane AM, Heyland DK. Nutrition support practices in critically ill head-injured patients: a global perspective. Crit Care. 2016;20:6. https://doi.org/10.1186/s13054-015-1177-1.
9. Carney N, Totten AM, O'Reilly C, et al. Guidelines for the management of severe traumatic brain injury, fourth edition. Neurosurgery. 2017;80(1):6–15. https://doi.org/10.1227/neu.0000000000001432.
10. Moonen HPFX, Beckers KJH, van Zanten ARH. Energy expenditure and indirect calorimetry in critical illness and convalescence: current evidence and practical considerations. J Intensive Care. 2021;9(1):8. https://doi.org/10.1186/s40560-021-00524-0.
11. Compher C, Bingham AL, McCall M, et al. Guidelines for the provision of nutrition support therapy in the adult critically ill patient: The American Society for Parenteral and Enteral Nutrition. J Parenter Enter Nutr. 2022;46(1):12–41. https://doi.org/10.1002/jpen.2267.
12. Matters K, Murray EJ, Mok V, Flower O. Protein requirements in traumatic brain injury: a systematic review. Australas J Neurosci. 2014;24(1):42–8.
13. Institute of Medicine (US). 2: Nutrition in clinical practice guidelines for traumatic brain injury. In: Erdman J, Oria M, Pillsbury L, editors. Nutrition and traumatic brain injury: improving acute and subacute health outcomes in military personnel. Washington: National Academies Press; 2011.
14. Alexopoulos AS, Fayfman M, Zhao L, et al. Impact of obesity on hospital complications and mortality in hospitalized patients with hyperglycemia and diabetes. BMJ Open Diabetes Res Care. 2016;4(1):e000200. https://doi.org/10.1136/bmjdrc-2016-000200.
15. Abhyankar S, Leishear K, Callaghan FM, Demner-Fushman D, McDonald CJ. Lower short- and long-term mortality associated with overweight and obesity in a large cohort study of adult intensive care unit patients. Crit Care. 2012;16(6):R235. https://doi.org/10.1186/cc11903.
16. Finkielman JD, Gajic O, Afessa B. Underweight is independently associated with mortality in post-operative and non-operative patients admitted to the intensive care unit: a retrospective study. BMC Emerg Med. 2004;4(1):3. https://doi.org/10.1186/1471-227x-4-3.
17. Dickerson RN, Andromalos L, Brown JC, et al. Obesity and critical care nutrition: current practice gaps and directions for future research. Crit Care. 2022;26(1):283. https://doi.org/10.1186/s13054-022-04148-0.
18. Farkas GJ, Sneij A, McMillan DW, Tiozzo E, Nash MS, Gater DR. Energy expenditure and nutrient intake after spinal cord injury: a comprehensive review and practical recommendations. Br J Nutr. 2022;128(5):863–87. https://doi.org/10.1017/s0007114521003822.
19. Thibault-Halman G, Casha S, Singer S, Christie S. Acute management of nutritional demands after spinal cord injury. J Neurotrauma. 2011;28(8):1497–507. https://doi.org/10.1089/neu.2009.1155.
20. Farkas GJ, Sneij A, Gater DR Jr. Energy expenditure following spinal cord injury: a delicate balance. Top Spinal Cord Inj Rehabil. 2021;27(1):92–9. https://doi.org/10.46292/sci20-00030.
21. National Institute for Health and Care Excellence. Erythromycin for gastroparesis (delayed stomach emptying). Bazian Ltd.; 2013. https://www.nice.org.uk/advice/esuom13/resources/erythromycin-for-gastroparesis-delayed-stomach-emptying-pdf-17474679493.
22. Moore FA, Moore EE, Poggetti R, et al. Gut bacterial translocation via the portal vein: a clinical perspective with major torso trauma. J Trauma. 1991;31(5):629–36; discussion 636-8. https://doi.org/10.1097/00005373-199105000-00006.

23. Kudsk KA, Croce MA, Fabian TC, et al. Enteral versus parenteral feeding. Effects on septic morbidity after blunt and penetrating abdominal trauma. Ann Surg. 1992;215(5):503–11; discussion 511-3. https://doi.org/10.1097/00000658-199205000-00013.
24. Hanscom M, Loane DJ, Shea-Donohue T. Brain-gut axis dysfunction in the pathogenesis of traumatic brain injury. J Clin Invest. 2021;131(12):43777. https://doi.org/10.1172/jci143777.
25. Katzenberger RJ, Ganetzky B, Wassarman DA. The gut reaction to traumatic brain injury. Fly. 2015;9(2):68–74. https://doi.org/10.1080/19336934.2015.1085623.
26. Bosscha K, Nieuwenhuijs VB, Vos A, Samsom M, Roelofs JM, Akkermans LM. Gastrointestinal motility and gastric tube feeding in mechanically ventilated patients. Crit Care Med. 1998;26(9):1510–7. https://doi.org/10.1097/00003246-199809000-00017.
27. Chaudhry R, Kukreja N, Tse A, et al. Trends and outcomes of early versus late percutaneous endoscopic gastrostomy placement in patients with traumatic brain injury: nationwide population-based study. J Neurosurg Anesthesiol. 2018;30(3):251–7. https://doi.org/10.1097/ANA.0000000000000434.
28. Coke A, Gilbert M, Hill S, Siddiqui F. Nasogastric feeding tube/dobhoff placement: a multidisciplinary approach to the management of malnutrition during radiation therapy in patients with head and neck cancer. Cureus. 2022;14(5):e24905. https://doi.org/10.7759/cureus.24905.
29. Nicholson FB, Korman MG, Richardson MA. Percutaneous endoscopic gastrostomy: a review of indications, complications and outcome. J Gastroenterol Hepatol. 2000;15(1):21–5. https://doi.org/10.1046/j.1440-1746.2000.02004.x.
30. Preclik G, Grüne S, Leser HG, et al. Prospective, randomised, double blind trial of prophylaxis with single dose of co-amoxiclav before percutaneous endoscopic gastrostomy. BMJ. 1999;319(7214):881–4. https://doi.org/10.1136/bmj.319.7214.881.
31. Pidala MJ, Slezak FA, Porter JA. Pneumoperitoneum following percutaneous endoscopic gastrostomy. Does the timing of panendoscopy matter? Surg Endosc. 1992;6(3):128–9. https://doi.org/10.1007/bf02309084.
32. Lee A, Kuo B. Metoclopramide in the treatment of diabetic gastroparesis. Expert Rev Endocrinol Metab. 2010;5(5):653–62. https://doi.org/10.1586/eem.10.41.
33. Yuan B, Lu XJ, Wu Q. Gut microbiota and acute central nervous system injury: a new target for therapeutic intervention. Front Immunol. 2021;12:800796. https://doi.org/10.3389/fimmu.2021.800796.

Chapter 16
Early Mobility—Multimodal Effects on Function

Julie Lanphere

Chapter Objectives

1. Understand the negative sequelae of bed rest and immobility.
2. Understand how immobility contributes to long-term cognitive impairments, poor healthcare outcomes, cost, and hospital length of stay.
3. Define immobility harm, its contributions to post-hospital syndrome, and functional impairments as a result of critical illness in diverse populations and how their vulnerability can be impacted.
4. Understand cognitive long-term outcomes in critically ill patients.
5. Understand how current studies demonstrate improved outcomes because of structured mobility programs, the importance of data, standardization, and multidisciplinary team rounding in early mobility programs for neurological and medically complex patients.
6. Understand the unique considerations for early mobility implementation and goal setting for the neurotrauma population.

Introduction

The negative effect of hospitalization on patient mobility has been recognized in the literature since the 1940s and is now identified as a potential impediment to recovery [1–4]. There is now a paradigm shift in care towards early mobility programs as hospitals work to improve clinical outcomes. Physical inactivity and bed rest in the hospitalized patient has long been viewed as a primary factor contributing to functional decline and a mitigating factor contributing to clinical complications and poorer outcomes [1, 5, 6]. Hospital-acquired physical impairments are associated with increased hospital length of stay (LOS), hospital-acquired complications, nursing facility and acute inpatient rehabilitation admissions, and impaired physical functioning months to years after

J. Lanphere (✉)
Intermountain Medical Center, Murray, UT, USA
e-mail: julie.lanphere@imail.org

A. K. Wagner, J. Weppner (eds.), *Acute Care Neuroconsultation and Neurorehabilitation Management*, https://doi.org/10.1007/978-3-031-42830-2_16

hospitalization [1]. Patients with traumatic brain injury (TBI), spinal cord injury (SCI), or stroke suffer impairments that require critical care and a focus on early spontaneous breathing and awakening trials, which is key to allowing for optimal neuro assessment, stimulating neuroplasticity, and promoting early mobilization towards recovery.

Mobility Culture Shift

There was an effort in the early 2000s to revolutionize immobility and sedation practices in the intensive care unit (ICU). The Herridge trials demonstrated 1- and 5-year outcomes in survivors with acute respiratory distress syndrome (ARDS)—including persistent physical and cognitive impairments post-discharge [7–11]. This work sparked a broader conversation and the introduction of the ABCDEF bundle into clinical care [12–14]—of which mobility is a key aspect [9]. The ABCDEF bundle is a framework for managing the care of critically ill patients in the ICU, consisting of six key components: awakening and breathing coordination, both spontaneous awakening trials and spontaneous breathing trials, choice of analgesia and sedation, delirium assessment, prevention, and management, early mobility and exercise, and family engagement and empowerment. Delirium is a common neuropsychiatric syndrome in acquired brain injury and is characterized by acute onset and fluctuating course, inattention, and altered level of consciousness. One of the potential complications of delirium is impaired mobility, which can lead to functional decline and further exacerbate the patient's overall health status. Research has shown that there is a bidirectional relationship between delirium and mobility [15, 16]. On the one hand, delirium can lead to decreased mobility due to the patient's altered level of consciousness, inattention, and overall weakness. On the other hand, impaired mobility can contribute to the development of delirium, as it can cause a decrease in cognitive stimulation and sensory input, leading to sensory deprivation and increased delirium risk [15, 17, 18]. A study by Inouye et al. found that patients with delirium had significantly lower mobility levels than those without delirium. The study also showed that the incidence of delirium was significantly higher among patients with impaired mobility compared to those without impaired mobility. These findings suggest that impaired mobility is not only a consequence of delirium but also a risk factor for its development [16]. Early mobilization can have a positive impact on preventing delirium and improving patient outcomes. A study by Balas et al. found that an early mobilization protocol led to a significant decrease in the incidence of delirium among critically ill patients. The study also showed that early mobilization improved patients' overall functional status and reduced the length of hospital stay [19].

The ABCDEF bundle is designed to promote better outcomes by reducing the duration of mechanical ventilation, improving cognitive function, and enhancing overall quality of life for critically ill patients. This bundle represents an evidence-based guide for clinicians to approach ICU patient recovery and outcomes with a variety of diagnoses. In Neuro ICUs and trauma centers, a major focus is placed on wakefulness and neuro exams. However, nursing and therapy-led early mobility programs have demonstrated there is room for improvement in these populations. For neurologically impaired patients, the focus around spontaneous breathing and awakening trials is beneficial for recovery and neuronal sprouting [14, 20–23]. Additionally, these strategies in the SCI population afford opportunities around diaphragm activation, strength assessment, respiratory muscle utilization, advocacy for skin integrity, and key functional assessments. Care coordination rounds in ICUs all over the world can prioritize mobility in their care plans, with a focus on early mobilization and rehabilitation for critically ill patients. Algorithmic considerations and key decision points in using the ABCDEF bundle include identifying appropriate patients for early mobilization and determining their level of mobility. The patient's medical condition, level of sedation, and presence of delirium are all important factors to consider when deciding whether to initiate early mobilization. If an institution does not have the ABCDEF bundle available, there are still ways to prioritize mobility when caring for critically ill patients. For example, consulting physiatrists implement and recommend early mobilization and rehabilitation programs, prioritize delirium screening and management, and collaborate with the ICU staff to minimize the use of sedatives and promote wakefulness. It is important to note, however, that the use of a structured approach like the ABCDEF bundle has been shown to improve patient outcomes, including reducing the duration of mechanical ventilation, reducing the incidence of delirium, and improving functional outcomes [15, 17, 18]. Institutions that have not yet implemented the ABCDEF bundle should consider doing so as part of their care coordination rounds. Physiatrists can play a key role in this process by promoting and facilitating the implementation of the ABCDEF bundle at their institution.

In addition to the benefits of early mobilization for reducing delirium and improving outcomes such as functional status and quality of life, there is growing recognition of the importance of addressing other specific needs of patients with TBI, SCI, and stroke. This includes implementing bowel and bladder programs contracture prevention programs, and seating and positioning interventions. By integrating these interventions into care coordination rounds, healthcare teams can provide more comprehensive and patient-centered care for critically ill patients with TBI, SCI, and stroke. Additionally, the ABCDEF bundle enables family engagement and empowerment, resulting in patients and families receiving more assistance with post-ICU syndrome management at discharge.

Speech-language pathologists (SLPs) and occupational therapists (OTs) are being utilized far more routinely, improving the standardization of testing and management plans and raising awareness among all providers caring for these patients about the impairments present. Awareness around the need for measurement, prospective randomized control trials, and observational studies are rising. The ABCDEF bundle has facilitated a conducive environment for research in neurocritical care, resulting in greater engagement from healthcare professionals across multiple disciplines, including nurses and therapists. ABCDEF bundle implementation has not only demonstrated its efficacy in improving patient outcomes in critical care but also promoted a collaborative culture among healthcare professionals, which is essential for delivering high-quality patient care. These developments have far-reaching implications, for critical illness populations and also for the healthcare system, emphasizing the importance of a multidisciplinary approach to care. Multidisciplinary care is becoming standard in ICUs and acute hospital units and is no longer limited to the inpatient rehabilitation setting—where a multidisciplinary approach is more readily implemented to improve healthcare-related outcomes. The acute care focus has been reoriented to prioritize the patient moving out of bed for meals, improved practices and protocols for orientation to day/time, improvement of muscle strength with gait and transfer activities, and other intentional activities to increase mobility.

Mobility Assessment

The impact of mobility on clinical outcomes requires a pragmatic use of the research data informing early mobility. Patients with neurologic disabilities have specific care needs, such as muscle weakness, spasticity, hemispatial neglect, and impulsivity, which therapy-driven care mobility initiatives may mitigate. Data is growing around hospital-wide mobility initiatives with scales and quality improvement metrics that are appropriate for all patient types, including neurologically impaired caseloads.

To provide comprehensive mobility care and management, it is crucial to consider a wide range of assessments, as immobility can have significant effects across multiple domains. Various assessments include Montreal Cognitive Assessment (MOCA), Repeatable Battery for the Assessment of Neuropsychological Status (RBANS), Mini-Mental State Examination (MMSE), and Saint Louis University Mental Status Examination (SLUMS), among others. In addition, delirium metrics such as Intensive Care Delirium Screening Checklist (ICDSC) and Confusion Assessment Method for the ICU (CAM-ICU) can also be implemented.

At the systems level, it is important for Neurorehabilitation Consultants to understand elements like fall culture, fall rates, and fall scales/scores. Safe patient handling should also be considered, taking into account the costs associated with staff and patient injuries. Ultimately, Neurorehabilitation Consultants can be important advocates for initiating early mobility activities and objective measures, such as Activity Measure for Post-Acute Care (AMPAC) and therapy outcome metrics, should be tracked to ensure that each patient's mobility care and management plan is effective and that functional status is improved [24].Several mobility assessments are currently being studied for efficacy, practicality, and ease of use that will translate to use between a multidisciplinary team of clinicians. These assessments focus on function with the aim to improve data flow and allow for more structured randomized control trials and cohort studies—see the Johns Hopkins HLM and Activity and Mobility Program (AMP) Scale [25, 26] (Fig. 16.1). The Functional Status Score for the ICU (FSS-ICU) has had much research published around its use and efficacy in the last several years. The Bedside Mobility Assessment Tool (BMAT)

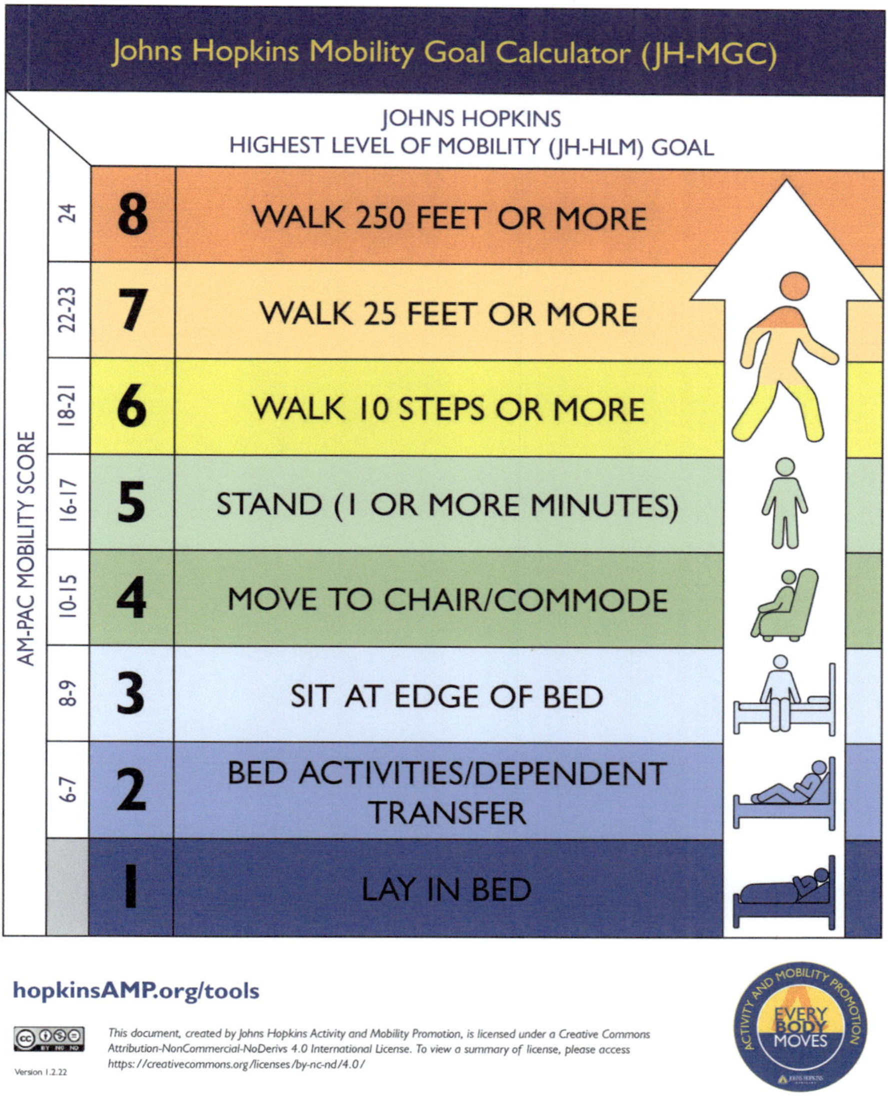

Fig. 16.1 Johns Hopkins HLM and activity and mobility program (AMP) scale [26]. Reproduced with permission

[27] has been used successfully in nursing lead initiatives focused on safe patient handling procedures that reduce injuries (Fig. 16.2).

Several quality improvement initiatives in ICUs and acute care hospital settings are underway looking at ways to address mobility needs in a value-based care environment to improve functional, quality, safe patient handling, and disposition outcomes. The aim is to demonstrate the effects of early mobility on healthcare

TEST	DESCRIPTION	PASS RESPONSE	PASS/FAIL
Assessment Level 1 Assessment of: ▪ Sitting balance ▪ Upper extremity and core strength ▪ Orthostatic response to sitting ▪ Ability to follow directions	**Assessment Level 1 – Sit and Shake – verifies hemodynamic stability and sitting balance.** **Sit and Shake:** From semi-reclined or sitting position, ask patient to sit upright for up to 1 minute (as indicated based on concern for orthostatic hypotension or postural intolerance); then reach across midline and shake hands with caregiver – repeat with other hand. (Patient's feet may or may not be flat on the floor) **Safe Mode:** Use sling and lift to assist to side of bed or complete in bed with HOB raised and patient leaning forward or with bed in chair mode.	**Sit and Shake:** • Able to follow commands and sit unsupported (by sling or surface) for up to 1 minute. • Able to maintain seated balance while reaching across midline of trunk with one or both hands and shaking caregiver's hand. *NOTE: If patient has "strict bed rest" orders, or is hemodynamically unstable, patient is a Mobility Level 1. Do not proceed with the assessment.* 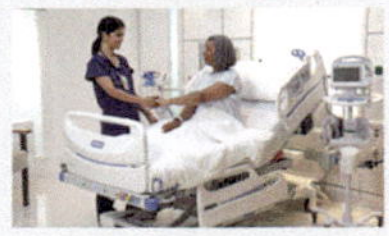	**FAIL = Mobility Level 1** Goal: Avoid complications of immobility 1. EOB dangling with sling and lift; calf pump exercises 2. Bed in Fowlers or chair position 3. Lift and repo sheet – boosting and turning 4. Lift and Multistraps – turning and limb holding 5. Lift and sling – bed to chair/ commode transfers 6. Friction Reducing Device (FRD) for AROM/PROM PASS – Proceed to Assessment Level 2
Assessment Level 2 Assessment of: ▪ Lower extremity strength in preparation for weight bearing ▪ Foot drop	**Assessment Level 2 – Stretch – verifies some lower extremity strength.** **Patient demonstrates Level 1 function and lower extremity strength.** **Stretch:** While sitting upright unsupported, extend leg by straightening knee, then point toes/ pump ankle between dorsiflexion/plantar flexion 3 times. Knee remains below hip level. **Safe Mode:** Use seated sling with lift (mobile or overhead) or bed in chair position.	**Stretch:** Able to extend leg and straighten knee to engage quadriceps; then able to pump ankle for 3 repetitions to engage lower leg muscles and assist with venous return/fluid shift. 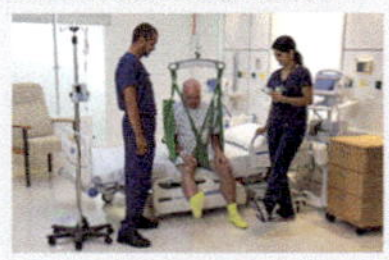	**FAIL = Mobility Level 2** Goal: Avoid Complications of Immobility 1. FRD: partial squats and leg AROM exercises 2. Lift and repo sheet – boosting and turning 3. Lift and Multistraps™ – turning and limb holding 4. Lift and sling – bed to chair/ commode transfers 5. Ankle pumps **PASS** – Proceed to Assessment Level 3
Assessment Level 3 Assessment of: ▪ Ability to perform sit to stand transfer ▪ Static standing balance ▪ Orthostatic response to standing	**Assessment Level 3 – Stand – verifies patient has adequate strength, physiological stability and balance to stand.** **Stand:** With feet flat on the floor about shoulder width apart, ask patient to shift weight forward and come to standing position. Stand for a minimum of 5 seconds and up to 1 minute if there is concern for orthostatic hypertension or syncope. **Safe Mode:** Use sit-to-stand lift or ambulation vest/pants with lift.	**Stand:** Able to rise, maintain standing position for up to 1 minute. *NOTE: The majority of patients who exhibit orthostatic hypotension do so within the first minute of standing.* May use walker, cane, crutches or prosthetic leg(s) as appropriate. 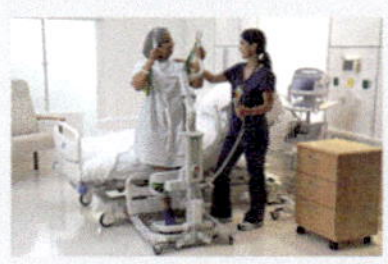	**FAIL = Mobility Level 3** Goal: Strengthen, assist fluid shifts, avoid falls 1. Sit-to-stand lift – stand for 1-2 minutes, weight shift side to side and forward/ back, 2-3 deep breaths 2. Squats using FRD with bed in tilt position 3. Lifts and Multistraps™: limb holding 4. Sit-to-stand lift (powered or non-powered) chair/ commode transfers 5. Progress to standing with sit-to-stand lift to standing with aid. **PASS** – Proceed to Assessment Level 4
Assessment Level 4 Assessment of: ▪ Pre-ambulation weight shifting ▪ Dynamic standing balance ▪ Motor planning and ability to follow directions	**Assessment Level 4 – Step – verifies adequate leg strength, balance and control to lift foot off floor and advance forward/back prior to walking.** **Step:** 1. March or step in place (not high marching) 2. Step forward with one foot, weight bear/ shift weight onto foot and return to starting position; repeat with other foot. **Safe Mode:** Use ambulation vest/pants and lift. Always default to Safe Mode if concerned regarding orthostatic hypotension/syncope or falls.	**Step:** Able to perform both marching-in-place and step forward/back with each leg. May use walker, cane, crutches, or prosthetic leg(s) as appropriate. 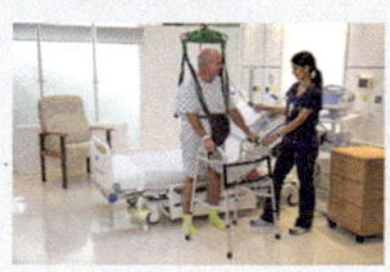	**FAIL = Mobility Level 4** Goal: Improve standing tolerence, balance; avoid falls; consider mobility goals 1. Ambulation vest/pants and lift for standing, pre-gait and ambulation activities 2. Set ambulance distance and frequency goals after passing 'Step' 3. If using aid to pass 'Step,' assure that aid is always accessible and used **PASS** – Pass BMAT Assessment; Proceed through Discharge Planning; Continue to complete once per shift and with change in condition

Adapted from Boynton, et al., T. (2020). The Bedside Mobility Assessment Tool 2.0. American Nurse Journal, 15(2).

Fig. 16.2 Bedside mobility assessment tool (BMAT). Reproduced with permission of Hill-Rom Services, Inc

outcomes and patient quality, change the immobility culture, educate patients, caregivers, and providers about the harms of immobility, and provide resources to perform movement safely and effectively with the healthcare team. Multidisciplinary rounds across the country have also improved with input from all providers. Care needs can be addressed for vulnerable groups, including neurologically impaired patients. Although these patients often receive most therapy resources, better mobility prevention allows therapists to work with neurological populations efficiently, and impact their outcomes.

Immobility Harm

Immobility harm widely contributes to increased delirium and confusion, pressure ulcers, deep vein thrombosis, urinary tract complications, constipation, increased fall rates and risks, depression, and anxiety [2]. Neurologically impaired patients are immobilized by their injuries, and for those without neurological impairments immobility harm has profound effects even after discharge. Post-discharge, patients may experience intensive care unit (ICU)-acquired weakness and post-hospital syndrome—an acquired period of vulnerability for adverse health events [3]. Previous studies have suggested immobility and impaired functional status may be a predictor of hospital readmission and/or hospital-acquired complications. However, until recently, most studies did not consider functional status as a focus unless a patient population (i.e., stroke) warranted investigating these outcomes.

Kortebein et al. assessed the physiologic effects in healthy older adults after 10 days of bed rest and showed a loss of almost 1 kg of lean tissue in the lower extremities, 16% decline in isokinetic knee extensor strength, and significant aerobic capacity decline. Similar bed rest studies in younger healthy patients also noted a significant decline in aerobic capacity in addition to loss of strength [1, 5]. Coupled with TBI, SCI, and stroke, neurological impairment adds profound immobility burden, often by increasing hospital and rehabilitation time. Despite strides made with early mobility, there is a substantial decline in function among vulnerable patient groups associated with immobility. It is imperative that neurologically impaired patients are mobilized early, as they are a far more vulnerable population functionally. They require passive and active range of motion (ROM), positioning, contracture prevention, skin breakdown prevention, and stimulation. The Neurorehabilitation Consultant may also consider early pharmacological interventions to address sleep, arousal and cognitive deficits associated with neurological injuries that require a prolonged ICU hospital course.

In a multicenter, prospective cohort study, Pandharipande et al. studied a diverse population of patients in general medical and surgical ICUs and found that one in four patients had cognitive impairment 12 months after critical illness that was similar in severity to that of patients with mild Alzheimer's disease, and one in three had impairment typically associated with moderate TBI [28]. Impairments affected a broader array of neuropsychological domains than is characteristically seen in Alzheimer's disease, but were similar to those observed after moderate TBI. A validated instrument that assessed baseline cognitive status showed that only 6% of patients had evidence of mild-to-moderate cognitive impairment before ICU admission, indicating that these profound cognitive deficits were new in most patients. Long-term cognitive impairment affected both old and young patients, regardless of the burden of coexisting conditions at baseline [16]. A longer duration of delirium was associated with worse long-term global cognition and executive function, an association that was independent of sedative or analgesic medication use, age, preexisting cognitive impairment, burden of coexisting conditions, and ongoing organ failures during ICU care [16]. Certain ICU populations, such as patients with acute respiratory distress syndrome (ARDS), have a higher prevalence of cognitive impairment compared with mixed ICU populations. This difference in prevalence may be attributed to varying pathophysiological mechanisms responsible for ICU-related cognitive impairment between ICU populations. Research suggests that patients with ARDS have a mean prevalence of 82% cognitive impairment at ICU discharge, whereas mixed ICU populations have a mean prevalence of 48% at ICU discharge. Also, ICU-related cognitive impairment appears to persist in a substantial number of ICU survivors, even at 1 and 2 years after ICU discharge (mean prevalence of 42% and 46%, respectively) [17]. Taken together, the Neurorehabilitation Consultant may find these populations appropriate for acute inpatient neurorehabilitation and may also consider acute care pharmacotherapies addressing sleep, arousal and cognition as useful adjuncts to early mobility in addressing.

Immobility and Function

Much of the literature around early mobility programs exists in ICUs exploring the harms of sedation practices, delirium, and immobility. The focus of literature is now shifting towards success and prevention by looking at outcome measures to reflect the care. There has been extensive research in the last 10 years around cognitive dysfunction and studies addressing the long-term outcomes of critical illness and prevention. The Critical Illness, Brain Dysfunction, and Survivorship (CIBS) Center is a collaboration of Vanderbilt University, the Monroe Carell Jr. Children's Hospital at Vanderbilt, the Nashville Veterans Affairs Hospital, and investigators at external institutions across the United States. The CIBS is composed of an interprofessional group of physicians, nurses, psychologists, biostatisticians, pharmacists, physical and occupational therapists, support staff, and trainees. The Center's team members work with patients who are, or have been, critically ill and have suffered from delirium and are at risk for long-term cognitive, functional, and neuropsychological impairments. Actionable results will emerge, important to neurorehabilitation consultation care, as they look at evidence-based practice and data-driven outcomes around ICU level of care in all cohorts.

Specialized Neuro and Trauma ICUs focus on less sedation, mostly due to different comorbidities and management needs, but the literature growth around cognitive dysfunction is notable for this population given TBI patients are far more sensitive to these effects. Sedation practices and delirium are thought to be the main comorbidity drivers, and practices embedded in the ABCDEF Bundle, are steps towards prevention and functional preservation.Yen et al. evaluated a revised progressive early mobilization protocol for patients with moderate to severe TBI and demonstrated that the intervention cohort at ICU discharge showed significantly improved Perme ICU Mobility Scores with no change in LOS [29, 30]. The AVERT Trial Collaboration group assessed early mobilization and how it promotes the recovery of physical function and quality of life in the stroke population [31–34]. Klein et al.

introduced a nursing-driven early mobility program to a large Neuro ICU using a prospective, pre-post-intervention design, and the study suggests significantly higher mobility levels, lower hospital and ICU LOS, and a higher likelihood of being discharged home in patients receiving the early mobility program [11].

Prior studies suggest that functional impairments can represent limitations in physiologic reserves that lead to vulnerabilities and readmissions [2]. Maintenance and efforts to improve functional status during acute care hospitalizations may be important modifiable risk factors affecting hospital LOS, readmission, and reduction of complication rates [35]. Neurotrauma and medical critical care units are starting to utilize data collected from assessments to make decisions around care and management. Examples of scales used for data collection include: the Confusion Assessment Method for the ICU (CAM-ICU), Glasgow Coma Scale (GCS), Ranchos Los Amigos Scale, and Richmond Agitation-Sedation Scale (RASS), which are assessments that provide data from which patient-specific care and management plans are based.

As a consulting physiatrist, it is crucial to consider the unique challenges that patients in the ICU face when implementing early mobilization interventions. Reid et al. conducted a scoping review that identified several key recommendations for physical rehabilitation interventions in the ICU [36]. To start, it is important to assess the patient's physical and cognitive status regularly. This includes evaluating their level of consciousness and ability to follow commands, which can inform decisions around appropriate mobilization techniques. Weight-bearing status and precautions must also be considered when developing a rehabilitation plan. The use of assistive devices or specialized equipment may be necessary to support the patient during standing and walking exercises. Furthermore, consideration must be given to the patient's hemodynamic status, as early mobilization may exacerbate conditions such as orthostatic hypotension or dysautonomia. To manage these conditions during standing exercises, strategies such as lower extremity compression stockings and abdominal binders may be necessary. Patients with spasticity may require tailored interventions to manage tone and improve range of motion. This may involve incorporating specific exercises or using specialized equipment such as dynamic splints.

Consulting physiatrists must work closely with the interdisciplinary ICU team, including nurses, respiratory therapists, and physical therapists, to ensure that rehabilitation interventions are integrated into the patient's overall care plan and are implemented safely and effectively. In the ICU, therapy teams can also focus on simple but important engaging tasks that can also address visual impairments, diplopia, arousal/stimulation for wakefulness, paresis of extraocular muscles, visual scanning, postural control, interaction with the environment using vision and cognition, head and neck alignment/control, cognitive tasks, self-feeding, dysphagia, and activities of daily living (ADL) functions. By considering these key recommendations, consulting physiatrists can develop individualized rehabilitation plans that optimize functional outcomes and minimize the risk of complications for patients in the ICU.

Physiatrists play a vital role in the ICU care of patients with TBI, SCI, and stroke. In these patient populations, physiatrists provide consultation to the interdisciplinary team regarding the rehabilitation and management of patients with functional deficits caused by critical illness or injury. Neurorehabilitation Consultants can have a significant impact on these patients' outcomes by implementing early rehabilitation interventions that focus on optimizing functional outcomes and reducing disability. Early mobilization, physical therapy, and cognitive rehabilitation have been shown to improve outcomes in TBI, SCI, and stroke patients, including shorter ICU and hospital length of stay, reduced incidence of delirium, and improved functional status upon discharge [36]. Additionally, physiatrists can assist in identifying patients who may benefit from post-ICU rehabilitation services and provide guidance on developing rehabilitation plans that address patients' specific needs and goals. Moreover, physiatrists can provide education and training to other members of the ICU team on functional assessment, rehabilitation interventions, and preventing functional decline in TBI, SCI, and stroke patients. By promoting a multidisciplinary approach to patient care, physiatrists can help improve the quality of care and outcomes for patients in these populations.

Case illustration

A 50-year-old male with a history of hypertension and hyperlipidemia was admitted to the ICU following a motor vehicle accident resulting in multiple traumatic injuries, including a TBI and multiple fractures and was non-weight bearing to the right lower extremity. Upon admission, the patient was intubated and mechanically ventilated due to respiratory failure.

The interdisciplinary ICU team utilized the ABCDEF ICU bundle to guide patient care and optimize outcomes. An important component of this framework was early mobilization and rehabilitation, which prompted a consultation with a physiatrist to assess the patient's functional status and provide recommendations for interventions.

The physiatrist performed a comprehensive evaluation, including the CAM-ICU, and determined that the patient was at high risk for functional decline due to prolonged bed rest and immobility. To address this, the physiatrist recommended early mobilization and physical therapy to optimize the patient's functional status and reduce the risk of complications such as pressure injury, deep vein thrombosis, and pulmonary embolism. Bedside exercises, such as ankle pumps, knee bends, and shoulder shrugs, were performed to maintain range of motion while lying in bed. Additionally, the physical therapist implemented bedside sitting exercises to work on seated balance, as well as sit-to-stand transfers, to promote early mobilization while complying with weight-bearing restrictions. Additionally, the patient was experiencing orthostatic hypotension, which made it difficult to maintain a standing position. The interdisciplinary ICU team, in collaboration with the physiatrist, devised a modified rehabilitation plan that incorporated several interventions to address the patient's complex needs. This included standing frame use under the supervision of the physical therapist, as well as the use of lower extremity compression stockings and an abdominal binder to manage the patient's orthostatic hypotension during standing exercises.

The CAM-ICU assessment identified that the patient was experiencing delirium, indicating a need for urgent intervention to address the patient's confusion. The physiatrist worked closely with the ICU team to develop a multifaceted approach to address the patient's delirium. This included discontinuing sedative medications such as benzodiazepines and reducing the dose of opioids to minimize their impact on the patient's cognitive function. The physiatrist also recommended environmental modifications to promote sleep and reduce stimulation, such as adjusting the lighting and noise levels in the patient's room. The patient demonstrated improved cognitive function and resolution of delirium symptoms, which allowed for more meaningful engagement with the rehabilitation process. Ultimately, the patient was able to successfully complete inpatient rehabilitation and was discharged home with a rehabilitation plan to continue improving his functional status.

Key Points

- Immobility harm contributes to hospital-acquired physical impairments that are associated with increased hospital LOS, hospital-acquired complications, nursing facility and acute inpatient rehabilitation admissions, and impaired cognitive and physical functioning. Neurologically impaired patients with acute spinal cord, stroke, or traumatic brain injuries have added layers of complexity and risk associated with these harms and need special considerations of focus for prevention.
- There are real physical, cognitive, emotional, and physiologic consequences that affect hospitalized patients, and immobility contributes to these consequences. Structured programs around mobility are demonstrating improvements in outcome measures, quality of studies, implementation successes, and multidisciplinary team participation. Programs are safe, feasible, and standardized around multidisciplinary team care, which are now therapy and/or nursing initiatives.
- There is growing literature with quality improvement projects and nationwide initiatives in critical care settings around early mobility and cognitive programs around diverse ICU populations including stroke, spinal cord, and traumatic brain injury. Neurorehabilitation Consultants can help lead and implement these initiatives.

References[1]

1. Kortebein P, Ferrando A, Lombeida J, Wolfe R, Evans WJ. Effect of 10 days of bed rest on skeletal muscle in healthy older adults. JAMA. 2007;297(16):1772–4. https://doi.org/10.1001/jama.297.16.1772-b.
2. Hoyer EH, Friedman M, Lavezza A, et al. Promoting mobility and reducing length of stay in hospitalized general medicine patients: a quality-improvement project. J Hosp Med. 2016;11(5):341–7. https://doi.org/10.1002/jhm.2546.

[1] Key References [2, 3, 6, 35].

3. Krumholz HM. Post-hospital syndrome–an acquired, transient condition of generalized risk. N Engl J Med. 2013;368(2):100–2. https://doi.org/10.1056/NEJMp1212324.
4. Dock W. The evil sequelae of complete bed rest. J Am Med Assoc. 1944;125(16):1083–5. https://doi.org/10.1001/jama.1944.02850340009004.
5. Kortebein P, Symons TB, Ferrando A, et al. Functional impact of 10 days of bed rest in healthy older adults. J Gerontol A Biol Sci Med Sci. 2008;63(10):1076–81. https://doi.org/10.1093/gerona/63.10.1076.
6. Covinsky KE, Palmer RM, Fortinsky RH, et al. Loss of independence in activities of daily living in older adults hospitalized with medical illnesses: increased vulnerability with age. J Am Geriatr Soc. 2003;51(4):451–8. https://doi.org/10.1046/j.1532-5415.2003.51152.x.
7. Wilcox ME, Herridge MS. Lung function and quality of life in survivors of the acute respiratory distress syndrome (ARDS). Presse Med. 2011;40(12):595–603. https://doi.org/10.1016/j.lpm.2011.04.024.
8. Wilcox ME, Herridge MS. Long-term outcomes in patients surviving acute respiratory distress syndrome. Semin Respir Crit Care Med. 2010;31(1):55–65. https://doi.org/10.1055/s-0029-1246285.
9. Wilcox ME, Patsios D, Murphy G, et al. Radiologic outcomes at 5 years after severe ARDS. Chest. 2013;143(4):920–6. https://doi.org/10.1378/chest.12-0685.
10. Wilcox ME, Rivera MP, Sassoon C, Ware LB, Wunsch H, Herridge MS. Clinical year in review II: mechanical ventilation, acute respiratory distress syndrome, critical care, and lung cancer. Proc Am Thorac Soc. 2012;9(4):190–6. https://doi.org/10.1513/pats.201206-033TT.
11. Herridge MS, Cheung AM, Tansey CM, et al. One-year outcomes in survivors of the acute respiratory distress syndrome. N Engl J Med. 2003;348(8):683–93. https://doi.org/10.1056/NEJMoa022450.
12. Liang S, Chau JPC, Lo SHS, Li S, Gao M. Implementation of ABCDEF care bundle in intensive care units: a cross-sectional survey. Nurs Crit Care. 2021;26(5):386–96. https://doi.org/10.1111/nicc.12597.
13. Marra A, Ely EW, Pandharipande PP, Patel MB. The ABCDEF bundle in critical care. Crit Care Clin. 2017;33(2):225–43. https://doi.org/10.1016/j.ccc.2016.12.005.
14. Morandi A, Piva S, Ely EW, et al. Worldwide survey of the "Assessing pain, both spontaneous awakening and breathing trials, choice of drugs, delirium monitoring/management, early exercise/mobility, and family empowerment" (ABCDEF) bundle. Crit Care Med. 2017;45(11):e1111–22. https://doi.org/10.1097/CCM.0000000000002640.
15. Devlin JW, Skrobik Y, Gelinas C, et al. Clinical practice guidelines for the prevention and management of pain, agitation/sedation, delirium, immobility, and sleep disruption in adult patients in the ICU. Crit Care Med. 2018;46(9):e825–73. https://doi.org/10.1097/CCM.0000000000003299.
16. Inouye SK, Westendorp RG, Saczynski JS. Delirium in elderly people. Lancet. 2014;383(9920):911–22. https://doi.org/10.1016/s0140-6736(13)60688-1.
17. Seo Y, Lee HJ, Ha EJ, Ha TS. 2021 KSCCM clinical practice guidelines for pain, agitation, delirium, immobility, and sleep disturbance in the intensive care unit. Acute Crit Care. 2022;37(1):1–25. https://doi.org/10.4266/acc.2022.00094.
18. Mart MF, Williams Roberson S, Salas B, Pandharipande PP, Ely EW. Prevention and management of delirium in the intensive care unit. Semin Respir Crit Care Med. 2021;42(1):112–26. https://doi.org/10.1055/s-0040-1710572.
19. Balas MC, Vasilevskis EE, Burke WJ, et al. Critical care nurses' role in implementing the "ABCDE bundle" into practice. Crit Care Nurse. 2012;32(2):35–8, 40-7; quiz 48. https://doi.org/10.4037/ccn2012229.
20. Girard TD, Kress JP, Fuchs BD, et al. Efficacy and safety of a paired sedation and ventilator weaning protocol for mechanically ventilated patients in intensive care (awakening and breathing controlled trial): a randomised controlled trial. Lancet. 2008;371(9607):126–34. https://doi.org/10.1016/s0140-6736(08)60105-1.

21. Hsieh SJ, Otusanya O, Gershengorn HB, et al. Staged implementation of awakening and breathing, coordination, delirium monitoring and management, and early mobilization bundle improves patient outcomes and reduces hospital costs. Crit Care Med. 2019;47(7):885–93. https://doi.org/10.1097/ccm.0000000000003765.
22. Jeffery AD, Werthman JA, Danesh V, Dietrich MS, Mion LC, Boehm LM. Assess, prevent, and manage pain; both spontaneous awakening and breathing trials; choice of analgesia/sedation; delirium: assess, prevent, and manage; early mobility; family engagement and empowerment bundle implementation: quantifying the association of access to bundle-enhancing supplies and equipment. Crit Care Expl. 2021;3(9):e0525. https://doi.org/10.1097/cce.0000000000000525.
23. Hooper MH, Girard TD. Sedation and weaning from mechanical ventilation: linking spontaneous awakening trials and spontaneous breathing trials to improve patient outcomes. Crit Care Clin. 2009;25(3):515–25. https://doi.org/10.1016/j.ccc.2009.04.002.
24. Huang M, Chan KS, Zanni JM, et al. Functional status score for the ICU: an international clinimetric analysis of validity, responsiveness, and minimal important difference. Crit Care Med. 2016;44(12):e1155–64. https://doi.org/10.1097/CCM.0000000000001949.
25. Johns Hopkins Medicine. Activity and mobility promotion (JH-AMP). https://www.hopkinsmedicine.org/physical_medicine_rehabilitation/education_training/amp/toolkit.html. Accessed 3 January 2023.
26. McLaughlin KH, Friedman M, Hoyer EH, et al. The Johns Hopkins activity and mobility promotion program: a program to increase activity and mobility among hospitalized patients. J Nurs Care Qual. 2022. https://doi.org/10.1097/NCQ.0000000000000678.
27. Boynton T, Kumpar D, Van Glider C. The bedside mobility assessment tool 2.0. Am Nurse J. 2020;15(7):18–22.
28. Pandharipande P, Shintani A, Peterson J, et al. Lorazepam is an independent risk factor for transitioning to delirium in intensive care unit patients. Anesthesiology. 2006;104(1):21–6. https://doi.org/10.1097/00000542-200601000-00005.
29. Perme C, Nawa RK, Winkelman C, Masud F. A tool to assess mobility status in critically ill patients: the perme intensive care unit mobility score. Methodist Debakey Cardiovasc J. 2014;10(1):41–9. https://doi.org/10.14797/mdcj-10-1-41.
30. Yen HC, Han YY, Hsiao WL, et al. Functional mobility effects of progressive early mobilization protocol on people with moderate-to-severe traumatic brain injury: a pre-post intervention study. NeuroRehabilitation. 2022;51(2):303–13. https://doi.org/10.3233/nre-220023.
31. AVERT Trial Collaboration group. Efficacy and safety of very early mobilisation within 24 h of stroke onset (AVERT): a randomised controlled trial. Lancet. 2015;386(9988):46–55. https://doi.org/10.1016/s0140-6736(15)60690-0.
32. Bernhardt J, Churilov L, Ellery F, et al. Prespecified dose-response analysis for a very early rehabilitation trial (AVERT). Neurology. 2016;86(23):2138–45. https://doi.org/10.1212/wnl.0000000000002459.
33. Bernhardt J, Dewey H, Thrift A, Collier J, Donnan G. A very early rehabilitation trial for stroke (AVERT): phase II safety and feasibility. Stroke. 2008;39(2):390–6. https://doi.org/10.1161/strokeaha.107.492363.
34. Langhorne P, Wu O, Rodgers H, Ashburn A, Bernhardt J. A very early rehabilitation trial after stroke (AVERT): a phase III, multicentre, randomised controlled trial. Health Technol Assess. 2017;21(54):1–120. https://doi.org/10.3310/hta21540.
35. Hoyer EH, Needham DM, Atanelov L, Knox B, Friedman M, Brotman DJ. Association of impaired functional status at hospital discharge and subsequent rehospitalization. J Hosp Med. 2014;9(5):277–82. https://doi.org/10.1002/jhm.2152.
36. Reid JC, Unger J, McCaskell D, Childerhose L, Zorko DJ, Kho ME. Physical rehabilitation interventions in the intensive care unit: a scoping review of 117 studies. J Intensive Care. 2018;6:80. https://doi.org/10.1186/s40560-018-0349-x.

Chapter 17
Geriatric Considerations: Medical Comorbidities and Principles of Medical Management

Shanti M. Pinto

Chapter Objectives

1. Summarize common medical comorbidities in the geriatric population with acquired neurologic injury.
2. Discuss the considerations for pharmacologic management among older adults with acquired neurologic injury.
3. Review the impact of acquired neurologic disability on the aging process.

Introduction

Older individuals have a greater number and severity of comorbid medical conditions than younger individuals. These medical comorbidities and associated treatments have an important impact on the patient's overall rehabilitation outcomes. Chapter 11 provides an overview of age-related functional changes with special focus on how aging impacts the patient's overall rehabilitation goals. For the acute care neurorehabilitation consultant, this chapter focuses on common medical comorbidities and principles of medical management in the geriatric population with acquired neurologic injury requiring neurorehabilitation care during their acute hospitalization.

S. M. Pinto (✉)
Department of Physical Medicine and Rehabilitation, University of Texas - Southwestern, Dallas, TX, USA
e-mail: shanti.pinto@utsouthwestern.edu

A. K. Wagner, J. Weppner (eds.), *Acute Care Neuroconsultation and Neurorehabilitation Management*, https://doi.org/10.1007/978-3-031-42830-2_17

Common Medical Comorbidities in the Geriatric Population

Cardiac

In the heart, autonomic tissues become fibrotic, leading to conduction abnormalities, such as atrial fibrillation, sick sinus syndrome, or bundle branch blocks. Blood vessels stiffen, leading to elevated systolic blood pressure (SBP) and lower diastolic blood pressure (DBP) [1, 2]. Additionally, older individuals are at increased risk for orthostatic hypotension due to altered baroreceptor activation in response to large artery stiffness [1]. Typical SBP goal is under 130 mmHg to prevent secondary cardiovascular complications in otherwise healthy community-dwelling older adults [3]; however, older adults are more susceptible to adverse antihypertensive drug effects, e.g., postural hypotension, cognitive impairments, and fatigue [4]. Careful evaluation should be taken of the antihypertensive medications with consideration of the risks and benefits in treating older adults with functional and cognitive decline [1].

Respiratory

Older adults have a decline of forced vital capacity by 14–30 cc/year and forced expiratory capacity of roughly 30 cc/year in males due to decreased chest wall compliance, respiratory muscle strength, and lung elasticity [2]. Patients with a history of cigarette smoking are at increased risk for development of chronic obstructive pulmonary disease (COPD), which is characterized by chronic airflow obstruction and accelerated decline in pulmonary function [5]. This decline in respiratory function worsens with active smoking, greater number of years of smoking, and increasing age [6, 7]. Furthermore, cigarette smoking has been linked to multiple adverse health outcomes, namely peripheral vascular disease [8], stroke [9], cardiovascular disease [10], Alzheimer's dementia [11], and cancer [12]. For those with neurotrauma, cigarette smoking has been associated with worse cognitive recovery following mild traumatic brain injury (TBI) [13]; however, no difference in global functional outcomes was noted in patients over a range of TBI severity [14]. Cigarette smoking may lead to increased spinal cord edema in the acute period, but no difference has been identified in motor recovery following spinal cord injury (SCI) [15]. Nonetheless, education on smoking cessation is important to address the adverse effects of cigarette smoking on medical comorbidities. Older adults more frequently require mechanical ventilation and typically have more difficulties weaning from the ventilator than younger adults due to poorer premorbid pulmonary status [2, 16].

Renal

Nephrosclerosis is a set of histologic findings characterized as glomerulosclerosis, tubular atrophy, interstitial fibrosis, and arteriosclerosis [17]. The rate of nephrosclerosis increases with aging and is associated with an age-related decline in the glomerular filtration rate (GFR) of roughly 45% by age 80 [2, 17]. More pronounced GFR declines occur in those with poorly controlled diabetes mellitus and hypertension. Serum creatinine remains relatively stable due to concurrent decline in muscle mass; therefore, serum creatinine may not be a reliable estimate of the degree of renal impairment in older adults [2]. It is important to periodically monitor renal function as the dose of renally cleared medications should be adjusted in patients with renal insufficiency [2, 18]. Specific GFR thresholds for adjustments differ based on the medication utilized, and close communication with the hospital-based pharmacist can help with drug selection and clinical decision-making.

Pain Management

Older patients frequently have chronic pain disorders, typically resulting from musculoskeletal disease, and pain management should be addressed cautiously in older adults due to an increased risk of medication side effects. Acetaminophen is the first-line treatment for mild to moderate pain in older adults [19, 20]. Elevations of liver enzymes while taking acetaminophen are typically mild and do not lead to liver failure in patients taking less than the maximum dose of 3 g/day [20]. Acetaminophen is less effective than nonsteroidal anti-inflammatory drugs (NSAIDs) in the treatment of inflammatory conditions; however, NSAIDs are associated with higher risk of adverse events in older patients. Gastric side effects and peptic ulcers typically occur due cyclooxygenase-1 (COX-1) inhibition, decreasing protection of the gastric mucosal lining. The selective COX-2 inhibitor, celecoxib, is generally better tolerated, but gastrointestinal side effects can still occur [19–21]. NSAIDs are associated with an increased risk of major vascular events, such as myocardial infarction, coronary artery disease, and stroke. One meta-analysis found that naproxen and ibuprofen were not associated with an increased risk of these cardiovascular events; however, individuals taking these medications still were at an increased risk of congestive heart failure and gastrointestinal bleeding [21]. Overall, NSAIDs are not associated with an increased risk of intracranial hemorrhage, except for individuals prescribed oral diclofenac or meloxicam [22] or when NSAIDs are used concurrently with antidepressant medications [23]. More research is needed to determine when NSAIDs would be safe to start following intracranial hemorrhage from either traumatic or non-traumatic causes. Topical NSAIDs, such as diclofenac gel, can be used for local areas of inflammation with decreased rate of systemic effects [20]. Current evidence does not support the concern that NSAIDs lead to delayed healing or non-union in humans following orthopedic trauma or surgery

[24–26], particularly when used in low dose and for a short duration of less than 14 days [24, 27]. Further studies are needed to determine whether the risk of delayed healing or non-union is greater for older adults and those with osteoporosis. Opiates can be used for persistent moderate to severe pain following acute traumatic injury [19, 20, 26], but evidence regarding long-term efficacy is lacking [20, 26]. Caution should be taken when using opiate pain medications in older adults due to an increased risk of delirium [28] and falls [29, 30]. Furthermore, opiate pain medications are associated risk of falls in older adults when used with other centrally acting medications [31]. Neuropathic pain can be treated with the use of antiepileptic medications. Gabapentin is widely utilized as adjunctive treatment for pain [26], but dose must be lowered in those with renal insufficiency [19, 20, 32]. Tricyclic antidepressants (TCAs) are not recommended for use in the geriatric population due to increased anticholinergic effects—notably cognitive impairments, constipation, and urinary retention [19, 20, 32].

Cognitive Impairments

Adults reach peak intellectual capacity between the third and fourth decades. This peak capacity persists in healthy adults until the middle of the ninth decade when a rapid decline is noted [2]. Structurally, the brain undergoes significant increase in white matter volume for the first six decades followed by a rapid decline. Decline in periventricular white matter is associated with age-related cognitive decline [33]. Mild cognitive impairment (MCI) refers to the presence of cognitive impairments greater than expected for chronological age without significant deficits in normal daily living [34]. Patients with MCI, characterized by memory impairments, are at increased risk for progression to dementia [34]. Dementia presents with more severe cognitive impairments that impact multiple cognitive domains and impair daily functioning. Dementia rates increase with advanced age, increasing from 1.5% at age 65 to 25% in those over 85 years old [2]. It is important for the acute care consultant to screen older individuals for history of pre-existing cognitive dysfunction because it can have a major impact on ability to participate in therapy and return to independent living following acquired neurologic injury. Donepezil is an acetyl cholinesterase inhibitor that can be used for the treatment of dementia and MCI [34, 35]. Donepezil may also aid in improvements in cognitive functioning for those with a history of TBI [36] and mild to moderate vascular dementia due to stroke [37]. Two small studies suggest that donepezil may improve language function in those with aphasia due to stroke [38, 39].

Patients with dementia are at increased risk for delirium, a transient state of altered consciousness and cognition, during acute medical illness and hospitalization. Patients have significant impairment in attention, and cognition fluctuates throughout the day. Agitation and refusal to participate in medical care are common features; however, patients may also present with apathy and decreased arousal. Increased delirium risk occurs with advancing age, premorbid cognitive and/or functional impairment, TBI, increased medical comorbidities, prior alcohol abuse, prolonged surgical interventions of at least 3 h, and increased time of pharmacologic sedation [40–42]. Multiple causes of delirium have been identified, and work-up should include careful evaluation of medications, evaluation for infection, and laboratory testing. Laboratory testing may include electrolytes, liver function testing with serum ammonia level, thyroid stimulating hormone, and vitamin B12 and folate levels. Evaluation of medications should be undertaken with careful attention to any new medications. Medications most frequently associated with delirium include anticholinergic medications, benzodiazepines, opiate medications, and sedative medications. Benzodiazepine use should be limited to cases of acute alcohol withdrawal, and dose and duration should be determined using an objective symptom scale such as the Clinical Institute Withdrawal Assessment for Alcohol (CIWA-Ar) [43]. Acetylcholinesterase inhibitors, such as donepezil, generally do not prevent or treat delirium [44, 45]. Acetylcholinesterase inhibitors are generally well tolerated; however, adverse events, such as increased mortality, were noted in a few studies [44].

Medical Comorbidities and Impact on Papers on SCI Outcomes

Older adults have greater medical complexity than younger adults, which is associated with greater mortality risk and poor outcomes after traumatic injury. Older adults frequently have comorbid arthritis, hypertension, cardiovascular disease, diabetes mellitus, and respiratory disease [46–51] and are more likely to develop medical complications, such as pneumonia, sepsis, gastrointestinal bleed, pulmonary embolism, renal failure, cardiac complications, and delirium [16, 50, 52, 53]. Importantly, those with pre-existing medical comorbidities and medical complications have a higher rate of mortality following blunt force trauma [16, 51, 53]. Older patients are more likely to be prescribed antiplatelet or anticoagulant medications for the treatment of pre-existing conditions, which are associated with increased mortality rates and poor outcomes following traumatic intracranial hemorrhage [54, 55] but not trauma without intracranial injury [56]. Those with greater medical comorbidity burden during acute hospitalization for TBI have prolonged time of post-traumatic amnesia, longer inpatient rehabilitation length of stay, and higher rehospitalization rates over the first year following discharge [57]. Furthermore, those with higher comorbidity burden have poorer functional outcomes at 1 year post-injury [57] as well as worse trajectories of functional change up to 10 years post-injury [58]. Furthermore, recent evidence has suggested that certain medical comorbidities, namely hypertension, cardiac disease, depression, and drug/alcohol abuse, may negatively impact recovery over the first 5 years post-TBI, with the effect of the medical comorbidity on functional outcomes varying based on time since injury [59].

In persons with geriatric SCI, the most common co-morbidities include elevated blood pressure, back pain, and high levels of cholesterol. The occurrence of multiple co-morbidities was notably higher among individuals aged ≥76 years (average: 2.0; range: 0–12) [60]. In an analysis of acute SCI injuries in individuals over 60 years old, secondary complications such as infections, mood disorders, pressure injuries, and cardiovascular events were more prevalent compared to those under 60 [61]. These findings imply that strict adherence to acute SCI care principles and timely physiatry consultations might help alleviate the increased vulnerability to secondary complications among the elderly. This underscores the vital importance of implementing a multidisciplinary approach led by physiatrists in treating acute spinal cord injuries among older patients to reduce or prevent these subsequent complications effectively.

It is important to consider medical comorbidity burden when providing recommendations for rehabilitation programming and discharge disposition. Acute inpatient rehabilitation facilities are more equipped to manage these pre-existing and co-occurring medical comorbidities than subacute rehabilitation due to the requirements of at least 3 day/week physician rounds and around the clock physician oversight. At the same time, it is important to ensure that the patient can tolerate the intensive rehabilitation program as they might be limited due (for example) to poor endurance from cardiopulmonary disease or pain from pre-existing arthritis. Additional need for frequent medical procedures, such as chronic hemodialysis, can impact the ability to participate in the required daily and/or weekly therapy thresholds and should be considered when determining the most appropriate setting for post-acute rehabilitation.

Medication Prescription

Principles of Prescription of Medications for Geriatric Patients

Aging triggers multiple physiologic changes that impact pharmacokinetics. There is a decrease in lean body mass, decrease in total body water, and increase in body fat with aging. As a result, hydrophilic medications have lower volume of distribution; therefore, low doses will lead to higher body concentration. Liver size and blood flow decrease with increased age, resulting in either (1) decreased first-pass metabolism and increased bioavailability of medications with extensive first-pass metabolism or (2) inactivation and decreased bioavailability of medications with extensive first-pass activation [18]. As noted above, renal clearance decreases with increased age, leading to higher serum concentration of renally cleared medications. Patients who are acutely ill or malnourished have lower serum albumin levels and associated increases in free serum drug concentrations [18]. Older adults can exhibit different responses to the same dose and bioavailability of medications compared to younger patients. For example, histamine type-2 receptor blockers (H2 blockers), such as famotidine, are commonly used for gastrointestinal prophylaxis during hospitalization for acute traumatic injury or severe medical illness; however, they are associated with increased rate of delirium and altered mental status in older adults [32]. In general, benzodiazepines should be avoided following acute neurologic trauma as they can impair cognitive recovery and cause paradoxical agitation. However, they may be used acutely for management of alcohol withdrawal or anxiety. Older adults are more susceptible to the sedative and cognitive side effects of these medications compared to younger adults, even with equal serum concentrations [18].

Polypharmacy

Polypharmacy refers to the use of multiple medications by a single patient. Medication use increases with age. Roughly one-third of older adults report polypharmacy, typically defined as use of at least five medications simultaneously [18, 62, 63]. In one study of a cohort of community-dwelling adults aged 62–85 years old, the rate of polypharmacy increased from 30.6% in 2004–2005 to 35.8% in 2010–2011 [63]. Those taking at least five medications are more likely to have decreased functional performance of instrumental activities of daily living and cognitive impairments [64]. In one prospective cohort, >10 prescription medications were associated with worse nutritional status, cognition, and performance of instrumental activities of daily living over a 3-year follow-up period [65]. Drug-drug interaction rates increase with an increased number of medications taken and is particularly notable when at least one medication impacts the hepatic cytochrome P450 system. The rate of drug-drug interactions can be up to 13% in patients taking two medications and ~80% in those taking >5 medications [18, 64].

A careful review of the medication list should be undertaken at the time of initial acute care consultation and again prior to admission to inpatient rehabilitation as patients with acquired neurologic disorders are at increased risk for polypharmacy and associated adverse outcomes. Polypharmacy is more common in adults with SCI and is associated with an increased risk of adverse drug reactions [66, 67]. Psychotropic medications are frequently utilized during TBI rehabilitation [68]. Pre-injury polypharmacy is associated with increased TBI-associated mortality [69], and the risk of falling post-TBI is greater for those taking a higher number of medications post-injury [70]. There are no studies investigating how polypharmacy specifically impacts outcomes in persons with acquired neurologic injury; however, older adults are likely at increased risk for these adverse events based on the literature in the general population.

Medications to Avoid or Use with Caution in Geriatric Patients

Adverse drug reactions are a frequent cause of hospitalization in the elderly population and may lead to cognitive impairments and increased fall risk [18, 31, 32]. A comprehensive summary of medications to use with caution in older adults can be found in the most updated Beers Criteria for Potentially Inappropriate Medication Use in Older Adults by the American Geriatrics Society [32]. Medications with a narrow therapeutic window are centrally acting, affect blood pressure, and have anticholinergic effects that frequently cause adverse events in older adults [18, 20, 31]. Many medications can mimic or precipitate medical conditions in older adults. For example, Parkinsonian features can occur in patients taking metoclopramide for gastroparesis, and cognitive impairments can occur in patients taking antihistamines [18]. Careful assessment of the patient's medication regimen should be undertaken during evaluation of new symptoms.

Psychotropic medications are associated with high adverse event rates among older adults, and they have been associated with a high rate of falls. Antipsychotic medications are associated with the highest rate of falls even when controlling for Parkinsonian effects of the medications [31]. Atypical antipsychotic medications are less likely to cause extra-pyramidal effects than typical antipsychotic medications, but there is no difference in the risk of falls with atypical antipsychotics [18, 31]. Antipsychotic medications have been utilized frequently for the treatment of delirium in the hospital. This practice is no longer recommended due to adverse effects of these medications and limited evidence of their efficacy [32]. Antidepressant medications, particularly TCAs and selective serotonin reuptake inhibitors (SSRIs), are next most likely psychotropic medications to cause falls. Additionally, SSRIs are associated with an increased risk of fracture due to decrease in bone mineral density [31]. It is recommended to avoid benzodiazepine use except for active seizures and alcohol or benzodiazepine withdrawal because they are associated with a high rate of central nervous system side effects. There is no difference in risk of falls based on half-life of the medication, but there is a higher rate of falls with increased benzodiazepine dose. Fall risks remain elevated for at least 30 days after starting benzodiazepines, suggesting that older adults do not acclimate to these drugs' effects on the central nervous system [31]. Also, antihistamine use is not recommended in older adults as they are more susceptible to their associated anticholinergic side effects [31, 32].

Aging with Disability

As noted in Chap. 11, persons with disability are living longer due to advances in health care. Persons aging with disability exhibit earlier signs of aging in the musculoskeletal, endocrine, and cardiovascular systems than age-matched controls. Accelerated aging can manifest as earlier onset of cardiovascular disease, osteoarthritis, degenerative spine disease, and chronic pain conditions [71, 72]. Those aging with developmental disabilities have earlier onset of osteoporosis, cardiovascular disease, hypertension, diabetes mellitus, depression, and dental abnormalities [73]. Higher rates of pressure ulcers, venous thromboembolism, depression, and nephrolithiasis have been observed with an increased time since the onset of disability [71, 74]. A sedentary lifestyle, coupled with poor nutrition and lower access to medical services, often accounts for the earlier onset of these chronic medical conditions. Patients with disability are more likely to be obese due to lower physical activity levels and diets that are high in fat and low in fruits and vegetables [72, 73]. Reduced access to medical services is due to multiple factors including lower financial resources for health care [72, 73] and less likelihood of completing routine physician visits due to cost, even after controlling for annual household income [75]. Other factors associated with decreased access to physician services include lower rate of private insurance, poor social support, and lack of transportation [72, 73]. It is important for the rehabilitation consultant to be aware of these unique challenges facing individuals with premorbid disabilities when planning for post-discharge services. These individuals are at increased risk for further functional decline during hospitalization and may benefit from post-acute rehabilitation services and/or alternative forms of service, such as telehealth visits [76].

Case Illustrations

The two cases highlighted in Chap. 11 are revisited below to focus on medical management. The first case discusses an elderly man with acute TBI as a result of fall. The second case focuses on the medical complications experienced by a patient aging with SCI.

TBI in Geriatric Patient

A 95-year-old male with a history of hypertension, osteoarthritis, and mild cognitive impairments suffers mild TBI due to a fall. CT scan showed small intracranial hemorrhage and left zygomaxillary fracture, both nonoperatively managed. He had no medical complications during his initial hospitalization and was admitted to inpatient rehabilitation (IPR) on day seven post-injury.

Prior to admission his blood pressure was controlled on lisinopril 20 mg daily and atenolol 50 mg daily. He complained of lightheadedness that limited ambulation. His SBP was consistently in the 110s, and his heart rate would be as low as the upper 50s early in the morning. His atenolol was discontinued with improved orthostatic symptoms, but he developed an elevated resting heart rate, for which he was started on metoprolol 12.5 mg twice daily. As for his osteoarthritis, he complained of right knee pain that limited ambulation. His therapist incorporated exercises for lower extremity strengthening and stretching, and his pain was treated with topical diclofenac gel with symptom improvement. During acute hospitalization, he had periods of confusion concerning for delirium. Work-up included thyroid stimulating hormone, vitamin B12, and ammonia levels, which were unremarkable. He was diagnosed with urinary tract infection (UTI) and started on antibiotics. His delirium improved with UTI treatment, but he continued to have cognitive impairments, particularly with memory and executive functioning.

Prior to IPR transfer, the neurorehabilitation consultant discussed with the patient and family about the goals for inpatient rehabilitation. Based on his cognitive impairment, it was stressed that he would need consistent supervision at discharge and would not be able to return to his prior home environment without in-home support. Rehabilitation was also discussed, and both the acute care therapists and neurorehabilitation consultant felt that he could tolerate 3 h of therapy daily if he was provided rest breaks during and between the therapy sessions.

During his rehabilitation admission, he was started on donepezil nightly and underwent speech therapy with memory improvements documented. Behaviorally, he was calm and cooperative during the day but would have periods of agitation towards staff every evening. This improved on risperidone 0.5 mg with dinner, and he slept better during the night. He was discharged to home with his daughter and son-in-law after 22 days in IPR. He was continued on the donepezil 10 mg nightly and risperidone 0.5 mg with dinner. His blood pressure was well controlled on lisinopril 20 mg daily and metoprolol 12.5 mg twice daily. At outpatient follow-up, his daughter reported no agitation in the evenings, and his cognition improved to premorbid status based on family report and structured outpatient speech therapy evaluations. Both risperidone and donepezil were discontinued.

Aging with SCI

A 68-year-old man with a history of C6 ASIA A SCI 50 years ago presents to the hospital with atrial fibrillation with a rapid ventricular rate. He was started on metoprolol 25 mg twice daily for atrial fibrillation, but he developed hypotension and was treated with midodrine 10 mg three times daily. He was also started on warfarin for stroke prevention. Due to his SCI history, the neurorehabilitation consultant was called to evaluate this patient. He reported that he was healthy prior to SCI. Over the past few years, he noted worsening of lower back discomfort. X-rays showed multilevel degenerative changes with facet arthropathy. He tried oxycodone as needed for his pain, but this caused constipation, requiring increased laxatives for his bowel program. When initially injured, he used reflex voiding into a condom catheter for bladder management. Six months ago, he experienced urinary retention and required emergency care Foley catheter placement due to age-related prostate changes. He tried tamsulosin but developed hypotension and discontinued the medication. He could not perform clean intermittent catheterization due to poor hand control and started using a suprapubic catheter. He then developed a stage II sacral decubitus pressure ulcer that required home healthcare nursing. As a result of this acute care consultation, this patient was referred for pressure mapping as an outpatient to identify the appropriate seating surface while in his wheelchair.

Summary/Key Points

There is a high rate of comorbid medical conditions in older adults that can impact outcomes. Older adults have changes in drug metabolism and may be more sensitive to medication side effects; therefore, prescription medications should be carefully reviewed. Also, those aging with premorbid disability develop chronic medical conditions at an earlier age than able-bodied individuals. With the aging of the population, it is important for treating clinicians to be aware of their unique challenges.

References[1]

1. Benetos A, Petrovic M, Strandberg T. Hypertension management in older and frail older patients. Circ Res. 2019;124(7):1045–60. https://doi.org/10.1161/CIRCRESAHA.118.313236.
2. Rosenthal RA, Kavic SM. Assessment and management of the geriatric patient. Crit Care Med. 2004;32(4):S92–105.
3. Whelton PK, Carey RM, Aronow WS, et al. 2017 ACC/AHA/AAPA/ABC/ACPM/AGS/APhA/ASH/ASPC/NMA/PCNA guideline for the prevention, detection, evaluation, and management of high blood pressure in adults: executive summary: a report of the American College of Cardiology/American Heart Association Task Force on clinical practice guidelines. Hypertens Dallas Tex. 2018;71(6):1269–324. https://doi.org/10.1161/HYP.0000000000000066.
4. Ayan M, Pothineni NV, Siraj A, Mehta JL. Cardiac drug therapy-considerations in the elderly. J Geriatr Cardiol. 2016;13(12):992–7. https://doi.org/10.11909/j.issn.1671-5411.2016.12.008.
5. Prevention (US) C for DC and, Promotion (US) NC for CDP and H, Health (US) O on S and pulmonary diseases. Centers for Disease Control and Prevention (US); 2010. https://www.ncbi.nlm.nih.gov/books/NBK53021/. Accessed 1 May 2020.
6. Kim EJ, Yoon SJ, Kim YE, Go DS, Jung Y. Effects of aging and smoking duration on cigarette smoke-induced COPD severity. J Korean Med Sci. 2018;34(1):e90. https://doi.org/10.3346/jkms.2019.34.e90.
7. Kohansal R, Martinez-Camblor P, Agustí A, Buist AS, Mannino DM, Soriano JB. The natural history of chronic airflow obstruction revisited: an analysis of the Framingham offspring cohort. Am J Respir Crit Care Med. 2009;180(1):3–10. https://doi.org/10.1164/rccm.200901-0047OC.
8. Lu L, Mackay DF, Pell JP. Meta-analysis of the association between cigarette smoking and peripheral arterial disease. Heart Br Card Soc. 2014;100(5):414–23. https://doi.org/10.1136/heartjnl-2013-304082.
9. Pan B, Jin X, Jun L, Qiu S, Zheng Q, Pan M. The relationship between smoking and stroke: a meta-analysis. Medicine. 2019;98(12):e14872. https://doi.org/10.1097/MD.0000000000014872.
10. Prevention (US) C for DC and, Promotion (US) NC for CDP and H, Health (US) O on S and. Cardiovascular diseases. Centers for disease control and prevention (US); 2010. https://www.ncbi.nlm.nih.gov/books/NBK53012/. Accessed 1 May 2020.
11. Durazzo TC, Mattsson N, Weiner MW. Alzheimer's disease neuroimaging initiative. Smoking and increased Alzheimer's disease risk: a review of potential mechanisms. Alzheimers Dement J Alzheimers Assoc. 2014;10(3):122–45. https://doi.org/10.1016/j.jalz.2014.04.009.

[1] Key References [2, 18, 31, 32, 69].

12. Prevention (US) C for DC and, Promotion (US) NC for CDP and H, Health (US) O on S and Cancer. Centers for Disease Control and Prevention (US); 2010. https://www.ncbi.nlm.nih.gov/books/NBK53010/. Accessed 1 May 2020.
13. Durazzo TC, Abadjian L, Kincaid A, Bilovsky-Muniz T, Boreta L, Gauger GE. The influence of chronic cigarette smoking on neurocognitive recovery after mild traumatic brain injury. J Neurotrauma. 2013;30(11):1013–22. https://doi.org/10.1089/neu.2012.2676.
14. Ostberg A, Tenovuo O. Smoking and outcome of traumatic brain injury. Brain Inj. 2014;28(2):155–60. https://doi.org/10.3109/02699052.2013.860468.
15. Kai FZ, Cao Y, Lv G, Song WY, Peng GZ. The effect of cigarette smoke exposure on spinal cord injury in rats. J Neurotrauma. 2013;30(6):473–9. https://doi.org/10.1089/neu.2012.2574.
16. DeVivo MJ, Kartus PL, Rutt RD, Stover SL, Fine PR. The influence of age at time of spinal cord injury on rehabilitation outcome. Arch Neurol. 1990;47(6):687–91. https://doi.org/10.1001/archneur.1990.00530060101026.
17. O'Sullivan ED, Hughes J, Ferenbach DA. Renal aging: causes and consequences. J Am Soc Nephrol. 2017;28(2):407–20. https://doi.org/10.1681/ASN.2015121308.
18. Boparai MK, Korc-Grodzicki B. Prescribing for older adults. Mt Sinai J Med N Y. 2011;78(4):613–26. https://doi.org/10.1002/msj.20278.
19. Burris JE. Pharmacologic approaches to geriatric pain management. Arch Phys Med Rehabil. 2004;85(7):45–9; quiz S50-51.
20. Gloth FM. Pharmacological management of persistent pain in older persons: focus on opioids and nonopioids. J Pain Off J Am Pain Soc. 2011;12(3):14–20. https://doi.org/10.1016/j.jpain.2010.11.006.
21. Bhala N, Emberson J, et al. Vascular and upper gastrointestinal effects of non-steroidal anti-inflammatory drugs: meta-analyses of individual participant data from randomised trials. Lancet Lond Engl. 2013;382(9894):769–79. https://doi.org/10.1016/S0140-6736(13)60900-9.
22. Ungprasert P, Matteson EL, Thongprayoon C. Nonaspirin nonsteroidal anti-inflammatory drugs and risk of hemorrhagic stroke: a systematic review and meta-analysis of observational studies. Stroke. 2016;47(2):356–64. https://doi.org/10.1161/STROKEAHA.115.011678.
23. Shin JY, Park MJ, Lee SH, et al. Risk of intracranial haemorrhage in antidepressant users with concurrent use of non-steroidal anti-inflammatory drugs: nationwide propensity score matched study. BMJ. 2015;351:h3517. https://doi.org/10.1136/bmj.h3517.
24. Borgeat A, Ofner C, Saporito A, Farshad M, Aguirre J. The effect of nonsteroidal anti-inflammatory drugs on bone healing in humans: a qualitative, systematic review. J Clin Anesth. 2018;49:92–100. https://doi.org/10.1016/j.jclinane.2018.06.020.
25. Dodwell ER, Latorre JG, Parisini E, et al. NSAID exposure and risk of nonunion: a meta-analysis of case-control and cohort studies. Calcif Tissue Int. 2010;87(3):193–202. https://doi.org/10.1007/s00223-010-9379-7.
26. Hsu JR, Mir H, Wally MK, Seymour RB, Orthopaedic Trauma Association Musculoskeletal Pain Task Force. Clinical practice guidelines for pain management in acute musculoskeletal injury. J Orthop Trauma. 2019;33(5):e158–82. https://doi.org/10.1097/BOT.0000000000001430.
27. Wheatley BM, Nappo KE, Christensen DL, Holman AM, Brooks DI, Potter BK. Effect of NSAIDs on bone healing rates: a meta-analysis. J Am Acad Orthop Surg. 2019;27(7):e330–6. https://doi.org/10.5435/JAAOS-D-17-00727.
28. Clegg A, Young JB. Which medications to avoid in people at risk of delirium: a systematic review. Age Ageing. 2011;40(1):23–9. https://doi.org/10.1093/ageing/afq140.
29. Seppala LJ, van de Glind EMM, Daams JG, et al. Fall-risk-increasing drugs: a systematic review and meta-analysis: III. Others. J Am Med Dir Assoc. 2018;19(4):372. https://doi.org/10.1016/j.jamda.2017.12.099.
30. Huang AR, Mallet L, Rochefort CM, Eguale T, Buckeridge DL, Tamblyn R. Medication-related falls in the elderly: causative factors and preventive strategies. Drugs Aging. 2012;29(5):359–76. https://doi.org/10.2165/11599460-000000000-00000.

31. Enderlin C, Rooker J, Ball S, et al. Summary of factors contributing to falls in older adults and nursing implications. Geriatr Nurs N Y N. 2015;36(5):397–406. https://doi.org/10.1016/j.gerinurse.2015.08.006.
32. American Geriatrics Society 2015 Beers Criteria Update Expert Panel. American Geriatrics Society 2015 updated beers criteria for potentially inappropriate medication use in older adults. J Am Geriatr Soc. 2015;63(11):2227–46. https://doi.org/10.1111/jgs.13702.
33. Liu H, Yang Y, Xia Y, et al. Aging of cerebral white matter. Ageing Res Rev. 2017;34:64–76. https://doi.org/10.1016/j.arr.2016.11.006.
34. Gauthier S, Reisberg B, Zaudig M, et al. Mild cognitive impairment. Lancet. 2006;367(9518):1262–70. https://doi.org/10.1016/S0140-6736(06)68542-5.
35. Knopman DS, DeKosky ST, Cummings JL, et al. Practice parameter: diagnosis of dementia (an evidence-based review). Report of the Quality Standards Subcommittee of the American Academy of Neurology. Neurology. 2001;56(9):1143–53.
36. Ballesteros J, Güemes I, Ibarra N, Quemada JI. The effectiveness of donepezil for cognitive rehabilitation after traumatic brain injury: a systematic review. J Head Trauma Rehabil. https://doi.org/10.1097/01.HTR.0000319935.99837.96.
37. Malouf R, Birks J. Donepezil for vascular cognitive impairment. Cochrane Database Syst Rev. https://doi.org/10.1002/14651858.CD004395.pub2.
38. Berthier ML, Hinojosa J, Martin M, Fernandez I. Open-label study of donepezil in chronic poststroke aphasia. Neurology. 2003;60(7):1218–9.
39. Tanaka Y, Miyazaki M, Albert ML. Effects of increased cholinergic activity on naming in aphasia. Lancet. https://doi.org/10.1016/S0140-6736(05)61820-X.
40. American Geriatrics Society Expert Panel on Postoperative Delirium in Older Adults. Postoperative delirium in older adults: best practice statement from the American Geriatrics Society. J Am Coll Surgeons. https://doi.org/10.1016/j.jamcollsurg.2014.10.019.
41. Bryczkowski SB, Lopreiato L, Yonclas PP, Sacca JJ, Mosenthal AC. Risk factors for delirium in older trauma patients admitted to the surgical intensive care unit. J Trauma Acute Care Surg. https://doi.org/10.1097/TA.0000000000000427.
42. Chow WB, Rosenthal RA, Merkow RP, Ko CY, Esnaola NF; American College of Surgeons National Surgical Quality Improvement Program. Optimal preoperative assessment of the geriatric surgical patient: a best practices guideline from the American College of Surgeons National Surgical Quality Improvement Program and the American Geriatrics Society. J Am Coll Surgeons. https://doi.org/10.1016/j.jamcollsurg.2012.06.017.
43. Taheri A, Dahri K, Chan P, Shaw M, Aulakh A, Tashakkor A. Evaluation of a symptom-triggered protocol approach to the management of alcohol withdrawal syndrome in older adults. J Am Geriatr Soc. https://doi.org/10.1111/jgs.12932.
44. Tampi RR, Tampi DJ, Ghori AK. Acetylcholinesterase inhibitors for delirium in older adults. Am J Alzheimer's Dis Other Dementias. https://doi.org/10.1177/1533317515619034.
45. Yu A, Wu S, Zhang Z, et al. Cholinesterase inhibitors for the treatment of delirium in non-ICU settings. Cochrane Database Syst Rev. https://doi.org/10.1002/14651858.CD012494.pub2.
46. Bean JF, Vora A, Frontera WR. Benefits of exercise for community-dwelling older adults. Arch Phys Med Rehabil. 2004;85(7):31–42; quiz S43-44.
47. Coronado VG, Thomas KE, Sattin RW, Johnson RL. The CDC traumatic brain injury surveillance system: characteristics of persons aged 65 years and older hospitalized with a TBI. J Head Trauma Rehabil. 2005;20(3):215–28.
48. Devivo MJ. Epidemiology of traumatic spinal cord injury: trends and future implications. Spinal Cord. 2012;50(5):365–72. https://doi.org/10.1038/sc.2011.178.
49. Kumar RG, Juengst SB, Wang Z, et al. Epidemiology of comorbid conditions among adults 50 years and older with traumatic brain injury. J Head Trauma Rehabil. 2017. https://doi.org/10.1097/HTR.0000000000000273.
50. Marion TE, Rivers CS, Kurban D, et al. Previously identified common post-injury adverse events in traumatic spinal cord injury-validation of existing literature and relation to selected

potentially modifiable comorbidities: a prospective Canadian cohort study. J Neurotrauma. https://doi.org/10.1089/neu.2016.4933.
51. Thompson HJ, Dikmen S, Temkin N. Prevalence of comorbidity and its association with traumatic brain injury and outcomes in older adults. Res Gerontol Nurs. 2012;5(1):17–24. https://doi.org/10.3928/19404921-20111206-02.
52. Arul K, Ge L, Ikpeze T, Baldwin A, Mesfin A. Traumatic spinal cord injuries in geriatric population: etiology, management, and complications. J Spine Surg. https://doi.org/10.21037/jss.2019.02.02.
53. Taylor MD, Tracy JK, Meyer W, Pasquale M, Napolitano LM. Trauma in the elderly: intensive care unit resource use and outcome. J Trauma. 2002;53(3):407–14. https://doi.org/10.1097/01.TA.0000020257.29911.70.
54. Nishijima DK, Shahlaie K, Sarkar K, Rudisill N, Holmes JF. Risk of unfavorable long-term outcome in older adults with traumatic intracranial hemorrhage and anticoagulant or antiplatelet use. Am J Emerg Med. 2013;31(8):1244–7. https://doi.org/10.1016/j.ajem.2013.04.035.
55. Peck KA, Calvo RY, Schechter MS, et al. The impact of preinjury anticoagulants and prescription antiplatelet agents on outcomes in older patients with traumatic brain injury. J Trauma Acute Care Surg. 2014;76(2):431–6. https://doi.org/10.1097/TA.0000000000000107.
56. Ott MM, Eriksson E, Vanderkolk W, Christianson D, Davis A, Scholten D. Antiplatelet and anticoagulation therapies do not increase mortality in the absence of traumatic brain injury. J Trauma. 2010;68(3):560–3. https://doi.org/10.1097/TA.0b013e3181ad6600.
57. Kumar RG, Olsen J, Juengst SB, et al. Comorbid conditions among adults 50 years and older with traumatic brain injury: examining associations with demographics, healthcare utilization, institutionalization, and 1-year outcomes. J Head Trauma Rehabil. https://doi.org/10.1097/HTR.0000000000000470.
58. Kumar RG, Ketchum JM, Corrigan JD, Hammond FM, Sevigny M, Dams-O'Connor K. The longitudinal effects of comorbid health burden on functional outcomes for adults with moderate to severe traumatic brain injury. J Head Trauma Rehabil. https://doi.org/10.1097/HTR.0000000000000572.
59. Corrigan JD, Zheng T, Pinto SM, et al. Effect of preexisting and co-occurring comorbid conditions on recovery in the 5 years after rehabilitation for traumatic brain injury. J Head Trauma Rehabil. https://doi.org/10.1097/HTR.0000000000000521
60. Tallqvist S, Kauppila AM, Vainionpää A, et al. Prevalence of comorbidities and secondary health conditions among the Finnish population with spinal cord injury. Spinal Cord. 2022;60(7):618–27. https://doi.org/10.1038/s41393-021-00704-7.
61. Krassioukov AV, Furlan JC, Fehlings MG. Medical comorbidities, secondary complications, and mortality in elderly with acute spinal cord injury. J Neurotrauma. 2003;20(4):391–9. https://doi.org/10.1089/089771503765172345.
62. Kaufman DW, Kelly JP, Rosenberg L, Anderson TE, Mitchell AA. Recent patterns of medication use in the ambulatory adult population of the United States: the Slone survey. JAMA. 2002;287(3):337–44.
63. Qato DM, Wilder J, Schumm LP, Gillet V, Alexander GC. Changes in prescription and over-the-counter medication and dietary supplement use among older adults in the United States, 2005 vs 2011. JAMA Intern Med. 2016;176(4):473–82. https://doi.org/10.1001/jamainternmed.2015.8581.
64. Maher RL, Hanlon J, Hajjar ER. Clinical consequences of polypharmacy in elderly. Expert Opin Drug Saf. 2014;13(1):57–65. https://doi.org/10.1517/14740338.2013.827660.
65. Jyrkkä J, Enlund H, Lavikainen P, Sulkava R, Hartikainen S. Association of polypharmacy with nutritional status, functional ability and cognitive capacity over a three-year period in an elderly population. Pharmacoepidemiol Drug Saf. https://doi.org/10.1002/pds.2116.
66. Hand BN, Krause JS, Simpson KN. Polypharmacy and adverse drug events among propensity score matched privately insured persons with and without spinal cord injury. Spinal Cord. https://doi.org/10.1038/s41393-017-0050-2.

67. Kitzman P, Cecil D, Kolpek JH. The risks of polypharmacy following spinal cord injury. J Spinal Cord Med. https://doi.org/10.1179/2045772314Y.0000000235.
68. Hammond FM, Barrett RS, Shea T, et al. Psychotropic medication use during inpatient rehabilitation for traumatic brain injury. Arch Phys Med Rehabil. https://doi.org/10.1016/j.apmr.2015.01.025.
69. Catapano JS, Chapman AJ, Horner LP, Lu M, Fraser DR, Fildes JJ. Pre-injury polypharmacy predicts mortality in isolated severe traumatic brain injury patients. Am J Surg. https://doi.org/10.1016/j.amjsurg.2016.07.010.
70. Murphy MP, Carmine H, Kolakowsky-Hayner S. Modifiable and nonmodifiable risk factors for falls after traumatic brain injury: an exploratory investigation with implications for medication use. Rehabil Nurs. https://doi.org/10.1002/rnj.89.
71. Jensen MP, Molton IR, Groah SL, et al. Secondary health conditions in individuals aging with SCI: terminology, concepts and analytic approaches. Spinal Cord. 2012;50(5):373–8. https://doi.org/10.1038/sc.2011.150.
72. LaPlante MP. Key goals and indicators for successful aging of adults with early-onset disability. Disabil Health J. 2014;7(1):44–50. https://doi.org/10.1016/j.dhjo.2013.08.005.
73. Heller T, Sorensen A. Promoting healthy aging in adults with developmental disabilities. Dev Disabil Res Rev. 2013;18(1):22–30. https://doi.org/10.1002/ddrr.1125.
74. DeVivo MJ. Sir Ludwig Guttmann lecture: trends in spinal cord injury rehabilitation outcomes from model systems in the United States: 1973-2006. Spinal Cord. 2007;45(11):713–21. https://doi.org/10.1038/sj.sc.3102026.
75. Lee JC, Heinemann AW. Forgoing physician visits because of cost: a source of health disparities for elderly people with disabilities? Arch Phys Med Rehabil. 2010;91(9):1319–26. https://doi.org/10.1016/j.apmr.2010.06.007.
76. Galea MD. Telemedicine in rehabilitation. Phys Med Rehabil Clin N Am. 2019;30(2):473–83. https://doi.org/10.1016/j.pmr.2018.12.002.

Chapter 18
Patient Prognostication in Traumatic Spinal Cord Injury and Brain Injury

Michelle Didesch, Justin Weppner, and Gary Galang

Chapter Objectives

1. Review key factors and testing in determining prognosis after traumatic spinal cord injury.
2. Review key factors and testing in determining prognosis after traumatic brain injury.
3. Understand differences in expected outcomes between traumatic brain injury and anoxic brain injury.
4. Build a framework for family meetings.
5. Understand key concepts through case illustrations.

Introduction

Amidst the intensity of events in acute care, patients and family members inevitably inquire about prognosis after a traumatic event. Information provided is often challenging to process and can be perceived as lacking detail, making it difficult to set

M. Didesch
Confluence Health, Central Washington Hospital and Clinics Campus, Wenatchee, WA, USA
e-mail: Michelle.Didesch@confluencehealth.org

J. Weppner (✉)
Virginia Tech Carilion School of Medicine, Edward Via College of Osteopathic Medicine, Roanoke, VA, USA
e-mail: jlweppner@carilionclinic.org

G. Galang
Department of Physical Medicine and Rehabilitation, University of Pittsburgh School of Medicine, Pittsburgh, PA, USA
e-mail: galangg@upmc.edu

A. K. Wagner, J. Weppner (eds.), *Acute Care Neuroconsultation and Neurorehabilitation Management*, https://doi.org/10.1007/978-3-031-42830-2_18

expectations for recovery [1]. An expert consultant serves as a resource for patients, family members, as well as other clinicians to provide a better understanding of prognosis and outcomes. The purpose of this chapter is to help guide these discussions. However, it is important to note that each patient is different and has their own set of circumstances. Outcomes data, while helpful in guiding clinical management, is imperfect. Therefore, this information should be used to provide anticipatory guidance, while acknowledging that individuals may either surpass or fall short of an expected outcome. The length of time it will take for an individual to make their recovery is variable. Ensuring quality care to prevent secondary complications such as spasticity and pressure injuries is essential in maximizing long-term functional independence.

Prognostic Factors in Traumatic Spinal Cord Injury

The most important prognostic factor for recovery after a traumatic spinal cord injury (SCI) is distinguishing between a complete versus incomplete injury [2]. This is determined by clinical examination using the International Standards for Neurological Classification of SCI (ISNCSCI) [3, 4]. The details of how to perform this exam are provided in Chap. 3.

A complete SCI is classified as American Spinal Injury Association (ASIA) Impairment Scale (AIS) A, which is defined as "no sensory or motor function is preserved in the sacral segments S4-5 [3, 4]". An incomplete injury is classified as ASIA Impairment Scale B-D, indicating that there is some sensory or motor sparing at the most distal spinal cord segments [3, 4]. Performing a neurological exam early after SCI is important as it helps determine treatment options and serves to monitor evolution of the neurologic injury. However, early exams can be affected by confounding factors such as patient participation, medical stability, and sedative medications [2, 5]. Furthermore, SCI can evolve with time and after surgical intervention. Therefore, recommendations are to use the ISNSCI exam starting at 72 h to 1 week to provide improved prognostic accuracy [5, 6]. That being said, early and periodic neurological exams using the ISNSCI standards are important to assess baseline neurological status and monitor for changes [5].

Recovery tends to be fastest in the first few months, with slower gains after 3–6 months [5]. Most of the expected recovery tends to occur by around 1–1.5 years after injury [2]. However, neurological improvement past this time point has been reported [5]. A patient with complete tetraplegia will usually recover at least one motor level, with some degree of improvement within two to three levels below the baseline neurologic level of injury [2, 7]. This can make a substantial difference in level of independence. For example, gaining a level from C3 to C4 may be the difference needed to wean off mechanical ventilation; gaining a level from C6 to C7 may allow for independent functional transfers [8]. Recovery of the "most rostral key muscle" that is less than 3/5 strength is correlated with initial strength [5]. If that muscle initially has at least some strength (1/5 or 2/5), it has a 90% likelihood of recovery at 1 year; whereas if the muscle initially has no strength (0/5), it has a

45% likelihood of recovery at 1 year [5]. Unfortunately, those whose injuries remain complete at their one-month exam have a poor prognosis for recovery of lower extremity strength [2, 9]. In complete paraplegia, functional neurological level tends to be more stagnant [2, 10].

Conversion from a complete to an incomplete injury varies depending on literature from 4 to 30% [2], but the consensus is that about 80–90% remain complete injuries [5, 9]. Of note, conversion to incomplete includes conversion to ASIA Impairment Scale B. Although technically an injury classified as ASIA Impairment Scale B is incomplete, only 20–50% will ultimately regain the ability to ambulate at 1 year [2]. For those with AIS B classifications, preservation of sharp/dull discrimination using pin prick, particularly in bilateral sacral dermatomes, is associated with a better prognosis for improvement in lower extremity strength than preservation of light touch only [5, 11, 12]. In addition, the ability to feel deep anal pressure has the weakest association with prognosis for ambulation when compared to the other sensory modalities at S4–S5 dermatomes or presence of voluntary anal contraction [2, 13]. On the other hand, ambulation potential with AIS C or D injury is higher with 28–75% reported with AIS C injuries and 67–100% reported for AIS D injuries [2, 5]. Of note, the term ambulation includes the use of assistive devices and braces if needed [5].

Recovery rates tend to be better after incomplete injuries as compared to complete injuries [5, 14]. Older age is associated with worse outcomes, including increased dependence on mobility and self-care, more medical complications, rehospitalizations, and discharge to a nursing home [15, 16]. In regard to specific incomplete syndromes, anterior cord syndrome has the poorest prognosis for motor recovery whereas Brown Sequard syndrome has the most favorable prognosis for ambulation potential [2, 17]. Rehabilitation outcomes and goals based on neurological level of injury are described in Table 18.1 and the Consortium Guidelines [5]. These expected outcomes can help guide goals in rehabilitation.

Spinal Shock

Spinal shock occurs acutely after traumatic SCI and is defined as the loss or decrease in spinal reflexes [18]. Return of reflexes is not an all-or-nothing phenomenon. Reflexes return sequentially, and the speed at which they return has prognostic value. The first reflex to return is called the deep plantar reflex. To evoke this reflex, the sole of the patient's foot is stroked the same way as done for a Babinski sign but with slightly more pressure [19]. However, rather than a quick plantar flexion response or an upgoing toe, in the delayed plantar reflex there will be a delayed, slow toe flexion and relaxation. Typically, as spinal shock resolves, this is replaced by the Babinski sign, although at times they can occur simultaneously. The bulbocavernosus reflex is the next reflex to return. A persistent delay in plantar reflex response is a poor prognostic sign for transition from a complete to incomplete injury [2, 18–20].

Table 18.1 Expected functional outcomes following SCI [5]

	C1-4	C5	C6	C7-8	T1-9	T10-S5
Respiratory	C1–C3 – Ventilator dependent – Inability to clear secretions C4 – May be able to breath without the ventilator	Low endurance and vital capacity secondary to paralysis of intercostals; may require assist to clear secretions	Low endurance and vital capacity secondary to paralysis of intercostals; may require assist to clear secretions	Low endurance and vital capacity secondary to paralysis of intercostals; may require assist to clear secretions	Compromised vital capacity and endurance	Intact respiratory function
Bowel	Total assist	Total assist	Some assist to independent with equipment	Some assist to independent with equipment	Independent	Independent
Bladder	Total assist	Total assist	Some assist to independent with equipment	Independent with equipment	Independent	Independent
Bed mobility	Total assist	Some assist	Some assist	Independent to some assist	Independent	Independent
Transfers	Total assist	Total assist	Level: some assist to independent Uneven: some to total assist	Level: independent Uneven: independent to some assist	Independent	Independent
Pressure relief/ positioning	Total assist—may be independent with equipment	Independent with equipment	Independent with equipment and/or adapted techniques	Independent	Independent	Independent
Eating	Total assist	Total assist with setup; then independent eating with equipment	Independent with or without equipment; except cutting, which is total assist	Independent	Independent	Independent
Dressing	Total assist	Lower extremity: total assist Upper extremity: some assist	Lower extremity: some assist to total assist Upper extremity: independent	Lower extremity: independent to some assist Upper extremity: independent	Independent	Independent

Grooming	Total assist	Some to total assist	Some assist to independent with equipment	Independent	Independent	Independent
Bathing	Total assist	Total assist	Lower body: some assist to total assist Upper body: independent	Lower body: independent to some assist Upper body: independent	Independent	Independent
Wheelchair propulsion	Manual: total assist Power: independent with equipment	Power: independent Manual: independent to some assist indoors on non-carpet level surface; some to total assist outdoors	Power: independent with standard arm drive on all surfaces Manual: independent indoors; some to total assist outdoors	Manual: independent on all indoor surfaces and level outdoor surfaces; some assist with uneven outdoor surfaces	Independent	Independent
Standing/ ambulation	Standing: total assist Ambulation: not indicated	Standing: total assist Ambulation: not indicated	Standing: total assist Ambulation: not indicated	Standing: independent to some assist Ambulation: not indicated	Standing: independent Ambulation: typically not functional	Standing: independent Ambulation: functional, some assist to independent
Transportation	Total assist	Independent with highly specialized modified equipment; some assist with accessible public transportation; total assist for attendant-operated vehicle	Independent driving from wheelchair	Independent in car if independent with transfer and wheelchair loading/ unloading; independent driving with modified van from captain's seat	Independent in car, including loading and unloading wheelchair	Independent in car, including loading and unloading wheelchair
Assist required	24-h attendant care	– Personal care: 10 hours/day – Homecare: 6 hours/day	– Personal care: 6 h/day – Homecare: 4 h/day	– Personal care: 6 h/ day – Homecare: 2 h/day	Homecare: 3 h/ day	T10-L1 Homecare: 2 h/day L2-S5 Homecare: 0–1 h/day

Assessments

Imaging Findings

Evidence of intramedullary spinal cord hemorrhage is a poor prognostic indicator [21–23]. Hemorrhagic areas are correlated with spinal cord necrosis [2]. Often, hemorrhage and edema co-occur; if there is spinal cord edema alone without hemorrhage, this finding holds a better prognosis than when there is evidence of blood [2, 23].

Neurophysiological Testing

Evoked potentials in the form of somatosensory evoked potentials (SSEPs) and motor evoked potentials (MEPs) are not necessary to diagnose traumatic SCI but can provide additional information [17, 24]. There are unique circumstances where this information can be particularly useful. This includes patients who are in a comatose state or for determining conversion disorder or malingering [2, 17]. For individuals with complete tetraplegia, tibial and pudendal SSEPs will generally be absent; among individuals with incomplete injury, these SSEP's will have prolonged latencies and decreased amplitudes [2]. The presence of tibial SSEPs indicates better prognosis for ambulation [17]. With motor evoked potentials, abductor digiti minimi is used to provide information on hand function while the tibialis anterior is used to provide prognosis for ambulation [2, 17]. Electromyographic (EMG) and nerve conduction studies can also be performed on peripheral nerves to rule out concomitant peripheral nerve injuries. If there are concomitant nerve injuries, these studies can provide more information on prognosticating peripheral nerve recovery [2, 17]. One important point to make is that SCI itself can also manifest with a low compound muscle action potential amplitude if there is motor neuron degeneration [2].

Case Illustration

A 25-year-old male is in a motor vehicle accident and has a flexion extension injury of his cervical spine. Initial MRI shows unilateral facet dislocation at C4–C5 spine level with associated hemorrhage and edema in the spinal cord. He is taken emergently to the operating room for stabilization of his spine. At 72 h, you complete an ISNCSCI neurologic exam and determine that he has a C4 ASIA Impairment Scale A classification SCI. His zone of partial preservation includes some strength in his bilateral biceps, wrist extensors, and right triceps. His family asks about his prognosis. What would you say?

Unfortunately, this patient has suffered a complete SCI and rate of recovery is limited when compared to incomplete injuries. With a C4 ASIA Impairment Scale A classification injury, he is expected to gain at least one motor level (C5), which means at least anti-gravity strength of the biceps. Because he has some strength remaining in his wrist extensors and triceps, we expect him to get some return of those muscles with time and rehabilitation. While his prognosis for ambulation is poor, we are hopeful that with the return of these key muscles in his upper extremities, he will be able to gain more functional independence. He should be referred to a specialized SCI rehabilitation center after his acute hospital stay to maximize his functional outcomes.

Prognostic Factors in Traumatic Brain Injury

Favorable long-term functional outcomes after severe traumatic brain injury (TBI) are underestimated, and a recent study demonstrated that severe TBI survivors have significant improvement in functional outcomes from 3 to 24 months after injury. At 2 years, three-fourths of survivors had a favorable outcome on the Glasgow Outcome Scale Extended (GOS-E) (Table 18.2) as defined as upper severe disability or better

Table 18.2 GOS-E [25]

Score	Description	
1	Death	
2	Vegetative state	
3	Severe disability—lower	– Patient requires frequent help or someone to be around most of the time
4	Severe disability—upper	– Does not need frequent help and is able to be at home alone for 8 hours at a time – Not able to shop without assistance – Not able to travel locally without assistance
5	Moderate disability—lower	– Not able to work or only able to work in a sheltered noncompetitive position – Unable to participate in regular social or leisure activities outside home – Daily disruption of family relationships or friendships due to psychological problems
6	Moderate disability—upper	– Able to work or study but at a reduced capacity – Participates less than half as often in regular social and leisure activities outside of the home – Frequent but tolerable disruption of family and relationships or friendships due to psychological problems
7	Good recovery—lower	– Participates at least half as often as before injury in regular social and leisure activities outside of the home – Occasional disruption of family and relationships or friendships due to psychological problems – Symptoms related to TBI affect daily life
8	Good recovery—upper	– Able to work at pre-TBI capacity – Able to resume regular social and leisure activities outside of the home – No psychological problems resulting in ongoing family disruption or disruption of friendships

Table 18.3 Summary of predictor variables in adults with severe TBI

Variable	Summary
Age	– Linear association between advancing age and poorer functional outcome with older age associated with a worse outcome Threshold values – Good recovery is unlikely when age is older than 65 years
GCS	– Lower admission GCS scores, and in particular, the lower motor response is associated with a worse patient outcome
MRI	– Bilateral brainstem lesions make a good recovery unlikely on GOS – Anterior and non-hemorrhagic lesions on MRI showed the highest positive predictive value for good outcome on the GOS Threshold values – Good recovery is unlikely when MRI indicates a bilateral brainstem lesion
Duration of coma	– Duration of coma has been shown to have a near linear relationship with duration of recovery time Threshold values – Length of coma greater than 4 weeks makes good recovery unlikely – Severe disability is unlikely when duration of coma is less than 2 weeks
Duration of PTA	– The longer the duration of PTA, the worse the patient outcome Threshold values – Severe disability is unlikely when PTA is less than 2 months – Good recovery is unlikely when duration of PTA is greater than 3 months
SSEP	– Bilaterally normal SSEPs usually imply a good outcome – Bilaterally absent SSEPs are strongly predictive of poor outcome – SSEPs provide valuable complementary information to assist with the prediction of outcome in patients with severe TBI

GCS Glasgow coma scale, *GOS* Glasgow outcome scale, *PTA* post-traumatic amnesia, *SSEP* somatosensory evoked potentials

(GOS-E score of 4–8) demonstrating long-term prognosis in severe TBI is better than broadly appreciated [26]. There are several key factors used to help determine prognosis after TBI (Table 18.3). In particular, these factors below are helpful in guiding families and the clinical team in the setting of more severe injuries.

Glasgow Coma Scale

The Glasgow Coma Scale (GCS) is commonly used to provide a general assessment on a patient's neurological status. It is divided into motor, verbal, and visual components [27]. The total score ranges from 3 to 15, with initial GCS of 3–8 correlating with severe brain injury, 9–12 with moderate brain injury, and 13–15 with mild brain injury. As expected, low initial GCS scores are associated with poorer outcomes [28–30]. However, these correlations are not linear [28]. GCS scores are influenced by other medical factors including intubation, sedation, and paralytics. The GCS score provides a measure of the severity of brain injury but should not be used alone as a prognostic tool.

Table 18.4 Glasgow outcome scale [25]

Score	Description	
1	Death	
2	Vegetative state	
3	Severe disability	– Unable to live alone and requires the daily assistance of another person at home
4	Moderate disability	– Modified independent at home – Able to utilize public transportation – Able to work in a supported environment
5	Good recovery	– Able to resume normal occupational and social activities – There may be minor residual physical or psychological deficits

Length of Coma

The term coma duration has variable definitions in literature but is generally described as the duration of time before command following [30]. Prolonged coma is associated with worse outcomes, in particular if the coma extends past one month [30–34]. Duration of coma is also correlated with the duration of post-traumatic amnesia [32].

Post-traumatic Amnesia

Post-traumatic amnesia (PTA) is defined as the inability to build new memories after TBI [35, 36]. Prolonged duration of post-traumatic amnesia is associated with worse outcomes including employment [30, 32–34, 36]. PTA lasting longer than 3 months is associated with poor outcome based on the Glasgow Outcome Scale (GOS) (Table 18.4) whereas PTA lasting less than two months is associated with decreased likelihood of severe disability [30].

Assessments

Imaging Findings

A CT scan can provide a quick emergent assessment of bony injury, hemorrhage, edema, and herniation after TBI. However, when able, magnetic resonance imaging (MRI) is recommended to evaluate the extent of neural injury. The centripetal model of closed TBI explains that stronger forces result in deeper shear lesions in the brain [37]. The shear lesions that occur with trauma are also known as diffuse axonal injury [37]. Therefore, deeper lesions seen on MRI, especially brainstem lesions, are correlated with more severe injuries, longer duration of coma, and worse outcomes [37–39]. Bilateral brainstem lesions are associated with poor prognosis for good recovery based on the GOS [30].

Electrophysiological Testing

In severe brain injury, electroencephalograms (EEGs) are used to rule out underlying seizures as a cause of neurological dysfunction. Malignant patterns can be correlated with poor outcomes [40].

SSEPs can provide more information regarding prognosis in patients in a comatose or unresponsive wakefulness syndrome. In fact, some argue that SSEPs provide the best outcome prediction data [41]. Details of electrophysiological testing are covered in Chap. 4. Preservation of normal somatosensory evoked potentials and brainstem auditory evoked potentials is associated with an improved prognosis [40]. On the other hand, abnormalities in the brainstem auditory evoked potentials are associated with worse outcomes [40]. Bilateral cortical response loss is correlated with very poor prognosis of good recovery [42]. The timing of when to perform this study is unclear, although serial exams may be helpful as initial presence of bilateral cortical responses does not guarantee a good recovery, and evoked potentials can change with time [40, 42].

Special Populations

Traumatic Brain Injury in Elderly

Older age, especially after age 65, is associated with worse outcomes after TBI [30]. The medical picture is complicated by pre-existing medical and neurodegenerative comorbidities, including underlying cerebral atrophy and use of blood thinners. Older individuals have higher mortality rates after TBI [43, 44]. Even after mild injury, patients should be monitored closely as they can have delayed worsening of neurological status [44]. Unfortunately, they are also more likely to need assistance, have slower improvements in functional independence, and be discharged to a long-term care facility [45, 46]. That said, older adults can also have good recovery. Therefore, inpatient rehabilitation should be considered as this can help many elderly TBI survivors return safely to the community [30, 45].

Mild to Moderate Injuries

The above prognostic factors are helpful when caring for patients with severe brain injuries. Patients with mild to moderate injuries have better prognosis for good recovery. Patients are more likely to have moderate disability with older age, CT scan changes and worse GCS scores [30]. Longer PTA duration is also associated with worse outcomes [47]. Even for those with good recovery, there can be persistent difficulties with attention, memory, headache, behavior, and mood disorders. These can affect functional independence, quality of life, and employment, and these issues should be addressed early on with close follow-up [47].

Anoxic Brain Injury

Any patient surviving a cardiac arrest should be screened for evidence of anoxic brain injury as the duration of cardiac arrest does not always correlate with the amount of neurologic damage [48]. Consultants have the opportunity to help identify these patients and assist with treatment. Patients with anoxic brain injury are thought to have worse prognosis than patients with TBI; however, as cardiac arrest survival improves, researchers are still working to better understand this cohort [48–50]. Although the rate of functional improvement is slower in patents with anoxic brain injury, there are still significant gains made with rehabilitation [49]. Somatosensory evoked potentials can be helpful in determining prognosis after severe anoxic brain injury. In particular, bilateral N20 response loss with stimulation from the median nerve is associated with poor prognosis after anoxic brain injury (i.e., unresponsive wakefulness syndrome or death) [40, 51]. However, peripheral nerve injury and SCI must be ruled out before making this conclusion as these can affect the results of the study. In addition, recommendations are to hold off for a period of 12–24 h after injury before performing the study, as there may be transient loss of the N20 response that recovers after a hypoperfusion event. Of note, the absence of an N20 response is a less reliable predictor in TBI [40].

The basal ganglia, cerebellum, and hippocampus are particularly vulnerable to hypoxic injury. The consequences of anoxic brain injury correlate with the degree of damage to these vulnerable regions. Movement disorders can be seen after anoxic brain injury, ranging from tremors, myoclonus, chorea, and hemiballismus, which is consistent with injuries to the basal ganglia and cerebellum. Unlike the hypodopaminergic state seen in TBI [52], research shows that there may be a hyperdopaminergic state in anoxic brain injury, which is worsened with dopamine agonists typically used after brain injury [53]. On the other hand, there may be selective damage to GABAergic neurons, raising the potential of using medications such as donepezil and zolpidem to modulate and restore pallidal-thalamic

GABAergic outflow. The occipital lobe is also vulnerable to hypoxic injury and may result in cortical blindness. Patients are also at risk for ischemic injury to the optic nerve [48].

Case Illustration

An 18-year-old male is admitted to the intensive care unit (ICU) after a motor vehicle accident. He was a restrained driver that collided with another vehicle at an intersection. He required intubation at the scene and on admission to the emergency room his GCS score was 4T (1 for eye response; 1 for verbal response; 2 for decerebrate posturing to pain; T = intubated). CT imaging of the head revealed a small subdural and subarachnoid hemorrhage; MRI imaging also revealed small petechial areas of hemorrhage in bilateral frontal lobes, temporal lobes, and corpus callosum. He is now Day 3 after trauma and repeat CT scan is stable. Sedation was weaned to assess his neurological status; however, no improvements in his neurological status were noted. The ICU team inquires as to why this may be and if further testing would help guide prognosis. What would you say?

The mechanism of injury is consistent with a high velocity TBI. CT scan can miss evidence of diffuse axonal injury; however, the findings on MRI are consistent with this diagnosis. The depth of lesions seen on imaging (i.e., corpus callosum involvement) indicates very strong forces at the time of injury. Continuous EEG monitoring can be helpful to evaluate for electrographic evidence of sleep and to rule out underlying seizures as a cause of his neurological dysfunction. In addition, SSEPs and brainstem auditory evoked potentials can provide more detail regarding the severity of his injury, including assessment of brainstem involvement. Other causes of encephalopathy such as metabolic encephalopathy should be ruled out at the same time.

Building a Framework for Family Meetings

Family meetings around the care of a critically ill patient are complex, and physiatry consultants can provide valuable information regarding prognosis and next steps after acute care. The withdrawal of life-sustaining treatment is commonly made in the early phase of acute hospitalization with limited knowledge of the range of possible outcomes following severe acquired brain injury [54–58]. In addition, medical providers often present an overly pessimistic prognosis that negatively influences care decisions [59, 60]. Prior to a family meeting, it is prudent to meet with other members of the team to create a framework for the discussion [61]. The consulting physiatrist should advocate that impairments evident during the first 2 weeks post-injury should not be a definitive indicator of unfavorable long-term functional outcomes for persons with severe TBI. Clinicians should be cautious about suggesting a high likelihood of permanent severe disability within the first two weeks post-injury [62]. In part, the family meeting allows the medical team to provide the most up-to-date information regarding the care of their loved one. The medical provider must understand the implicit personal, social, religious, and cultural biases and their impact on the delivery of prognostic information [63, 64]. On the other hand, how that information is perceived depends not only on the delivery, but also on the readiness of the caregivers. Careful attention should be made to providing information gradually and frequently re-assessing caregivers' perception [61]. Simple strategies such as turning off cell phones and pagers and allocating a quiet space for discussion can make a significant difference. Providing information on resources available both in the hospital and for transitioning care is necessary [61]. Based on the current disorders of consciousness (DoC) clinical practice guidelines "when discussing prognosis with caregivers of patients with a DoC during the first 28 days postinjury, clinicians must avoid statements that suggest these patients have a universally poor prognosis" [65]. As training on how to conduct family meetings is not a usual part of medical education, providers should take time to review palliative care literature and proceedings of the Curing Coma Campaign NIH Symposium on this topic [61, 63, 66].

Summary and Key Points

- The most important factor in prognosis after traumatic SCI is determining complete versus incomplete injury.
- Expect at least one motor level recovery in complete tetraplegia with more stagnant progress in complete paraplegia.
- Incomplete spinal cord injury has a better prognosis for recovery.
- Preservation of sharp/dull discrimination is associated with improved outcomes for AIS B classification injuries.
- Intramedullary spinal cord hemorrhage is a poor prognostic indicator.
- Findings correlated with poor outcomes in TBI are low GCS score, coma >4 weeks, PTA >3 months, penetrating injuries, deeper lesions, and/or bilateral brainstem injuries on imaging.
- Abnormal brainstem auditory evoked potentials and loss of bilateral cortical responses on SSEP testing are correlated with poor outcomes in TBI.
- Older age is associated with worse outcomes after both TBI and SCI.
- The consulting physiatrist should advocate that impairments evident during the first two weeks post-injury should not be a definitive indicator of unfavorable long-term functional outcomes for persons with severe TBI. Clinicians should be cautious about suggesting a high likelihood of permanent severe disability within the first two weeks post-injury.
- When discussing prognosis with caregivers of patients with a DoC during the first 28 days post-injury, clinicians must avoid statements that suggest these patients have a universally poor prognosis.
- For those with mild-moderate brain injuries, longer duration of PTA, lower GCS scores, and changes on CT scan are associated with worse outcomes.
- Functional improvement after anoxic brain injury is slower but there can still be significant gains.

References[1]

1. Lefebvre H, Levert MJ. Breaking the news of traumatic brain injury and incapacities. Brain Inj. 2006;20(7):711–8. https://doi.org/10.1080/02699050600744244.
2. Burns AS, et al. Predicting outcome following traumatic spinal cord injury. In: Campagnolo DI, Kirshblum S, Nash MS, Heary RF, Gorman PH, editors. Spinal cord medicine. 2nd ed. Philadelphia: Lippincott Williams & Wilkins; 2011.
3. Kirshblum SC, Burns SP, Biering-Sorensen F, et al. International standards for neurological classification of spinal cord injury (revised 2011). J Spinal Cord Med. 2011;34(6):535–46. https://doi.org/10.1179/204577211X13207446293695.
4. American Spinal Injury Association ISCS. International standards for neurological classification of spinal cord injury (ISNCSCI). http://asia-spinalinjury.org/learning/. Accessed 26 September 2017.
5. Consortium for Spinal Cord Medicine. Outcomes following traumatic spinal cord injury: clinical practice guidelines for health-care professionals. J Spinal Cord Med. 2000;23(4):289–316.
6. Brown PJ, Marino RJ, Herbison GJ, Ditunno JF. The 72-hour examination as a predictor of recovery in motor complete quadriplegia. Arch Phys Med Rehabil. 1991;72(8):546–8.
7. Sabharwal S. Functional outcomes following SCI. Essentials of spinal cord medicine. New York: Demos Medical Publishing; 2014.
8. Kirshblum S, et al. Rehabilitation of spinal cord injury. In: Campagnolo DI, Kirshblum S, Nash MS, Heary RF, Gorman PH, editors. Spinal cord medicine. 2nd ed. Philadelphia: Lippincott Williams & Wilkins; 2011.
9. Waters RL, Adkins RH, Yakura JS, Sie I. Motor and sensory recovery following complete tetraplegia. Arch Phys Med Rehabil. 1993;74(3):242–7.
10. Waters RL, Yakura JS, Adkins RH, Sie I. Recovery following complete paraplegia. Arch Phys Med Rehabil. 1992;73(9):784–9.
11. Crozier KS, Graziani V, Ditunno JF, Herbison GJ. Spinal cord injury: prognosis for ambulation based on sensory examination in patients who are initially motor complete. Arch Phys Med Rehabil. 1991;72(2):119–21.
12. Waters RL, Adkins RH, Yakura JS, Sie I. Motor and sensory recovery following incomplete tetraplegia. Arch Phys Med Rehabil. 1994;75(3):306–11.
13. van Middendorp JJ, AJF H, Pouw MH, Van de Meent H, EM-SCI Study Group. Is determination between complete and incomplete traumatic spinal cord injury clinically relevant? Validation of the ASIA sacral sparing criteria in a prospective cohort of 432 patients. Spinal Cord. 2009;47(11):809–16. https://doi.org/10.1038/sc.2009.44.
14. Waters RL, Adkins RH, Yakura JS, Sie I. Motor and sensory recovery following incomplete paraplegia. Arch Phys Med Rehabil. 1994;75(1):67–72.
15. DeVivo MJ, Kartus PL, Rutt RD, Stover SL, Fine PR. The influence of age at time of spinal cord injury on rehabilitation outcome. Arch Neurol. 1990;47(6):687–91. https://doi.org/10.1001/archneur.1990.00530060101026.
16. Penrod LE, Hegde SK, Ditunno JF Jr. Age effect on prognosis for functional recovery in acute, traumatic central cord syndrome. Arch Phys Med Rehabil. 1990;71(12):963–8.
17. Curt A, Dietz V. Electrophysiological recordings in patients with spinal cord injury: significance for predicting outcome. Spinal Cord. 1999;37(3):157–65.
18. Ko HY, Ditunno JF Jr, Graziani V, Little JW. The pattern of reflex recovery during spinal shock. Spinal Cord. 1999;37(6):402–9. https://doi.org/10.1038/sj.sc.3100840.
19. Weinstein DE, Ko HY, Graziani V, Ditunno JF Jr. Prognostic significance of the delayed plantar reflex following spinal cord injury. J Spinal Cord Med. 1997;20(2):207–11.
20. Ditunno JF, Little JW, Tessler A, Burns AS. Spinal shock revisited: a four-phase model. Spinal Cord. 2004;42(7):383–95. https://doi.org/10.1038/sj.sc.3101603.

[1] Key References [5, 30, 52, 61, 64].

21. Cotler HB, Kulkarni MV, Bondurant FJ. Magnetic resonance imaging of acute spinal cord trauma: preliminary report. J Orthop Trauma. 1988;2(1):1–4.
22. Marciello MA, Flanders AE, Herbison GJ, Schaefer DM, Friedman DP, Lane JI. Magnetic resonance imaging related to neurologic outcome in cervical spinal cord injury. Arch Phys Med Rehabil. 1993;74(9):940–6.
23. Ramon S, Dominguez R, Ramirez L, et al. Clinical and magnetic resonance imaging correlation in acute spinal cord injury. Spinal Cord. 1997;35(10):664–73.
24. Jacobs SR, Yeaney NK, Herbison GJ, Ditunno JF. Future ambulation prognosis as predicted by somatosensory evoked potentials in motor complete and incomplete quadriplegia. Arch Phys Med Rehabil. 1995;76(7):635–41.
25. Wilson L, Boase K, Nelson LD, et al. A manual for the Glasgow outcome scale-extended interview. J Neurotrauma. 2021;38(17):2435–46. https://doi.org/10.1089/neu.2020.7527.
26. Wilkins TE, Beers SR, Borrasso AJ, et al. Favorable functional recovery in severe traumatic brain injury survivors beyond six months. J Neurotrauma. 2019;36(22):3158–63. https://doi.org/10.1089/neu.2018.6153.
27. Teasdale G, Jennett B. Assessment of coma and impaired consciousness. A practical scale. Lancet. 1974;2(7872):81–4.
28. Udekwu P, Kromhout-Schiro S, Vaslef S, Baker C, Oller D. Glasgow Coma Scale score, mortality, and functional outcome in head-injured patients. J Trauma. 2004;56(5):1084–9.
29. Kim YJ. A systematic review of factors contributing to outcomes in patients with traumatic brain injury. J Clin Nurs. 2011;20(11-12):1518–32. https://doi.org/10.1111/j.1365-2702.2010.03618.x.
30. Kothari S, DiTomasso C. Prognosis after severe traumatic brain injury: a practical, evidence-based approach. In: Zasler ND, Katz DI, Zafonte RD, editors. Brain injury medicine: principles and practice. 2nd ed. New York: Demos Medical Publishing; 2013.
31. Tate RL, Lulham JM, Broe GA, Strettles B, Pfaff A. Psychosocial outcome for the survivors of severe blunt head injury: the results from a consecutive series of 100 patients. J Neurol Neurosurg Psychiatry. 1989;52(10):1128–34.
32. Katz DI, Alexander MP. Traumatic brain injury. Predicting course of recovery and outcome for patients admitted to rehabilitation. Arch Neurol. 1994;51(7):661–70.
33. Ellenberg JH, Levin HS, Saydjari C. Posttraumatic amnesia as a predictor of outcome after severe closed head injury. Prospective assessment. Arch Neurol. 1996;53(8):782–91.
34. Sherer M, Yablon SA, Nakase-Richardson R, Nick TG. Effect of severity of post-traumatic confusion and its constituent symptoms on outcome after traumatic brain injury. Arch Phys Med Rehabil. 2008;89(1):42–7. https://doi.org/10.1016/j.apmr.2007.08.128.
35. Russell WR, Smith A. Post-traumatic amnesia in closed head injury. Arch Neurol. 1961;5:4–17.
36. Nakase-Richardson R, Sepehri A, Sherer M, Yablon SA, Evans C, Mani T. Classification schema of posttraumatic amnesia duration-based injury severity relative to 1-year outcome: analysis of individuals with moderate and severe traumatic brain injury. Arch Phys Med Rehabil. 2009;90(1):17–9. https://doi.org/10.1016/j.apmr.2008.06.030.
37. Levin HS. Prediction of recovery from traumatic brain injury. J Neurotrauma. 1995;12(5):913–22. https://doi.org/10.1089/neu.1995.12.913.
38. Levin HS, Williams D, Crofford MJ, et al. Relationship of depth of brain lesions to consciousness and outcome after closed head injury. J Neurosurg. 1988;69(6):861–6. https://doi.org/10.3171/jns.1988.69.6.0861.
39. Lagares A, Ramos A, Perez-Nunez A, et al. The role of MR imaging in assessing prognosis after severe and moderate head injury. Acta Neurochir. 2009;151(4):341–56. https://doi.org/10.1007/s00701-009-0194-8.
40. Guerit JM. Neurophysiological testing in neurocritical care. Curr Opin Crit Care. 2010;16(2):98–104. https://doi.org/10.1097/MCC.0b013e328337541a.
41. Carter BG, Butt W. Are somatosensory evoked potentials the best predictor of outcome after severe brain injury? A systematic review. Intensive Care Med. 2005;31(6):765–75. https://doi.org/10.1007/s00134-005-2633-1.

42. Amantini A, Grippo A, Fossi S, et al. Prediction of 'awakening' and outcome in prolonged acute coma from severe traumatic brain injury: evidence for validity of short latency SEPs. Clin Neurophysiol. 2005;116(1):229–35. https://doi.org/10.1016/j.clinph.2004.07.008.
43. McIntyre A, Mehta S, Aubut J, Dijkers M, Teasell RW. Mortality among older adults after a traumatic brain injury: a meta-analysis. Brain Inj. 2013;27(1):31–40. https://doi.org/10.3109/02699052.2012.700086.
44. Thompson HJ, McCormick WC, Kagan SH. Traumatic brain injury in older adults: epidemiology, outcomes, and future implications. J Am Geriatr Soc. 2006;54(10):1590–5. https://doi.org/10.1111/j.1532-5415.2006.00894.x.
45. Flanagan SR, Hibbard MR, Riordan B, Gordon WA. Traumatic brain injury in the elderly: diagnostic and treatment challenges. Clin Geriatr Med. 2006;22(2):449–68. https://doi.org/10.1016/j.cger.2005.12.011.
46. Testa JA, Malec JF, Moessner AM, Brown AW. Outcome after traumatic brain injury: effects of aging on recovery. Arch Phys Med Rehabil. 2005;86(9):1815–23. https://doi.org/10.1016/j.apmr.2005.03.010.
47. van der Naalt J. Prediction of outcome in mild to moderate head injury: a review. J Clin Exp Neuropsychol. 2001;23(6):837–51. https://doi.org/10.1076/jcen.23.6.837.1018.
48. Sawyer KN, Callaway CW, Wagner AK. Life after death: surviving cardiac arrest—an overview of epidemiology, best acute care practices, and considerations for rehabilitation care. Curr Phys Med Rehabil Rep. 2017;5(1):30–9. https://doi.org/10.1007/s40141-017-0148-7.
49. Fitzgerald A, Aditya H, Prior A, McNeill E, Pentland B. Anoxic brain injury: clinical patterns and functional outcomes. A study of 93 cases. Brain Inj. 2010;24(11):1311–23. https://doi.org/10.3109/02699052.2010.506864.
50. Cullen NK, Crescini C, Bayley MT. Rehabilitation outcomes after anoxic brain injury: a case-controlled comparison with traumatic brain injury. PM R. 2009;1(12):1069–76. https://doi.org/10.1016/j.pmrj.2009.09.013.
51. Stevens RD, Sutter R. Prognosis in severe brain injury. Crit Care Med. 2013;41(4):1104–23. https://doi.org/10.1097/CCM.0b013e318287ee79.
52. Wagner AK, Sokoloski JE, Ren D, et al. Controlled cortical impact injury affects dopaminergic transmission in the rat striatum. J Neurochem. 2005;95(2):457–65. https://doi.org/10.1111/j.1471-4159.2005.03382.x.
53. Nora GJ, Harun R, Fine DF, et al. Ventricular fibrillation cardiac arrest produces a chronic striatal hyperdopaminergic state that is worsened by methylphenidate treatment. J Neurochem. 2017;142(2):305–22. https://doi.org/10.1111/jnc.14058.
54. Nakase-Richardson R, Whyte J, Giacino JT, et al. Longitudinal outcome of patients with disordered consciousness in the NIDRR TBI model systems programs. J Neurotrauma. 2012;29(1):59–65. https://doi.org/10.1089/neu.2011.1829.
55. Whyte J, Nakase-Richardson R, Hammond FM, et al. Functional outcomes in traumatic disorders of consciousness: 5-year outcomes from the National Institute on Disability and Rehabilitation Research Traumatic Brain Injury Model Systems. Arch Phys Med Rehabil. 2013;94(10):1855–60.
56. Hammond FM, Giacino JT, Nakase Richardson R, et al. Disorders of consciousness due to traumatic brain injury: functional status ten years post-injury. J Neurotrauma. 2019;36(7):1136–46. https://doi.org/10.1089/neu.2018.5954.
57. Turgeon AF, Lauzier F, Burns KE, et al. Determination of neurologic prognosis and clinical decision making in adult patients with severe traumatic brain injury: a survey of Canadian intensivists, neurosurgeons, and neurologists. Crit Care Med. 2013;41(4):1086–93. https://doi.org/10.1097/CCM.0b013e318275d046.
58. Kowalski RG, Hammond FM, Weintraub AH, et al. Recovery of consciousness and functional outcome in moderate and severe traumatic brain injury. JAMA Neurol. 2021;78(5):548–57. https://doi.org/10.1001/jamaneurol.2021.0084.

59. Hammond F, Natarajan S, Toomer A, Huynh T, Norton J. Accuracy of predicting 6-month outcome at 48 hours following severe traumatic brain injury: a pilot study. J Neurotrauma. 2009;26(8):A1–101.
60. Izzy S, Compton R, Carandang R, Hall W, Muehlschlegel S. Self-fulfilling prophecies through withdrawal of care: do they exist in traumatic brain injury, too? Neurocrit Care. 2013;19(3):347–63. https://doi.org/10.1007/s12028-013-9925-z.
61. Hudson P, Quinn K, O'Hanlon B, Aranda S. Family meetings in palliative care: multidisciplinary clinical practice guidelines. BMC Palliat Care. 2008;7:12. https://doi.org/10.1186/1472-684X-7-12.
62. McCrea MA, Giacino JT, Barber J, et al. Functional outcomes over the first year after moderate to severe traumatic brain injury in the prospective, longitudinal TRACK-TBI study. JAMA Neurol. 2021;78(8):982–92. https://doi.org/10.1001/jamaneurol.2021.2043.
63. Mainali S, Aiyagari V, Alexander S, et al. Proceedings of the second curing coma campaign NIH symposium: challenging the future of research for coma and disorders of consciousness. Neurocrit Care. 2022;37(1):326–50. https://doi.org/10.1007/s12028-022-01505-3.
64. Silvennoinen K, Meretoja A, Strbian D, Putaala J, Kaste M, Tatlisumak T. Do-not-resuscitate (DNR) orders in patients with intracerebral hemorrhage. Int J Stroke. 2014;9(1):53–8. https://doi.org/10.1111/ijs.12161.
65. Giacino JT, Katz DI, Schiff ND, et al. Practice guideline update recommendations summary: disorders of consciousness: report of the guideline development, dissemination, and implementation subcommittee of the American Academy of Neurology; the American Congress of Rehabilitation Medicine; and the National Institute on Disability, Independent Living, and Rehabilitation Research. Arch Phys Med Rehabil. 2018;99(9):1699–709. https://doi.org/10.1016/j.apmr.2018.07.001.
66. Claassen J, Akbari Y, Alexander S, et al. Proceedings of the first curing coma campaign NIH symposium: challenging the future of research for coma and disorders of consciousness. Neurocrit Care. 2021;35(1):4–23. https://doi.org/10.1007/s12028-021-01260-x.

Chapter 19
Acute Discharge: Levels of Care, Education, and Transition Planning

Justin Weppner and Amy K. Wagner

Chapter Objectives

1. Define transitional care as it applies to persons with neurologic impairment.
2. Describe levels of care, including LTACHs, SNFs, IRFs, DoC programs, and home healthcare.

Introduction

Transitional care is a set of actions designed to ensure the coordination and continuity of healthcare when patients transfer between different locations or different levels of care [1–3]. Representative locations include hospitals, long-term acute care hospitals (LTACHs), skilled nursing facilities (SNFs), acute inpatient rehabilitation facilities (IRFs), the patient's home, primary and specialty care offices, and long-term care facilities. Transitional care is based on a comprehensive care plan and the latest information regarding the patient's goals, preferences, and clinical status. It includes logistical arrangements, patient and family education, and coordination among the health professionals involved in the transition; patient safety and care continuity are essential goals of care. Transitional care, encompassing both the sending and receiving aspects of patient transfer, is essential for persons with complex care needs. Poor transitions between acute inpatient and post-acute care can lead to adverse events, unmet needs, low satisfaction with care, and high rehospitalization rates for patients with traumatic brain injury (TBI) and spinal cord injury (SCI).

J. Weppner (✉)
Virginia Tech Carilion School of Medicine, Edward Via College of Osteopathic Medicine, Roanoke, VA, USA
e-mail: jlweppner@carilionclinic.org

A. K. Wagner
Department of Physical Medicine and Rehabilitation, University of Pittsburgh School of Medicine, Pittsburgh, PA, USA
e-mail: wagnerak@upmc.edu

A. K. Wagner, J. Weppner (eds.), *Acute Care Neuroconsultation and Neurorehabilitation Management*, https://doi.org/10.1007/978-3-031-42830-2_19

Transition of Care Evaluation

Informed planning for care transitions is essential to avoid adverse effects in patients with complex health care needs. Transition to post-acute care occurs for patients who are especially vulnerable and requires careful planning and support with complex health care needs after TBI and SCI. Acute care hospitals are often under pressure to transfer patients from intensive care units to wards and subsequently discharge them. Consequently, a limited scope of patient transitional needs assessment, often paired with rapid decision-making, may lead to inadequate transitional care planning and inappropriate care transitions.

Establishing the answers to these questions should allow the consulting provider to make appropriate post-acute care recommendations:

- Was the patient independent before the acute admission?
- How will this current episode of illness or injury impact the patient's independence?
- Are the impairments expected to be short-term or long-term?
- Does the patient have an adequate existing support network, and/or access to outside supportive care, to manage the loss of independence?
- Does the patient require round the clock supervision, and is this level of supervision available to the patient?
- Does the patient have adequate resources for post-acute discharge needs such as medications, durable medical equipment, rehabilitation, or follow-up treatment?
- Does the patient have physical barriers in the home that will limit community discharge, such as stairs, narrow doorways, or other environmental barriers?
- What are the patient's goals for rehabilitation, and are they motivated to participate in an intensive rehabilitation program?
- Does the patient require active and ongoing therapeutic intervention in multiple disciplines (physical therapy, occupational therapy, speech-language pathology, prosthetics/orthotics, or rehabilitation psychology)?
- Does the patient require post-acute physician supervision for medical management of co-morbidities?
- Is the patient expected to actively participate in and benefit significantly from an intensive rehabilitation therapy program and realistically meet their goals?

Acute Inpatient Rehabilitation Facility

IRFs are designed to provide intensive rehabilitation therapy in a resource-intensive inpatient hospital environment for patients who, due to the complexity of their nursing, medical management, and rehabilitation needs, require and can reasonably be expected to benefit from an inpatient stay and an interdisciplinary team approach to the delivery of rehabilitation care. The rehabilitation team consists of physicians specializing in rehabilitation providing daily oversight; rehabilitation nurses;

physical therapists (PT) who work on problems with movement, walking, balance, and coordination; occupational therapists (OT) who help patients regain independence with eating, bathing, dressing, writing, and other daily tasks; certified speech therapists (SLP) who help patients recover speech, language, cognitive, and swallowing skills; orthotic and prosthetic specialists; dieticians; case managers; social workers; and psychologists who focus on adjustment to disability, family dynamics, and for those with agitation and aggressive behaviors, comprehensive agitation management.

IRF services provide a multidisciplinary approach in hospital settings to restore or enhance function after an illness or injury. These services are appropriate for patients with complex nursing, medical management, and rehabilitation needs. The determination of whether inpatient rehabilitation facility services are reasonable and necessary must be based on assessing the individual care needs of each patient. The following criteria must be met at the time of admission for inpatient rehabilitation care to be considered reasonable and necessary [4]:

1. Requires active and ongoing intervention of multiple therapy disciplines (PT, OT, SLP, or prosthetics/orthotics), at least one of which must be physical or occupational therapy.
2. The patient must require an intensive rehabilitation therapy program. The program generally consists of at least three hours of therapy per day, at least 5 days/week, or in certain well-documented cases, at least 15 h of intensive rehabilitation therapy within a seven-consecutive day period, beginning with the date of admission to the inpatient rehabilitation facility.
3. The patient must reasonably be expected to actively participate in and benefit from the intensive rehabilitation therapy program at the time of admission to the acute inpatient rehabilitation facility. The patient can only be expected to benefit significantly from the intensive rehabilitation therapy program if the patient's condition and functional status are such that they can reasonably be expected to make measurable improvement, which will be of practical value to improve their functional capacity or adaptation to impairments as a result of the rehabilitation treatment, and if such improvement can be expected to be made within a prescribed period.
4. The patient must require physician supervision by a rehabilitation physician, defined as a licensed physician with specialized training and experience in inpatient rehabilitation. The requirement for medical supervision means that the rehabilitation physician must conduct face-to-face visits with the patient at least three days per week throughout the patient's stay in the inpatient rehabilitation facility to assess the patient both medically and functionally, as well as to modify the course of treatment as needed to maximize the patient's capacity to benefit from the rehabilitation process.
5. The patient must require an intensive and coordinated interdisciplinary approach to providing rehabilitation.

Extensive documentation is required to meet Medicare requirements for admission, and patients are expected to meet all conditions listed below at the time of admission. The patient's medical records at the IRF must contain the following documentation [5].

1. A comprehensive preadmission screening that meets all of the following requirements:
   (a) Preadmission screening (PAS) is conducted by a licensed or certified clinician designated by a rehabilitation physician within the 48 hours immediately preceding IRF admission.
   (b) It includes a detailed and comprehensive review of each patient's condition and medical history, including the patient's level of functioning before the event or condition that led to the need for intensive rehabilitation therapy, expected level of improvement, the expected length of time necessary to achieve that level of improvement, an evaluation of the patient's risk for clinical complications, the conditions that caused the need for rehabilitation, the treatments needed (i.e., PT, OT, SLP, or prosthetics/orthotics), and anticipated discharge destination.
   (c) It serves as the basis for the initial determination of whether or not the patient meets the requirements for an IRF admission to be considered reasonable and necessary.
   (d) It is used to inform a rehabilitation physician who reviews and documents their concurrence with the findings and results of the PAS before IRF admission.
   (e) It is retained in the patient's medical record at the IRF.
2. The rehabilitation physician is responsible for leading the interdisciplinary treatment team and developing a comprehensive care plan. An individualized overall care plan for the patient meets the following requirements:
   (a) A rehabilitation physician develops it with input from the interdisciplinary team within 4 days of the patient's admission to the IRF.
   (b) It is retained in the patient's medical record at the IRF.

A hallmark of IRF-level rehabilitation is an interdisciplinary team approach to care. The patient must require an interdisciplinary team approach to care, as evidenced by the documentation of the patient's medical records of weekly interdisciplinary team meetings that meet the following requirements.

1. A rehabilitation physician leads the team meetings comprising the entire interdisciplinary treatment team. All team members must have current knowledge of the patient's medical and functional status. The rehabilitation physician may lead the interdisciplinary team meeting remotely via a mode of communication such as video or telephone conferencing.
2. Team meetings occur at least once per week throughout the patient's stay to implement appropriate treatment services:
   (a) Review the patient's progress toward stated rehabilitation goals,

(b) Identify any problems that could impede progress toward those goals and, where necessary, reassess previously established goals considering impediments; revise the treatment plan considering new goals; and monitor continued progress toward those goals.

3. The results and findings of the team meetings and the concurrence of the rehabilitation physician with these results and conclusions are retained in the patient's medical record.

Research published by the American College of Surgeons compared treatment in IRF and SNF settings of patients who experienced traumatic incidents. The study shows that trauma patients who went to an IRF following acute care increased their functional independence significantly, improved their chances of going home, and had a lower risk of death than those who did not receive IRF care [6].

The research reveals that patients discharged from an acute care facility to an inpatient acute rehabilitation facility [6]:

1. Significantly improved their functional independence,
2. Were nine times more likely to go home after posthospital care than patients who did not receive IRF care,
3. Had a 40% lower risk of death a year later than patients who did not receive IRF care,
4. Seventy-six percent of IRF patients (vs. 31% of SNF residents) were walking independently at discharge 14 days after admission,
5. Seventy-nine percent of IRF patients (vs. 30% of SNF residents) were transferring independently 14 days after admission.

An analysis of 5364 clinically and demographically matched SNF and IRF treated patients with brain injury found that IRF-rehabilitated patients experienced better long-term clinical outcomes than the SNF population. The average length of rehabilitation stay for the IRF cohort was less than half that of the average SNF cohort (13.7 vs. 30.7 days; $p < 0.0001$). Following the IRF stay, compared to SNF-discharged patients with brain injury, IRF patients experienced on average [7]:

1. Sixteen percent lower all-cause mortality rate over a 2-year period,
2. 93.2-day difference in average days alive over a 2-year period,
3. 43.9 fewer emergency room visits per 1000 patients per year,
4. Ninety-five more days residing at home (i.e., not receiving facility-based care) over a 2-year period,
5. Cost $21.86 more, per day, over a 2-year period.

Furthermore, an analysis of 4068 clinically and demographically matched SNF and IRF patients with SCI revealed that IRF-rehabilitated patients also experienced superior long-term clinical outcomes. The average length of rehabilitation stay for the IRF cohort was 8.7 days shorter (13.5 vs. 22.2 days; $p < 0.0001$). Following the IRF stay, compared to SNF-discharged patients with spinal cord injury, IRF patients experienced on average [7]:

1. As much as 6.7% lower all-cause mortality rate over a 2-year period,
2. 45.3-day difference in average days alive over a 2-year period,
3. Approximately 80.3 fewer emergency room visits per 1000 patients per year,
4. Forty-one more days residing at home (i.e., not receiving facility-based care) over a 2-year period,
5. Cost $20.66 more per day over a 2-year period.

Long-Term Acute Care Hospital

Most patients who require inpatient hospital services are admitted to an acute care hospital for a relatively short stay, but some may require a longer hospital stay. Such LTACHs are certified as acute care hospitals but focus on patients who stay for more than 25 days on average. Many patients in LTACHs are transferred from intensive or critical care units. They have complex diagnoses including, but not limited to, TBI, SCI, conditions requiring prolonged mechanical ventilation, significant wound care, and other conditions resulting in organ failure and requiring a hospital level of care for an extended period. Medical complexity may include the need for respiratory therapy owing to ventilator or tracheostomy dependence, prolonged ventilator weaning, intensive respiratory care, parenteral feeding, dialysis, complex wound care, or multiple intravenous medications or transfusions. In addition, a three-day intensive care unit length of stay at the acute hospital immediately preceding LTACH admission or 96 h of mechanical ventilation services during LTACH admission is required for admission. While LTACHs provide rehabilitative therapies, their primary focus is on medical and nursing care for complex conditions, and there is no requirement regarding the amount of rehabilitation therapy provided at LTACHs. To qualify as a LTACH for Medicare payment, a facility must meet Medicare's conditions of participation in acute care hospitals and have an average length of stay greater than 25 days for Medicare patients. Medicare is a significant payer for most LTACHs, accounting for approximately two-thirds of LTACH discharge.

Skilled Nursing Facility

SNF care is a post-acute level of care that provides skilled services to patients following an acute hospitalization. Skilled care is nursing and therapy care that is so complex that it can be safely and effectively performed only by, or under the supervision of, skilled nursing and therapy professionals. Skilled nursing and therapy professionals include registered nurses, licensed practical and vocational nurses, physical therapists, occupational therapists, speech-language pathologists, and audiologists. For days 1–20, Medicare pays the full cost for covered services; for days 21–100, Medicare pays all but a daily coinsurance ($194.50 in 2022) for covered services; for days beyond 100, Medicare does not cover services, and the patient is responsible for the full cost of care.

Home Health Rehabilitation

Insurance companies provide home health services if specific qualifying criteria are met:

(a) Beneficiary is "homebound", and leaving the home must require a considerable and taxing effort for the patient,
(b) Beneficiary has a "skilled need" such as nursing, physical therapy, speech therapy, or occupational therapy,
(c) Beneficiary requires only "intermittent" care,
(d) Services are performed under a physician's order.

Nursing assessment, treatment, or teaching is skilled if it must be provided by a registered nurse, or a licensed practical nurse under the supervision of a registered nurse, to be safe and effective. If a service can be safely and effectively performed by a non-nurse without nurse training or oversight, it is not a skilled service.

Insurance providers cover home PT, speech therapy, or OT visits necessary to treat a patient's illness or injury, or restore function affected by illness or injury. For physical, occupational, or speech therapy visits to constitute a "skilled need," the patient must have "restorative potential," i.e., there must be an expectation that the patient will improve in a generally predictable period. If there is no restorative potential, insurance may cover visits to develop and establish a care plan to be carried out by a non-therapist, periodically reevaluate a care plan, or teach the patient or the patient's family or caregivers necessary techniques, exercises, or precautions. However, general exercises to promote overall fitness or provide general motivation do not constitute skilled therapy.

Disorders of Consciousness Program

Individuals with disorders of consciousness (DoC) who are in a coma, vegetative state, or a minimally conscious state remain at a high level of medical acuity after intensive care. Individuals with DoC recover over a longer period and may regain their ability to function independently. In those who survive severe brain injury, there is marked variability in long-term medical, cognitive, and physical needs. DoC programs determine the patient's level of consciousness and responsiveness, identify barriers preventing effective communication and environmental control, advise on medical stability for continued care, establish prognosis and monitor for recovery, optimize the medication regimen, identify long-term care needs, prevent secondary complications, and ensure that proper medical equipment is available.

Families are provided with comprehensive education and hands-on training with follow-up support are likely willing and able to provide care to medically stable persons with DoC at home. Patients may transition to mainstream inpatient rehabilitation programs once they emerge.

Peer-to-Peer Requests

The peer-to-peer process is usually a phone conversation offered by commercial and managed insurance plans when their medical director denies acute inpatient rehabilitation level of care. Once a medical director has rendered an adverse determination, the peer-to-peer may be requested, and below are some tips that may help neurorehabililitation consultants during the peer-to-peer process:

1. Be prepared for the peer-to-peer discussion. Review the case so that you understand all the essential elements.
2. Familiarize yourself with guidelines for inpatient rehabilitation, as discussed in this chapter. Although it may seem so, the payer's medical director does not arbitrarily issue a denial for lack of medical necessity. There is a clinical basis for the denial. To be successful, you must understand the medical director's perspective and use the guidelines to bolster your arguments for medical necessity further.
3. Don't be distracted. Don't take a peer-to-peer phone call in a distracted environment. If the medical director calls when you are not ready, respectfully ask for time to go to a more private location. Open the patient's chart in a private area without distractions.
4. Always ask what information the medical director has. The insurance company often has incomplete data and will issue the denial for inpatient rehabilitation based on this incomplete picture. Always begin the conversation by asking if the medical director has the most current therapy and clinical records.
5. Be respectful but stand your ground. While being respectful, if you believe that the patient meets the criteria for inpatient rehabilitation, calmly state your case and do not back down. These cases are sometimes reviewed because they are in the gray zone for inpatient rehabilitation admission, where reasonable professionals can disagree over the level of care. Have a discussion with the medical director, not a shouting match.
6. Sometimes, you will lose. It is always nice to "win" a peer-to-peer call. That said, there will be many times where the medical director is unmoved by your argument, however compelling and correct, and will uphold the denial.

Case Illustration

A 21-year-old male patient was admitted to the acute hospital due to a high-speed motor vehicle collision with an isolated severe TBI with disordered consciousness resulting in a minimally conscious state. The patient underwent tracheostomy for respiratory failure secondary to pneumonia, and a percutaneous gastrostomy tube for severe dysphagia. The patient could not be weaned from the ventilator throughout his acute hospitalization and was transferred to an LTACH for continued ventilator weaning. The physical medicine and rehabilitation consultation service followed the patient at LTACH to assist with neurostimulation, spasticity, and sleep-wake management. The patient remained in the LTACH for 26 days and was then discharged to a DoC program. On day 21 of the DoC program, the patient demonstrated emergence from disordered consciousness and transitioned to a TBI inpatient rehabilitation program at the same facility. Twenty-one days after his inpatient rehabilitation stay, he was ready for discharge from inpatient rehabilitation. He had made significant functional gains and was decannulated, but he still required round the clock supervision and supplemental tube feeds. The day before discharge, the patient's primary caregiver was admitted to an acute care hospital with COVID-19. The patient was discharged to the SNF for skilled nursing care while awaiting his caregiver's recovery. After a 32-day SNF stay, the patient successfully transitioned to home with home health therapies and support from caregivers.

Summary and Key Points
Transitional care incorporates a broad range of services and environments designed to promote the safe and timely passage of patients between healthcare levels and across care settings, with the goal of supporting functional recovery. In the USA, multiple levels of post-acute care are available, including LTACHs, SNFs, acute IRFs, and home healthcare. Each level of care mentioned above has specific admission criteria and payment models to control for costs. Many factors, such as poor communication, incomplete transfer of information, inadequate education of patients and family caregivers, limitations in access to essential services, and the absence of a primary person to ensure continuity of care, contribute to gaps in care during critical transitions. An acute hospital interdisciplinary treatment team led by neurorehabilitation rehabilitation consultants can determine the appropriate level of rehabilitation care after acute hospitalization and facilitate a safe transfer to post-acute care.

References [1]

1. Coleman EA. Falling through the cracks: challenges and opportunities for improving transitional care for persons with continuous complex care needs. J Am Geriatr Soc. 2003;51(4):549–55.

[1] Key References [1–3, 6, 7].

2. Coleman EA, Boult C, Committee AGSHCS. Improving the quality of transitional care for persons with complex care needs. J Am Geriatr Soc. 2003;51(4):556–7.
3. Naylor MD. Nursing intervention research and quality of care: influencing the future of healthcare. Nurs Res. 2003;52(6):380–5.
4. US Centers for Medicare and Medicaid Services. Chapter 1 - inpatient hospital services covered under part A. In: 100-02 medicare benefit policy manual. Baltimore: US Centers for Medicare and Medicaid Services; 2021.
5. US Centers for Medicare and Medicaid Services. Chapter 4. Subchapter 8. Part 412.622. In: Title 42 of the code of federal regulations: US Centers for Medicare and Medicaid Services. Washington: HHS; 2020.
6. Nehra D, Nixon ZA, Lengenfelder C, et al. Acute rehabilitation after trauma: does it really matter? J Am Coll Surg. 2016;223(6):755–63.
7. DaVanzo J, El-Gamil A, Li J, Shimer M, Manolov N, Dobson A. Assessment of patient outcomes of rehabilitative care provided. In: Inpatient rehabilitation facilities (IRFs) and after discharge. Vienna: Dobson DaVanzo & Associates; 2014.

Chapter 20
Neuro-Consultation from the Veterans and Military Perspective

Blessen C. Eapen, Selina Doncevic, and Amy O. Bowles

Chapter Objectives

1. Learn how the Military Trauma Combat Causality Care System provides continuity of medical and surgical care from the point-of-injury until the Service Member arrives at definitive care and is ready for rehabilitation services.
2. Understand how the VA and Department of Defense (DoD) work cohesively to provide a seamless transition of care and services for Service Members and Veterans.
3. Learn how the Defense Health Agency Traumatic Brain Injury Center of Excellence provides clinical care, research, education, surveillance and outreach to active duty military, beneficiaries, and veterans.
4. Overview the multi-tiered level of care the DoD provides for Service Members who sustain a TBI.

The views expressed in this article are those of the authors and do not reflect the official policy of the Department of Army, Department of Defense, Department of Veterans Affairs or the U.S. Government.

B. C. Eapen (✉)
Department of Physical Medicine and Rehabilitation, VA Greater Los Angeles Health Care System, Los Angeles, CA, USA

Division of Physical Medicine and Rehabilitation, Department of Medicine, David Geffen School of Medicine at UCLA, Los Angeles, CA, USA
e-mail: blessen.eapen2@va.gov

S. Doncevic
United States Department of Veterans Affairs, Washington, DC, USA

Walter Reed National Military Medical Center, Bethesda, MD, USA
e-mail: Selina.p.doncevic.civ@health.mil, selina.doncevic@va.gov

A. O. Bowles
Department of Rehabilitation Medicine, Brooke Army Medical Center (BAMC), Joint Base San Antonio, San Antonio, TX, USA

Department of Physical Medicine and Rehabilitation, Uniformed Services University of the Health Sciences, Bethesda, MD, USA
e-mail: amy.o.bowles.civ@health.mil

A. K. Wagner, J. Weppner (eds.), *Acute Care Neuroconsultation and Neurorehabilitation Management*, https://doi.org/10.1007/978-3-031-42830-2_20

5. Understand that the VA Polytrauma System of Care (PSC) and VA Spinal Cord Injury/Disorders (SCI/D) Centers are integrated rehabilitation care continuums providing comprehensive inpatient rehabilitation to outpatient rehabilitation services, often for lifelong care needs.
6. Appreciate that Service Members and Veterans are provided lifelong case management services through the VA.

Introduction

United States military operations in Iraq and Afghanistan, and subsequent military operations have resulted in an increasing number of service members returning with neurological injuries, including traumatic brain injuries (TBI), spinal cord injuries (SCI), and neurovascular complications of polytraumatic injuries [1–3]. In prior conflicts, these injuries would have been fatal but given the advances in combat casualty care including battlefield equipment, organizational innovations and damage control strategies, the survival rates and outcomes have significantly improved [4]. The United States Military Tactical Combat Casualty Care can be divided into three distinct phases-of-care including: "Care Under Fire, Tactical Field Care, and Combat Casualty Evacuation Care" and involves "5 Roles" or levels-of-care to provide an integrated system to "triage, treat, evacuate and return the casualty to duty in the most time-efficient manner" [5, 6]. Each role has a distinct function prior to movement to a higher "role" with the goal of getting to definitive care.

Role 1: Point of Injury Care or Battalion Aid Station
Occurs at the time of injury and medical care is typically provided by first responders (self, combat medics, or corpsman) and includes first aid and life-saving techniques.

Role 2: Area Support Medical Company
Includes basic primary care and may include surgical capabilities, behavioral health, basic radiology, dental, and optometry services with limited inpatient beds. A Forward Surgical Team is co-located with this company or platoon. Advanced trauma management and tactical combat casualty care including beginning resuscitation is continued, and if necessary, additional emergency measures are instituted, but they do not go beyond the measures dictated by immediate necessities.

Role 3: Combat Surgical Hospital
Includes a fully staffed and equipped medical treatment facility for all patients and can also provide support to local units without medical assets. This facility can provide initial resuscitation, initial trauma surgery care, and postoperative treatment. In addition, this can also provide care for medical stabilization for those who are unstable to travel to the next "role."

Role 4: (Definitive Care) Outside the Continental United States (OCONUS) and Continental United States (CONUS):
OCONUS military treatment facilities (MTF) include Landstuhl Regional Medical Center (LRMC) in Germany. Generally, flight of C-17 from LRMC to Andrews

Air Force Base, Maryland is the travel pattern. Severity of injury determines if a Service Member remains over night at Andrews and or moves to next "role."

Role 5: (Definitive Care) Continental United States (CONUS):

Major MTF in the CONUS include locations such as Walter Reed National Military Medical Center, Bethesda, MD, Brooke Army Medical Center, TX, and Naval Medical Center, San Diego, CA. At the major MTF's each branch of the military has specialized programming which provides personalized clinical and non-clinical coordination and case management of the wounded, ill, or injured Service member in the inpatient or outpatient settings.

The Joint Trauma System (JTS) was implemented across Iraq and Afghanistan in 2005, modeled after civilian trauma systems, it provides organizational structure, communication and continuity of care along the care continuum [6]. The vision of the JTS is "every Soldier, Marine, Sailor, or Airman injured on the battlefield or in the theater of operations has the optimal chance for survival and maximal potential for functional recovery" [7]. The Department of Defense (DoD) and Veterans Health Administration (VA) are united in weekly global JTS teleconferences to discuss new injures, roles, current medical status, as well as continuing trauma education for participants. In addition, the VA Polytrauma System of Care (PSC) present real-time updates on the JTS calls and provide current medical and rehabilitation progress, sharing stories of recovery and outcomes to providers who cared for these Service Members across the continuum of care thus providing insight to rehabilitation care and requirements, as well as a level of closure.

To provide a seamless transition between the VA and DoD, Public Law 108-422, November 2004, 108th Congress: Title 111: Section 302 (e) (A) [8] established VA Liaisons to support inpatient and outpatient referral support—so that Active Duty Service Members (ADSM) could transition to VA acute rehabilitation as well as outpatient services. Recognized soon after, was the role of a VA/DoD Polytrauma Rehabilitation Nurse Liaison. Utilizing trauma informed care, clinicians from both the DoD and VA collaborate to assure that fine details of injury and requirements, illness, or social dynamics are well communicated for this special population. The majority of severely injured or ill ADSMs transition to VA PSC, VA Spinal Cord Injury Centers (SCIC) or occasionally to private sector facilities for acute rehabilitation. For those ADSM who do not require the acute inpatient rehabilitation, the DoD provides outpatient rehabilitation services, at times in collaboration with the VA.

Polytrauma System of Care

The VA defines polytrauma as "two or more injuries to physical regions or organ systems, one of which may be life threatening, resulting in physical, cognitive, psychological, or psychosocial impairments and functional disability" [9]. In November 2004, the 108th Congress charged the Secretary of the VA to establish centers for research, education, and clinical activities on complex multi-trauma associated with combat injuries. Thus, the VA developed the PSC in response to the growing demand of returning war heroes with the complex medical, rehabilitation, and psychosocial needs [10]. The PSC is an integrated network addressing the full continuum of care and encompassing a broad range of rehabilitation services from comprehensive acute inpatient rehabilitation units and residential brain injury programs to outpatient brain injury programs [11, 12]. It is divided into four distinct levels-of-care:

Level 1: Polytrauma Rehabilitation Center
Level 2: Polytrauma Network Sites
Level 3: Polytrauma Support Clinic
Level 4: Polytrauma Points of Contact

Level 1: Polytrauma Rehabilitation Centers (PRC)

The PRC provide the highest echelon of comprehensive interdisciplinary medical and inpatient rehabilitative services for the most complex and severely injured Veterans and ADSM. There are 5 Level One PRCs strategically located across the USA, in Richmond, VA; Tampa, FL; San Antonio, TX; Palo Alto, CA; and Minneapolis, MN (Fig. 20.1) [13]. The PRCs are national leaders in polytrauma and TBI clinical care, research and advocacy. The PRCs also provide consultation, medical education, and program development for the VA. In addition, each PRC is accredited by Commission on Accreditation of Rehabilitation Facilities (CARF) and is staffed by a full interdisciplinary care team. Finally, each PRC has an affiliated Polytrauma Transitional Rehabilitation Program (PTRP), Disorders of Consciousness Program, Assistive Technology Center of Excellence, Spinal Cord Injury Center, Amputee System of Care, and VA Epilepsy Center of Excellence thus providing the most integrated and comprehensive rehabilitation programs in the USA. As of 2021, each PRC has implemented, or in plans to establish an intensive evaluation treatment program (IETP) for those Service Members and Veterans suffering from challenging symptoms of mild TBI, PTSD, and a multitude of chronic symptomatology after multiple deployments during their service.

Special Programs affiliated with Polytrauma Rehabilitation Center of Care Include

Emerging Consciousness Program

The VA PRC Emerging Consciousness Program (ECP) was developed at the PRCs in 2006 due the increased number of ADSM returning in a state of impaired consciousness [14]. The ECP is a 90-day neurorehabilitation program focused on promoting recovery from disorders of consciousness, preventing secondary medical complications and providing family education and training [15, 16].

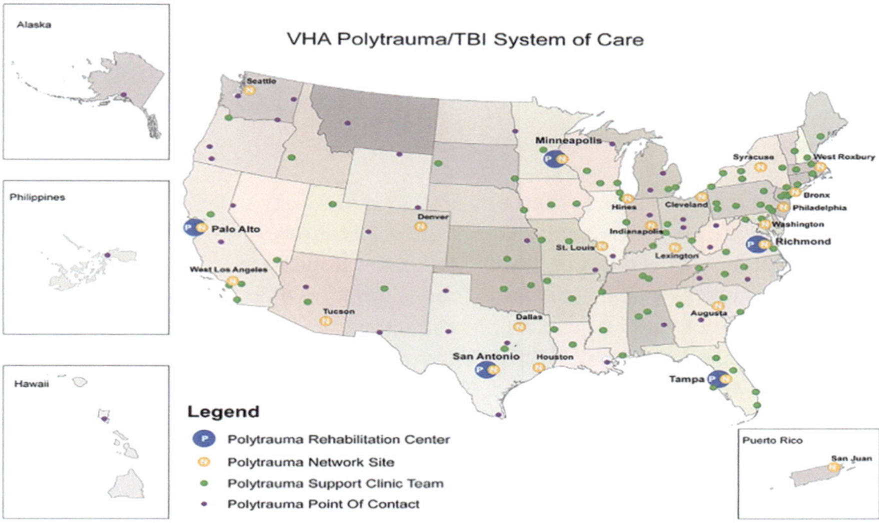

Fig. 20.1 VHA polytrauma system of care map

Polytrauma Transitional Rehabilitation Program (PTRP)

The Polytrauma Transitional Rehabilitation Program (PTRP) is a residential program designed to facilitate an optimal level of independence in the community for patients with moderate to severe disability related to acquired brain injury or other polytraumatic injuries [17]. The PTRP programming focuses on progressive return to independent living in the post-acute stages of rehabilitation and provides a holistic, ecologically-based program that addresses the individual needs, complex injuries and unique situations of each patient [18]. The PTRP programs place a strong emphasis on return to work or school, community navigation, self-management of complex life skills, interactive social skills, teamwork, and development of psychological adjustment and coping skills.

Amputee System of Care

The Amputation System of Care (ASoC) is an integrated continuum of care with expertise in amputation rehabilitation, incorporating the latest practices in medical rehabilitation management, rehabilitation therapies, and advanced prosthetic technology [19]. The ASoC is divided into four levels similar to the PSC. The highest level of specialized expertise in clinical care and technology is provided by Level I Regional Amputation Centers (RAC) who are capable of providing comprehensive rehabilitation care to the most complex amputation cases. At the other end of the spectrum are Level IV Amputation Points of Contact (APOC) where one person provides consultation and assessment as well as referrals to a facility capable of providing the level of services required.

TeleRehabilitation

The VA Telerehabilitation System of Care has rapidly expanded its footprint since 2017 to provide care for Veterans with TBI, amputations, and stroke [20]. In addition, the VA has utilized this modality for home safety assessments, specialty seating, power mobility clinics, and various rehabilitation therapies. Since the start of the pandemic, there has been an exponential growth in virtual care delivery and has shown tremendous value by reducing travel time to clinics, improving access to care, and decreasing drive times for rural Veterans and will be remain a primary mode of care delivery.

Physical Medicine and Rehabilitation Service NeuroRehabilitation Clinics

Robust outpatient teams dedicated to Neurorehabilitation are located throughout VHA, providing ongoing outpatient rehabilitation services for veterans with stroke, Amyotrophic Lateral Sclerosis, Multiple Sclerosis, Guillain-Barré Syndrome, and other neurological conditions. These interdisciplinary teams will often interface with other specialty programs such as Home-Based Primary Care or SCI Centers.

Level 2: Polytrauma Network Site (PNS)

There are currently 23 regional Level 2 PNS Clinics providing full range of comprehensive follow-on medical and rehabilitative services for patients recovering from polytrauma and TBI. These network sites support the polytrauma system of care by developing and supporting the patient's rehabilitation plan through a specialized comprehensive interdisciplinary team (IDT) [21]. At a minimum, each team consists of a Rehabilitation Medicine Physician, Registered Nurse, Social Worker, Speech-Language Pathologist, Physical Therapist, Occupational Therapist, Clinical Psychologist, Blind Rehabilitation Outpatient Specialist, and a Certified Prosthetist. This IDT meets on a regular basis to develop and monitor the Individualized Rehabilitation and Community Reintegration (IRCR) plan of care. Teams are tasked with providing the Comprehensive Traumatic Brain Injury Evaluation (CTBIE) for veterans of the recent conflicts identified through a screening process as possibly having sustained a traumatic brain injury [22]. These teams report to the Polytrauma Program Office annually and are tasked with monitoring outcomes to assess progress with community reintegration, using metrics such as the Mayo-Portland Participation Index (M2PI) [23]. PNS Clinics also serve as a regional resource for complex case consultation, a site for distribution of education and best practices, and a hub for coordination of services for TBI and polytrauma across the continuum.

Level 3: Polytrauma Support Clinic Team (PSCT)

There are currently 87 PSCTs, which provide and coordinate interdisciplinary rehabilitation services for Veterans and Service members within the catchment area of their medical facility. PSCTs also conduct comprehensive evaluations of patients with positive TBI screens and develop and implement rehabilitation and community reintegration plans. Referrals may be made to the assigned PNS team for patients requiring more complex evaluation or care.

Level 4: Polytrauma Point of Contact (PPOC)

At VA medical centers without a PSC program, the Transitional Care Manager ensures that Veterans and Service members needing specialized rehabilitation services are referred to a facility or program capable of providing the appropriate level of care. PPOCs serve as a local resource for assisting with continuation of care plan for patients transferring out of an inpatient setting or returning from evaluation by PNS or PSCT teams. While there are no mandatory staffing levels for PPOC, many of these sites will provide local services as available, such as physical or occupational therapy.

Department of Defense Traumatic Brain Injury Care

Between 2000 and 2020, the Defense Health Agency Traumatic Brain Injury Center of Excellence (TBICoE) estimate that Active Duty Service Members have sustained over 430,000 TBIs with over 85% being mild in severity [24]. As a result, mild TBI or concussion has been touted as the "signature injury" of our recent conflicts in Iraq and Afghanistan. Consequently, the DoD has committed a significant amount of resources to education, prevention, clinical management, and research. The DoD has many levels of care to treat individuals with TBI from TBI telehealth clinics to outpatient Brain Injury Clinics to the Intrepid Spirit Centers. Concussion is also a problem for troops at home, with a majority of concussions occurring at the home station ("in garrison"). Like the VA, the military has created a multi-tiered system of care with some level of service available at every military treatment facility. There are five Category 1 facilities located strategically around the country at major medical centers (Fort Gordon, GA, Joint Base Lewis McChord, WA, San Antonio Military Medical Center, TX, Landstuhl

Regional Medical Center, Germany, Tripler Army Medical Center, HI), and these facilities are able to provide care for the full spectrum of TBI from inpatient consultation to outpatient rehabilitation, although most defer inpatient rehabilitation to the VA or network providers.

Defense Health Agency Traumatic Brain Injury Center of Excellence (TBICoE)

TBICoE or formerly known as Defense and Veterans Brain Injury Center (DVBIC) is the TBI operational center for the Defense Centers of Excellence. TBICoE's supports a network of a network of multiple centers, operating out of military treatment facilities and VA Medical Centers with the overarching mission to provide clinical care, research, education surveillance and outreach to active duty military, their beneficiaries, and veterans.

National Intrepid Center of Excellence for Traumatic Brain Injury (NICoE) and Intrepid Spirit Centers (ISCs)

In 2007, Congress mandated that the DoD create a center to advance the understanding of the "invisible wounds" of recent wars, and to meet this request, the National Intrepid Center of Excellence (NICoE) was opened in Bethesda, MD, located on the campus of the Walter Reed National Military Medical Center (WRNMMC). The NICoE program is a four-week outpatient program for service members with complex co-morbid TBI and psychological health conditions who have not responded to traditional treatment. During the program, an interdisciplinary team of providers works with patients and their families to create a tailored treatment plan to meet their goals and achieve effective return-to-duty and community reintegration. Programming includes rehabilitation services, psychological services, and complementary and alternative medicine. Satellite Intrepid Spirit Centers (ISCs) have been established throughout the country to allow expansion of workspaces and improve access to this type of care at major troop centers. The ISCs serve ADSMs with two of posttraumatic stress disorder, chronic pain, and/or post-concussion complaints.

Spinal Cord Injury and Disorders (SCI/D) System of Care

The SCI/D system of care is an integrated network utilizing a hub and spoke model with 25 SCI/D Centers (hubs), 6 Spinal Cord Injury long-term care units and over 126 spoke sites (Fig. 20.2). The mission of the SCI/D programs is to promote and

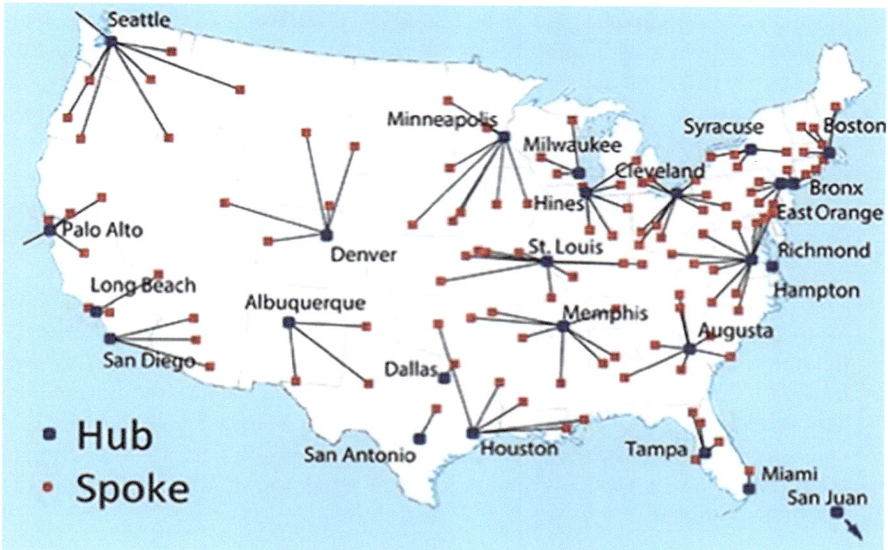

Fig. 20.2 Spinal cord injury system of care in a hub and spoke model of care

maintain the health, independence, quality of life, and productivity of individuals with SCI/D throughout their lives. The SCI/D centers provide Veterans and Service Members with acute and chronic SCI as well as neurological impairments of the spinal cord (e.g., myelopathy from spinal stenosis, multiple sclerosis and transverse myelitis, etc.) with an interdisciplinary care team. The SCI/D Centers provide medical, surgical, and all-levels of rehabilitation care (acute rehabilitation, subacute rehabilitation, ventilator management and weaning, and respite care) for this complex patient population.

VA and DoD Case Management

Three VA and joint VA/DoD programs seek to address the transition from DoD to VA health care facilities, which include:

1. Post-911 M2VA Case Management Program, formerly known as Transition and Care Management Program or OEF/OIF Care Management Program (www.oefoif.va.gov), is designed to serve returning injured or ill combat and post 9/11 Service Members as they transition into the VA or through standard discharge from their respective service back into the community. This program is comprised of case managers who triage referrals for those ADSMs with needs in transition, to those new Veterans who need monthly, quarterly or yearly follow-up. This is a national program with data tracking requirements, assuring standards of care management are met.

2. VA Liaison Program was established in 2003. VA Liaisons for Healthcare coordinate the transfer of healthcare for Service members needing continued care from the MTF to the VA Healthcare Facility closest to their assigned duty station, home of record or to the most appropriate VA facility for the specialized services required by the Service Member's medical condition. VA Liaisons educate Service Members and families about VA health care services and locations. Their role provides a warm handoff between VA and DoD healthcare systems. These VA Liaisons for Healthcare are nurses or social workers located at DoD Military Treatment Facilities.
3. Federal Recovery Coordination Program (FRCP) was established in 2008, assists in identifying and coordinating the medical and non-medical care, benefits and services needed to support the Service Members and Veterans as they transition through recovery, rehabilitation and reintegration into the community. The Federal Recovery Consultants (FRCs) provide enterprise-level longitudinal consultation and assistance to VA and DoD, providing clinical and non-clinical consultation about DoD, VA, other federal agencies, community, and other resources available.

References[1]

1. Risdall JE, Menon DK. Traumatic brain injury. Philos Trans R Soc Lond Ser B Biol Sci. 2011;366(1562):241–50. https://doi.org/10.1098/rstb.2010.0230.
2. Weaver FM, Burns SP, Evans CT, Rapacki LM, Goldstein B, Hammond MC. Provider perspectives on soldiers with new spinal cord injuries returning from Iraq and Afghanistan. Arch Phys Med Rehabil. 2009;90(3):517–21. https://doi.org/10.1016/j.apmr.2008.09.560.
3. White JM, Stannard A, Burkhardt GE, Eastridge BJ, Blackbourne LH, Rasmussen TE. The epidemiology of vascular injury in the wars in Iraq and Afghanistan. Ann Surg. 2011;253(6):1184–9. https://doi.org/10.1097/SLA.0b013e31820752e3.
4. Butler FK Jr, Blackbourne LH. Battlefield trauma care then and now: a decade of Tactical Combat Casualty Care. J Trauma Acute Care Surg. 2012;73(6 Suppl 5):S395–402. https://doi.org/10.1097/TA.0b013e3182754850.
5. Combat casualty care: lessons learned from OEF and OIF. Office of the Surgeon General, Department of the Army; 2012.
6. Berwick D, Downey A, Cornett E, (US) NAoSEaM, Sector CoMTCsLHSaITttC. A national trauma care system: integrating military and civilian trauma systems to achieve zero preventable deaths after injury. Washington: The National Academies Press; 2016.
7. Cubano M, Lenhart M, Institute B, Army OootSGU. Emergency war surgery. Washington: Government Printing Office; 2014.
8. Traumatic Brain Injury Act of 2008, Public Law 110-206, United States 110th Congress (2008). 2008/04/28/.
9. VHA Directive 1172.01, Polytrauma System of Care (2019).
10. Sigford BJ. "To care for him who shall have borne the battle and for his widow and his orphan" (Abraham Lincoln): the Department of Veterans Affairs polytrauma system of care. Arch Phys Med Rehabil. 2008;89(1):160–2. https://doi.org/10.1016/j.apmr.2007.09.015.

[1] Key References [4, 12, 13].

11. Eapen B, Jaramillo C, Tapia R, Johnson E, Cifu D. Rehabilitation care of combat related TBI: Veterans Health Administration polytrauma system of care. Curr Phys Med Rehabil Rep. 2013;1(3):151–8.
12. Cifu DX, Cohen SI, Lew HL, Jaffee M, Sigford B. The history and evolution of traumatic brain injury rehabilitation in military service members and veterans. Am J Phys Med Rehabil. 2010;89(8):688–94. https://doi.org/10.1097/PHM.0b013e3181e722ad.
13. Armstrong M, Champagne J, Mortimer DS. Department of Veterans Affairs Polytrauma Rehabilitation Centers: inpatient rehabilitation management of combat-related polytrauma. Phys Med Rehabil Clin N Am. 2019;30(1):13–27. https://doi.org/10.1016/j.pmr.2018.08.013.
14. McNamee S, Howe L, Nakase-Richardson R, Peterson M. Treatment of disorders of consciousness in the Veterans Health Administration polytrauma centers. J Head Trauma Rehabil. 2012;27(4):244–52. https://doi.org/10.1097/HTR.0b013e31825e12c8.
15. Eapen B. Emerging consciousness program. In: Kreutzer J, DeLuca J, Caplan B, editors. Encyclopedia of clinical neuropsychology. Cham: Springer; 2017.
16. Peterson M, Eapen BC, Himmler M, Galhotra P, Glazer D. Evolution of care for the veterans and active duty service members with disorders of consciousness. Phys Med Rehabil Clin N Am. 2019;30(1):29–41. https://doi.org/10.1016/j.pmr.2018.08.006.
17. Duchnick J, Ropacki S, Yutsis M, Petska K, Pawlowski C. Polytrauma transitional rehabilitation programs: comprehensive rehabilitation for community integration after brain injury. Psychol Serv. 2015;12(3):313–21.
18. Critchfield E, Bain KM, Goudeau C, Gillis CJ, Gomez-Lansidel MT, Eapen BC. A model of care for community reintegration: the polytrauma transitional rehabilitation program. Phys Med Rehabil Clin N Am. 2019;30(1):43–54. https://doi.org/10.1016/j.pmr.2018.08.009.
19. VHA HK 1172.03, Amputation System of Care.
20. Scholten J, Poorman C, Culver L, Webster JB. Department of Veterans Affairs Polytrauma Telerehabilitation: twenty-first century care. Phys Med Rehabil Clin N Am. 2019;30(1):207–15. https://doi.org/10.1016/j.pmr.2018.08.003.
21. Lew H, Cifu D, Sigford B, Scott S, Sayer N, Jaffee M. Team approach to diagnosis and management of traumatic brain injury and its comorbidities. J Rehabil Res Dev. 2007;44(7):7–9.
22. VHA Directive 2010-012, Screening and evaluation of possible traumatic brain injury in Operation Enduring Freedom (OEF) and Operation Iraqi Freedom (OIF) veterans (2010).
23. McCulloch K, Pastorek NJ, Miller BI, et al. Clinician versus veteran ratings on the Mayo-Portland participation index in veterans with a history of mild traumatic brain injury. J Head Trauma Rehabil. 2015;30(1):38–46. https://doi.org/10.1097/htr.0000000000000041.
24. Traumatic Brain Injury Center of Excellence. DOD numbers for traumatic brain injury worldwide - Totals. 2021.

Chapter 21
Resources and Advocacy

Shannon B. Juengst and Melissa Sutcliffe

Chapter Objectives
1. Provide basic information on community services and resources that promote and support community re-entry after both pediatric and adult patients with neurological conditions.
2. Identify specific resource considerations for pediatric versus adult patients, including focus on education and schooling versus vocational rehabilitation.
3. Present a list of organizations that provide resources and advocacy for individuals with neurological disabilities and their family members.

Introduction

Re-entry into the community after sustaining a neurological injury can be challenging for both patients and their families. While a thoughtful and comprehensive discharge plan can ease the transition back into the community from an acute medical setting, it is not possible to anticipate all of the needs that may arise over time. Family members of patients report a notable gap in the provision of information related to lifetime management planning, community integration and social belonging, management of cognitive, behavioral, and emotional issues, and availability of

S. B. Juengst (✉)
The Institute for Rehabilitation Research (TIRR), Memorial Hermann Hospital Brain Injury Research Center (BIRC), Houston, TX, USA
e-mail: shannon.juengst@memorialhermann.edu

M. Sutcliffe
Division of Pediatric Rehabilitation Medicine Center, Department of Physical Medicine and Rehabilitation, Children's Hospital of Pittsburgh of UPMC, Pittsburgh, PA, USA
e-mail: sternmk@upmc.edu

A. K. Wagner, J. Weppner (eds.), *Acute Care Neuroconsultation and Neurorehabilitation Management*, https://doi.org/10.1007/978-3-031-42830-2_21

resources [1–3]. Patients have reported that it is family members, rather than health-care professionals, that primarily help them to overcome barriers in rehabilitation [4]. However, independently managing challenging behavior, mental health, and other issues experienced by patients often results in substantial burden or emotional distress for family members or friends [5–12]. Therefore, it is especially important to provide resources for addressing issues that arise during transitions of care, to improve continuity of care and accessibility to important information as needed and to reduce caregiver burden on family members [3, 12–15].

Community Re-entry and Community Services

Community integration, including participation in productive and meaningful activities (e.g., school and work) and social integration (e.g., social activities and relationships), should be considered from multiple perspectives to identify potential barriers and supports to community re-entry after hospital discharge. This includes barriers and supports to reintegrating into the home environment, work or school environment, social settings, and outside clubs and activities (e.g., organized sports, religious activities). Preparing for community re-entry is a process that should involve care providers, family members, and members of the community [4, 16], and families should be thoroughly equipped through education and planning prior to rehabilitation discharge [3, 12, 14].

Community-based services can provide additional, ongoing support. Service providers can communicate directly with family members and teachers or employers regarding changes in a patient's functioning, so that those around the patient can best understand their abilities and needs [17, 18]. In some instances, documentation of these needs is required for eligibility for services (e.g., school-based services, vocational rehabilitation), reasonable accommodations (e.g., school, work), or participation in activities (e.g., adjusting expectations based on individual's needs). Alternative or adapted sports, for example, are available for interested individuals with disabilities. Participating in sports is a common pastime among children and adults, but many may be unable to participate in these previously enjoyed activities due to new functional limitations. Efforts should be made to provide resources for adaptive sports and exercise, as participation in these activities can improve health and overall quality of life [19, 20].

Education and Schooling

A main emphasis of discharge planning after pediatric injury is best placed on re-entry to the school environment. Preparing for re-entry into education and schooling should begin on rehabilitation admission [21–23]. Schooling is often referred to as a child's job as so much of the week is spent in that setting. Thus, planning for re-entry is a key component to the rehabilitation stay. This includes a multidisciplinary approach where all members of the treatment team work together to ensure that the needs of the child and family will be met once the child returns to the educational environment. Parents and adolescents tend to be more satisfied with this transition planning the more comprehensive and involved the hospital team can be with the school [17, 24]. This often includes participation in the process during and after discharge [24–26].

Contact should be made with the school or educational setting early in the child's stay. It is helpful to obtain a release of information from the family to receive the child's academic records such as any previous psychoeducational testing, current special educational service plans, and information on history [23]. With parental permission, the school should be made aware of the patient's current medical status so that they understand the severity of the situation and why the patient may be out of school for weeks to months.

As the child continues to improve functionally during their rehabilitation stay, they will be focusing on development of physical and cognitive skills, working with rehabilitation specialists to treat deficits associated with their injury. However, as the patient's awareness improves, they can benefit from working on some academic tasks, in conjunction with guidance from a school teacher or educational professional. This can help provide some casual information on the patient's level with respect to academic skills [23].

Planning for re-entry is a complex, step-down process. Firstly, prior to discharge, all members of the team should complete assessments to document functional or cognitive level in order to provide the school with this information [22]. This likely includes some focal neuropsychological assessment that can help prepare educators about what to expect for performance in the school environment, especially as there is concern that traditional achievement tests may not be sensitive to changes post-neurological injury [27]. Children who experience the need for inpatient rehabilitation have a high likelihood of needing special education services [27–29]. Research suggests that many children who should qualify based on injury are often missed by the system [29]. Thus, the opportunity for the rehabilitation team to ensure placement of needed services can be paramount to long-term outcomes, such as educational and employment achievement.

Some children may already receive special education services. However, for those who do not, they require evaluation for service eligibility [30]. This process, conducted by the school, can take some time, so it is important to begin the process at rehabilitation admission. If members of the team think there is a high possibility the child will need services, they should begin the process immediately. Children typically qualify under categories like "Other Health Impaired" or "Traumatic Brain Injury." These categories highlight the need for services based on a medical condition.

Children often are not ready to be fully immersed in the academic environment after discharge. Additional options are available, such as homebound education plans. Homebound education consists of an identified instructor traveling to the student's home to provide education when the student is unable to attend the physical school environment [31]. This differs from homeschooling, as it is run through the public school district and involves an educator employed by the district. Length of time spent in a homebound education setting often varies.

When children are ready to return to the physical school environment, gradual re-entry helps with acclimation and adjustment [23]. This process includes attending some half or partial days and slowly working up to the amount of time spent in school, based on the child's level of fatigue. Again, this step can vary in the amount of time needed based on each individual child.

When returning to academics, children often require a variety of services, including not only accommodations for cognitive and physical needs, but behavioral needs that can be common post-injury [22, 32]. Communication between the rehabilitation unit and school is key in this domain, as those who have intimately worked with the child for weeks to months are best able to provide recommendations on managing challenges. Prior to discharge, a meeting with members of the educational team should occur. Members of the rehabilitation team can provide suggestions at that time, including information on mobility, fine motor needs, language and communication, self-care, cognitive and learning needs, and medical needs. Providing information prior to discharge helps smooth the discharge transition [17, 24].

Research has demonstrated that family and educator satisfaction often improves when the team remains involved during the transition back to school, to help address any remaining or unforeseen needs and ensure that the child's services are adequate to address their limitations [17, 24]. Given that many children who should receive services often do not, this is a particularly necessary component [29].

Rehabilitation teams often have a unique opportunity to provide education on medical issues relating to a child's disability. Research indicates that teachers and other educators often do not receive training or formal education on disability categories, such as TBI [26, 28, 33], and can misattribute behaviors as willful or to lack of motivation, rather than to the injury itself. This information also empowers educators with the knowledge needed to be prepared to work with such populations [33], again reiterating the importance of communication between the team and the school.

Lastly, in addition to academic supports, some attention should be paid to the social needs of the child within the school setting itself. Children are at high risk for social difficulties after neurological injury [34], and many adolescents report difficulties with re-integration in this domain [17]. Thus some focus should be placed on identifying any difficulties in social communication and functioning, with a plan in place to provide appropriate supports, such as social skills training, peer in services, etc., to ease the transition.

Multidisciplinary Post-Acute Rehabilitation and Vocational Rehabilitation in Adults with Neurological Conditions

Rehabilitation centers or hospitals, academic institutions, and nonprofit service organizations provide multidisciplinary post-acute rehabilitation programs and interventions for adults with neurological conditions, though availability of these services varies greatly by location. Comprehensive, holistic day treatment programs, including integrated, intensive rehabilitative services that focus on cognitive rehabilitation and social functioning, are the most commonly studied, and have demonstrated some efficacy for improving productivity [35]. Multidisciplinary and community-based programs have also demonstrated efficacy for improving daily activities and social participation [36]. However, these programs, when available, do not typically address the challenging mental health and behavioral issues common after neurological injury that often require 24-h supervision from family members [37]. A systematic review of the literature on community-based interventions for patients with multiple morbidities found that focusing on management of specific areas of difficulty for individuals resulted in greater efficacy than broader interventions that focused on case management or changes in delivery of care [38]. Interventions that engaged healthcare providers were most effective [38], supporting the need for ongoing communication and engagement between healthcare providers and those affected by conditions associated with multimorbidity.

Vocational rehabilitation (VR), which involves services to support returning to work and maintaining employment, was first defined by the Rehabilitation Acts of 1973 [39]. VR services are available to any individual with a documented disability through state VR departments and to United States Veterans through the Department of Veterans Affairs (VA). VR counselors collect information from a variety of healthcare professionals to identify barriers and facilitators of return to or maintenance of competitive employment and work with individuals with disabilities to acquire necessary supportive services [40]. This process can include assessment (functional assessment, work capacity and interests, work site evaluation), career counseling, goal setting, case management, resource identification, service provision, and advocacy [40, 41].

VR counselors should meet with patients and/or their family members as early in the rehabilitation process as possible. Many inpatient rehabilitation facilities have a dedicated Vocational Rehabilitation Counselor who routinely meets with patients and their families. They can assist with identifying capacity to return to work, either returning to the same position or returning to competitive employment in a different position. VR counselors can help determine and advocate for reasonable accommodations and assistive technology. If a patient cannot return to pre-injury employment, VR counselors can identify transferable skills and other employment potential. If additional schooling or retraining is necessary, VR counselors can assist individuals by identifying necessary training, in some cases covering the cost of that training. Though VR is accessible and free of charge, it is only available to those with a documented disability who are seeking competitive employment.

Community-based nonprofit organizations often provide similar services to individuals unable to work to support productive and meaningful activity.

Website Resources on Community Services for Individuals with Neurological Injuries

https://www.ada.gov/: Website for the Americans with Disabilities Act, legislation relevant to civil rights of individuals with disabilities. This includes legal information on federal, private workplace, and school discrimination and on reasonable accommodations.

www.adaptedsports.org: Website for the American Association of Adapted Sports, providing information and links on adaptive sports.

http://www.strokeassociation.org/STROKEORG/: American Stroke Association, providing information on Stroke, including a Stroke Resource Center.

https://www.biausa.org/: The Brain Injury Association of America offers a variety of resources and Local Chapters (e.g. State, Regional) that help provide information, services, and advocacy to individuals with brain injuries.

www.brainline.org: Provides a variety of resources to individuals with TBI and their families, friends, or colleagues.

https://moveunitedsport.org/: Provides links and information about adaptive sports.

https://www2.ed.gov/parents/needs/speced/edpicks.jhtml: US Department of Education Website on Special Education Services.

https://askearn.org/state-vocational-rehabilitation-agencies/: Name, website, and contact information of every State Vocational Rehabilitation department.

http://idea.ed.gov/: Information on the Individuals with Disabilities Education Act, legislation relevant to the civil rights of school-aged children with disabilities.

http://www.msktc.org/: The Model Systems Knowledge Translation Center provides education through webinars, fact sheets, and resource links for individuals with traumatic brain injury, spinal cord injury, and burn injury and their family members.

https://www.parentcenterhub.org/: Educational Resources for parents of children in need of special education services

Case Illustration

Pediatric Case

Jane Smith was a previously healthy and typically developing 11-year-old girl who sustained a mild complicated TBI after falling off a horse unhelmeted. She had brief loss of consciousness (less than 1 min), emesis, and some brief confusion. She was taken to the Emergency Department where imaging revealed a small left fronto-temporal bleed and temporal skull fracture. She was admitted to the hospital for monitoring of her mental status, bleed, and consultation with neurosurgery. During her stay, neuropsychology was consulted on the floor. The neuropsychologist met with the family and provided psychoeducation regarding cognitive outcomes, appropriate environment for brain injury recovery, and planning for school re-entry. The neuropsychologist coordinated with the trauma team to ensure homebound education post-discharge due to healing skull fracture. Both physical and occupational therapy were consulted and also provided recommendations for ambulating in the community and at home after discharge given risks associated with skull fracture. The neuropsychologist completed screening testing which identified challenges with attention and processing speed. The neuropsychologist helped coordinate a follow-up comprehensive neuropsychological evaluation as an outpatient in 6 weeks, prior to returning to the physical school environment. After discharge at the 4 week mark, the child was seen briefly in the Acquired Brain Injury Clinic by a multidisciplinary team. The neuropsychologist there provided additional recommendations for schooling in the homebound setting, and confirmed follow-up appointment. Physical and occupational therapy provided some recommendations for transitioning between classes, and these recommendations were given to the family in clinic. Discussions regarding delaying a return to horseback riding supported parents in their hesitancy to allow this to occur just yet as the child had not been released from activity restrictions. After comprehensive testing, a formalized service plan was recommended for return to school to compensate for ongoing attention challenges. The family expressed appreciation and satisfaction with the multidisciplinary approach to helping transition back to school/community and the continuity of care across settings.

Adult Case

John Doe was a 33-year-old, high school educated man who worked full-time for a landscape company for 9 years. He was married and was an independent driver. John sustained a moderate TBI in a motor vehicle accident. After six days in acute care, John was discharged home with his wife. Though John was independent for basic activities of daily living, he required cues for memory and attention. He had difficulty in loud or crowded places, which he reported made his headaches worse and caused him to feel irritable. He also reported significant fatigue. As a result of having a seizure after injury, John was no longer able to drive or operate heavy machinery safely. John and his wife received information about VR services while he was in the hospital and scheduled a meeting with a VR counselor three months post-discharge. At that meeting, it was determined that John could not return to his pre-injury position, as a result of his physical symptoms (headache, fatigue) and safety concerns (operating machinery). Given John's long-standing history with his employer and the advocacy of his VR counselor, the landscape company agreed to bring John back as a part-time, office-based employee, to manage phone calls and scheduling; if successful, they would negotiate transitioning to a full-time position. John began his new position with a Job Coach, to assist with the transition and acquisition of new skills. A coworker provided transportation to and from work. John required a five-minute break each hour, to manage fatigue, and continued to work with his physiatrist to address his headaches and seizures. The VR counselor monitored John's progress, particularly as there was concern for how he would cognitively manage in the busy work environment and for behavioral issues noted by his wife. In addition, John and his wife attended the local TBI Support Group recommended by the Social Worker they met with during his acute care stay, to address his wife's concern over his anger management and depression. While John successfully returned to work, ongoing monitoring and support were necessary to maintain his success and/or provide support if and when his situation changed.

Summary/Key Points

Children and adults who have sustained a brain injury are often discharged with a variety of physical, cognitive, and emotional needs that can make the transition back to home challenging and stressful. Whether or not they are discharged from acute care to inpatient rehabilitation, to another facility, or to home varies based on multiple factors, ranging from injury severity or medical complexity to availability of family or personal preference to insurance status or availability of other resources. Planning for re-entry into the community after brain injury is a long and complicated process, requiring coordination of care across providers, caregivers, families, and community members. Research indicates that families are often the ones helping patients overcome barriers post-discharge, and discharge planning offers a unique opportunity to help patients and families be better prepared for these hurdles. Discharge planning should begin on hospital admission and include educational components, not only with the patient and family members themselves, but also with others in the patient's community, such as coworkers or supervisors, friends, teachers and school administrators, or organizers of extracurricular activities. Additionally, arming patients and families with a variety of advocacy and transition resources reduces the burden of transition to home. This may include providing information to patients and their family members on how to contact other agencies, such as vocational rehabilitation, or how to qualify a child for special education services at school or identifying other community-based resources that might support the patient and their family, such as support groups or adapted sports programs. What resources and transition needs are required will depend on the individual needs of the patient. However, what is clear is that patients and families can benefit from help learning about these services on admission, with continued follow-up post-discharge to help in obtaining these services to meet their needs and improve long-term health, functioning, and quality of life.

References[1]

1. Rotondi A, Sinkule J, Balzer K, Harris J, Moldovan R. A qualitative needs assessment of persons who have experienced traumatic brain injury and their primary family caregivers. J Head Trauma Rehabil. 2007;22(1):14–25.
2. Murphy M, Carmine H. Long-term health implications of individuals with TBI: a rehabilitation perspective. NeuroRehabilitation. 2012;31(1):85–94.
3. Kirk S, Fallon D, Fraser C, Robinson G, Vassallo G. Supporting parents following childhood traumatic brain injury: a qualitative study to examine information and emotional support needs across key care transitions. Child Care Health Dev. 2015;41(2):303–13.
4. Graff H, Christensen J, Poulsen I, Egerod I. Patient perspectives on navigating the field of traumatic brain injury rehabilitation: a qualitative thematic analysis. Disabil Rehabil. 2018;40(8):926–34.
5. Tam S, McKay A, Sloan S, Ponsford J. The experience of challenging behaviours following severe TBI: a family perspective. Brain Inj. 2015;29(7-8):813–21.
6. Arnould A, Rochat L, Azouvi P, Van der Linden M. Apathetic symptom presentations in patients with severe traumatic brain injury: assessment heterogeneity and relationship with psychosocial functions and caregivers' burden. Brain Inj. 2015;29(13-14):1597–603.
7. Manskow U, Sigurdardottir S, Roe C, et al. Factors affecting caregiver burden 1 year after severe traumatic brain injury: a prospective nationwide multicenter study. J Head Trauma Rehabil. 2015;30(6):411–23.
8. Kreutzer J, Rapport L, Marwitz J, et al. Caregivers' well-being after traumatic brain injury: a multicnter prospective investigation. Arch Phys Med Rehabil. 2009;90(6):939–46.
9. Pinquart M, Sorensen S. Associations of stressors and uplifts of caregiving with caregiver burden and depressive mood: a meta-analysis. J Gerontol B Psychol Sci Soc Sci. 2003;58(2):112–28.
10. Powell J, Wise E, Brockway J, Fraser R, Temkin N, Bell K. Characteristics and concerns of caregivers of adults with traumatic brain injury. J Head Trauma Rehabil. 2017;32(1):E33–41.
11. Wade S, Taylor H, Drotar D, Stancin T, Yeates K. Family burden and adaptation during the initial year after traumatic brain injury in children. Pediatrics. 1998;102(1):110–6.
12. Josie KL, Peterson CC, Burant C, et al. Predicting family burden following childhood traumatic brain injury: a cumulative risk approach. J Head Trauma Rehabil. 2008;23(6):357–68.
13. Lefebvre H, Levert M. The close relatives of people who have had a traumatic brain injury and their special needs. Brain Inj. 2012;26(9):1084–97.
14. Holland D, Shigaki C. Subject review: Educating families and caretakers of traumatically brain injured patients in the new health care environment: a three phase model and bibliography. Brain Inj. 2009;12(12):993–1009.
15. Gan C, Gargaro J, Brandys C, Gerber G, Boschen K. Family caregivers' support needs after brain injury: a synthesis of perspectives from caregivers, programs, and researchs. NeuroRehabilitation. 2010;27(1):5–18.

[1] Key References [2, 23, 30, 35, 38].

16. Anderson V, Catroppa C. Advances in postacute rehabilitation after childhood-acquired brain injury: a focus on cognitive, behavioral, and social domains. Am J Phys Med Rehabil. 2006;85(9):767–78.
17. Sharp N, Bye R, Llewellyn G, Cusick A. Fitting back in: Adolescents returning to school after severe acquired brain injury. Disabil Rehabil. 2006;28(12):767–78.
18. Chevignard M, Brooks N, Truelle J. Community integration following severe childhood traumatic brain injury. Curr Opin Neurol. 2010;23(6):695–700.
19. Zabriskie R, Lundberg N, Groff D. Quality of life and identity: the benefits of a community-based therapeutic recreation and adaptive sports program. Ther Recreat J. 2005;39(3):176–91.
20. Jennen C, Uhlenbruck G. Exercise and life-satisfactory-fitness: complementary strategies in the prevention and rehabilitation of illnesses. Evid Based Complement Alternat Med. 2004;1(2):157–65.
21. Savage RC, DePompei R, Tyler J, Lash M. Paediatric traumatic brain injury: a review of pertinent issues. Pediatr Rehabil. 2005;8(2):92–103.
22. Carney J, Porter P. School reentry for children with acquired central nervous systems injuries. Dev Disabil Res Rev. 2009;15(2):152–8.
23. Ylvisaker M, Hartwick P, Stevens M. School reentry following head injury: managing the transition from hospital to school. J Head Trauma Rehabil. 1991;6(1):10–22.
24. Roscigno CI, Fleig DK, Knafl KA. Parent management of the school reintegration needs of children and youth following moderate or severe traumatic brain injury. Disabil Rehabil. 2015;37(6):523–33.
25. Gillett J. The pediatric acquired brain injury community outreach program (PABICOP) - an innovative comprehensive model of care for children and youth with an acquired brain injury. NeuroRehabilitation. 2004;19(3):207–18.
26. Glang A, Tyler J, Pearson S, Todis B, Morvant M. Improving educational services for students with TBI through statewide consulting teams. NeuroRehabilitation. 2004;19(3):219–31.
27. Ewing-Cobbs L, Fletcher J, Levin H, Iovino I, Miner M. Academic achievement and academic placement following traumatic brain injury in children and adolescents: a two-year longitudinal study. J Clin Exp Neuropsychol. 1998;20(6):769–81.
28. Hawley CA, Ward AB, Magnay AR, Mychalkiw W. Return to school after brain injury. Arch Dis Child. 2004;89(2):136–42.
29. Glang A, Todis B, Thomas C, Hood D, Bedell G, Cockrell J. Return to school following childhood TBI: who gets services? NeuroRehabilitation. 2008;23(6):477–86.
30. 105th Congress. Individuals with Disabilities Act Amendments of 1997. 1997.
31. Deidrick K, Farmer J. School reentry following traumatic brain injury. Prev Sch Fail. 2010;49(4):23–33.
32. Schwartz L, Taylor H, Drotar D, Yeates K, Wade S, Stancin T. Long-term behavior problems following pediatric traumatic brain injury: prevalence, predictors, and correlates. J Pediatr Psychol. 2003;28(4):251–63.
33. Hartman L, Duncanson M, Farahat S, Lindsay S. Clinician and educator experiences of facilitating sutdents' transition back to school following acquired brain injury: a qualitative systematic review. Brain Inj. 2015;29(12):1387–99.
34. Ryan N, van Bijnen L, Catroppa C, et al. Longitudinal outcome and recovery of social problems after pediatric traumatic brain injury (TBI): contribution of brain insult and family environment. Int J Dev Neurosci. 2016;49:23–30.
35. Brasure M, Lamberty G, Sayer N, et al. Multidisciplinary postacute rehabilitation for moderate to severe traumatic brain injury in adults. Rockville: Agency for Healthcare Research and Quality; 2012.
36. Powell J, Rich T, Wise E. Effectivesness of occupation- and activity-based interventions to improve everyday activities and social participation for people with traumatic brain injury: a systematic review. Am J Occup Ther. 2016;70(3):1–9.

37. Centers for Disease Control and Prevention. Report to congress on traumatic brain injury in the United States: epidemiology and rehabilitation. Atlanta: National Center for Injury Prevention and Control; 2015.
38. Smith SM, Soubhi H, Fortin M, Hudon C, O'Dowd T. Managing patients with multimorbidity: systematic review of interventions in primary care and community settings. BMJ. 2012;345:e5205.
39. 93rd Congress. Public Law 93-112: Rehabilitation Act. 1973.
40. Rubin S, Roessler R, Rumrill P Jr. Foundations of the vocational rehabilitation process. 7th ed. Austin: Pro-Ed; 2016.
41. Lee G. Vocational rehabilitation for people with disabilities. In: Center for International Rehabilitation Research Information and Exchange (CIRRIE), editor. International encyclopedia of rehabilitation. Buffalo: CIRRIE; 2010.

Index

A. K. Wagner, J. Weppner (eds.), *Acute Care Neuroconsultation and Neurorehabilitation Management*, https://doi.org/10.1007/978-3-031-42830-2

MIX
Papier aus verantwortungsvollen Quellen
Paper from responsible sources
FSC® C105338

If you have any concerns about our products,
you can contact us on
ProductSafety@springernature.com

In case Publisher is established outside the EU,
the EU authorized representative is:
Springer Nature Customer Service Center GmbH
Europaplatz 3, 69115 Heidelberg, Germany

Printed by Libri Plureos GmbH
in Hamburg, Germany